High-Yield™ Systems
Gastrointestinal Tract

High-Yield™ Systems
Gastrointestinal Tract

Ronald W. Dudek, Ph.D
Professor
Brody School of Medicine
East Carolina University
Department of Anatomy and Cell Biology
Greenville, North Carolina

Lippincott Williams & Wilkins
a Wolters Kluwer business
Philadelphia • Baltimore • New York • London
Buenos Aires • Hong Kong • Sydney • Tokyo

Acquisitions Editor: Crystal Taylor
Product Manager: Sirkka E. Howes
Manufacturing Manager: Margie Orzech
Marketing Manager: Jennifer Kuklinski
Vendor Manager: Bridgett Dougherty
Design Coordinator: Teresa Mallon
Compositor: SPi

Cover images from Yamada T, Alpers DH, Laine L, et al. Textbook of Gastroenterology, vol 2, 3rd Ed. Philadelphia: Lippincott Williams & Wilkins, 1999:2956, 2959, 3103; Erkonen WE and Smith WL. Radiology 101: The Basics and Fundamentals of Imaging. 2nd Ed. Philadelphia: Lippincott Williams & Wilkins, 2005:91.

351 West Camden Street
Baltimore, MD 21201

530 Walnut Street
Philadelphia, PA 19106

Printed in China

9 8 7 6 5 4 3 2 1

Library of Congress Cataloging-in-Publication Data

Dudek, Ronald W., 1950-
High-yield systems gastrointestinal tract / Ronald W. Dudek.
p. ; cm. — (High-yield systems)
Includes index.
ISBN 978-0-7817-8337-8 (alk. paper)
1. Gastrointestinal system—Outlines, syllabi, etc. I Title. II. Series: High-yield systems.
[DNLM: 1. Gastrointestinal Tract—Outlines. 2. Gastrointestinal Diseases—Outlines. WI 18.2 D845h 2009]
QP151.D83 2009
612.3'2—dc22

2009019061

DISCLAIMER

Care has been taken to confirm the accuracy of the information present and to describe generally accepted practices. However, the authors, editors, and publisher are not responsible for errors or omissions or for any consequences from application of the information in this book and make no warranty, expressed or implied, with respect to the currency, completeness, or accuracy of the contents of the publication. Application of this information in a particular situation remains the professional responsibility of the practitioner; the clinical treatments described and recommended may not be considered absolute and universal recommendations.

The authors, editors, and publisher have exerted every effort to ensure that drug selection and dosage set forth in this text are in accordance with the current recommendations and practice at the time of publication. However, in view of ongoing research, changes in government regulations, and the constant flow of information relating to drug therapy and drug reactions, the reader is urged to check the package insert for each drug for any change in indications and dosage and for added warnings and precautions. This is particularly important when the recommended agent is a new or infrequently employed drug.

Some drugs and medical devices presented in this publication have Food and Drug Administration (FDA) clearance for limited use in restricted research settings. It is the responsibility of the health care provider to ascertain the FDA status of each drug or device planned for use in their clinical practice.

To purchase additional copies of this book, call our customer service department at **(800) 638-3030** or fax orders to **(301) 223-2320**. International customers should call **(301) 223-2300**.

Visit Lippincott Williams & Wilkins on the Internet: http://www.lww.com. Lippincott Williams & Wilkins customer service representatives are available from 8:30 am to 6:00 pm, EST.

Preface

A Focused Curriculum is a curriculum in which students are immersed in one basic science discipline (e.g., Histology) for a concentrated period of time when Histology is covered from A to Z. A Systems-based Curriculum is a curriculum wherein students are immersed in one system (e.g., urinary system) for a concentrated period of time when all basic science disciplines of the Urinary system are covered (e.g., Embryology, Histology, Physiology, Pharmacology, and so forth).

The *High-Yield Systems* series addresses a problem endemic to medical schools in the United States and medical students using a Focused Curriculum. After completing a Focused Curriculum, the medical student is faced with the daunting task of integrating and collating all the basic science knowledge accrued from the Focused Curriculum into the various systems. For example, a medical student wanting to review everything about the kidney will find the information scattered in his or her embryology notes, histology notes, physiology notes, pharmacology notes, and so forth. The *High-Yield Systems* series eliminates this daunting task for the medical student by bringing together the embryology, gross anatomy, radiology, histology, physiology, microbiology, and pharmacology of the kidney all in one clear concise book.

The *High-Yield Systems* series has great utility for the following users:

1. First-year medical students in a Focused Curriculum, who want to get a head start on the inevitable process of integrating and collating all the information learned in a Focused Curriculum into systems
2. First-year medical students in a Systems-based Curriculum, who will find this series a natural textbook for such an approach
3. Medical students preparing for Step 1 of the USMLE in which the questions are becoming increasingly more systems-based than discipline-based
4. Second-year medical students for whom the curriculum is much more systems-based, as pathology covers the pathology of each system as a block (e.g., pathology of the lung, pathology of the heart, and pathology of the kidney)
5. Senior medical students who may want to quickly review all aspects of kidney function before starting a rotation in nephrology, for example
6. Recent medical graduates who may want to quickly review all aspects of kidney function before starting a residency in nephrology, for example

In the *High-Yield Systems* series, the student will find the same painstaking attention given to including high-yield information as found in other *High-Yield* books. However, the breadth of information has been expanded somewhat to cover some baseline information without which a complete understanding of the system would be difficult.

The *High-Yield* books based on the presentation of high-yield information that is likely to be asked on the USMLE have clearly been an asset to the medical student. After writing many *High-Yield* books, however, I have found that high-yield information can also be presented in a high-efficiency manner. In the *High-Yield Systems* series, the student now gets the benefit of both high yield and high efficiency in his or her studies.

I appreciate any feedback and can be contacted at dudekr@ecu.edu.

Contents

Chapter 1

Embryology

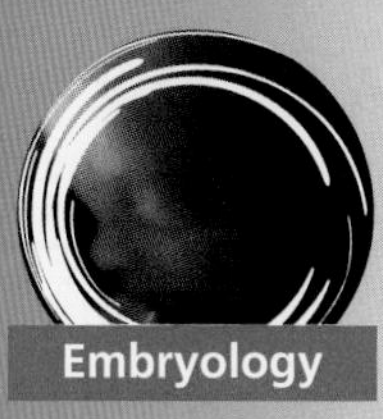

I Primitive Gut Tube *(Figure 1-1)*

The **primitive gut tube** is formed from the incorporation of the dorsal part of the yolk sac into the embryo due to the craniocaudal folding and lateral folding of the embryo. The primitive gut tube extends from the **oropharyngeal membrane** to the **cloacal membrane** and is divided into the **foregut**, **midgut**, and **hindgut**. The primitive gut tube is composed of two layers: an inner layer of **endoderm** that lines the lumen and an outer layer of **visceral mesoderm**. Histologically, the general plan of the adult gastrointestinal tract consists of a **mucosa** (epithelial lining and glands, lamina propria, and muscularis mucosae), **submucosa**, **muscularis externa**, and **adventitia** or **serosa**. Embryologically, the epithelial lining and glands of the mucosa are derived from endoderm, whereas the other components are derived from visceral mesoderm. Early in development, the epithelial lining of the gut tube proliferates rapidly and obliterates the lumen. Later in development, **recanalization** occurs.

II Foregut Derivatives

The foregut derivatives are the esophagus, stomach, liver, gallbladder, pancreas, and upper duodenum. The foregut ends gross anatomically at the **ampulla of Vater**. The foregut derivatives are supplied by the **celiac artery**. The exception to this is the esophagus, wherein the intra-abdominal portion of the esophagus is supplied by the celiac trunk, but the intrathoracic portion is supplied by other branches of the aorta.

A. Esophagus *(Figure 1-2)*

1. **Formation**. The foregut is divided into the esophagus dorsally and the trachea ventrally by the **tracheoesophageal folds**, which fuse to form the **tracheoesophageal septum**. The esophagus is initially short but lengthens as it descends with the heart and lungs. During development, the endodermal lining of the esophagus proliferates rapidly and obliterates the lumen; later recanalization occurs. At week 13, mature ganglion cells are found in the myenteric plexus of Auerbach but the onset of motor activity does not begin until ≈week 17. Human fetal swallowing has been observed as early as week 17.
2. **Clinical correlations**
   a. **Esophageal atresia** occurs when the tracheoesophageal septum deviates too far dorsally, causing the esophagus to end as a closed tube. About 33% of patients with esophageal atresia also have other congenital defects associated with the VATER or VACTERL syndromes. It is associated clinically with polyhydramnios (fetus is unable to swallow amniotic fluid) and a tracheoesophageal fistula.
   b. **Esophageal stenosis** usually involves the midesophagus and occurs when the lumen of the esophagus is narrowed. The stenosis may be caused by submucosal/muscularis externa hypertrophy, remnants of the tracheal cartilaginous ring within the wall of the esophagus, or a membranous diaphragm obstructing the lumen probably because of incomplete recanalization.
   c. **Esophageal duplication** occurs most commonly because of a congenital esophageal cyst, which is usually found (60% of the cases) in the lower esophagus. Duplication cysts may lie on the posterior aspect of the esophagus

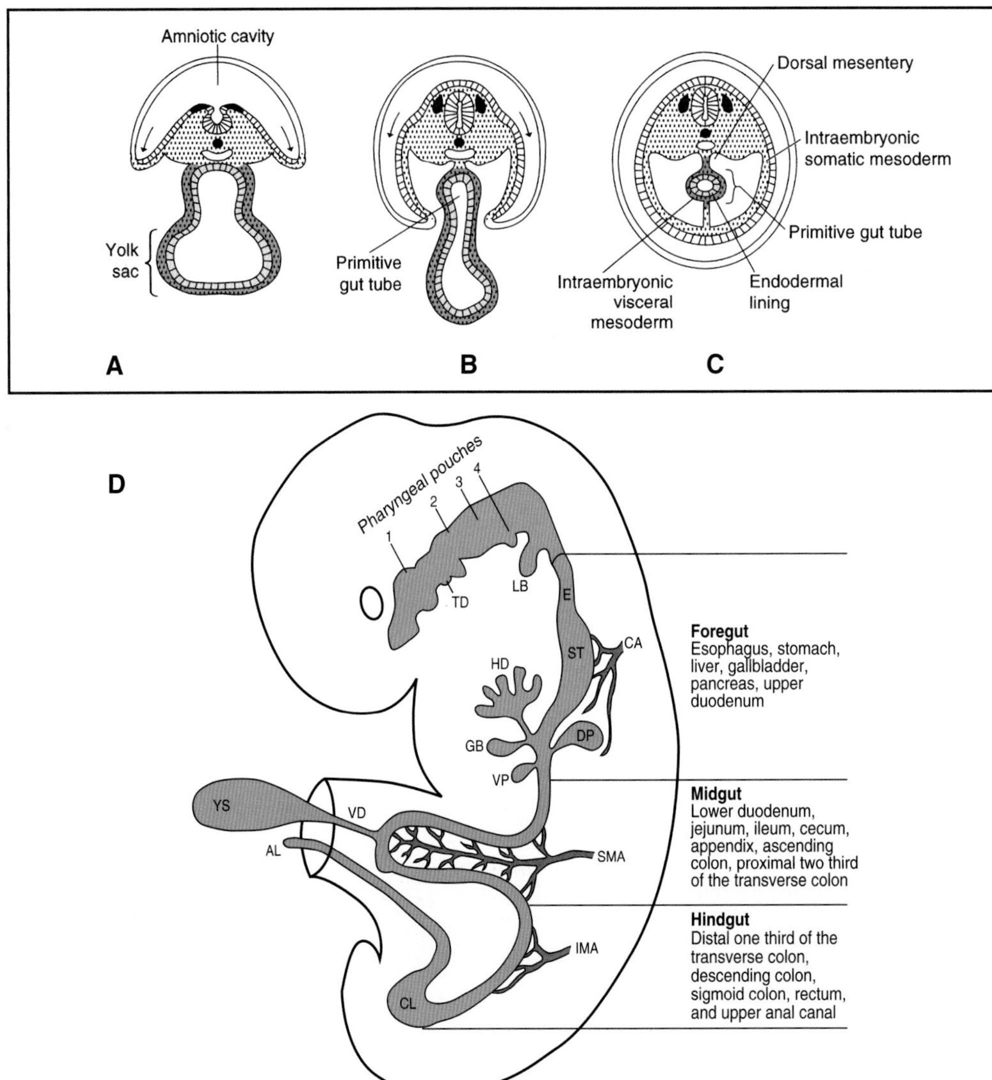

FIGURE 1-1. **Primitive Gut Tube. (A–C) Cross Sections of an Embryo Showing the Formation of the Primitive Gut Tube.** Note that as the lateral body folds fuse in the midline to form the ventral body wall, the yolk sac consisting of endoderm and visceral mesoderm is incorporated into the intraembryonic coelom. **(D) Development of Gastrointestinal Tract Showing the Foregut, Midgut, and Hindgut Along with the Adult Derivatives.** The entire length of the endodermal gut tube is shown from the mouth to the anus. The fate of the lung bud (LB), pharyngeal pouches (1,2,3,4), and thyroid diverticulum (TD) are related to head and neck development and will not be considered here.

where they protrude into the posterior mediastinum or within the wall of the esophagus (i.e., intramural).

d. **Vascular compression of the esophagus** occurs when there is an abnormal origin of the **right subclavian artery** because of developmental anomalies of the aortic arches. The anomalous right subclavian artery passes from the aortic arch behind the esophagus and may cause dysphagia ("dysphagia lusoria").

e. **Tracheoesophageal fistula** is an abnormal communication between the trachea and esophagus that results from improper division of the foregut by the tracheoesophageal septum. It is generally associated with **esophageal atresia** and **polyhydramnios**. Clinical findings include excessive accumulation of saliva or mucus in the nose and mouth, episodes of gagging and cyanosis after swallowing milk, abdominal distention after crying, and reflux of gastric contents into lungs, causing pneumonitis. Diagnostic findings include inabil-

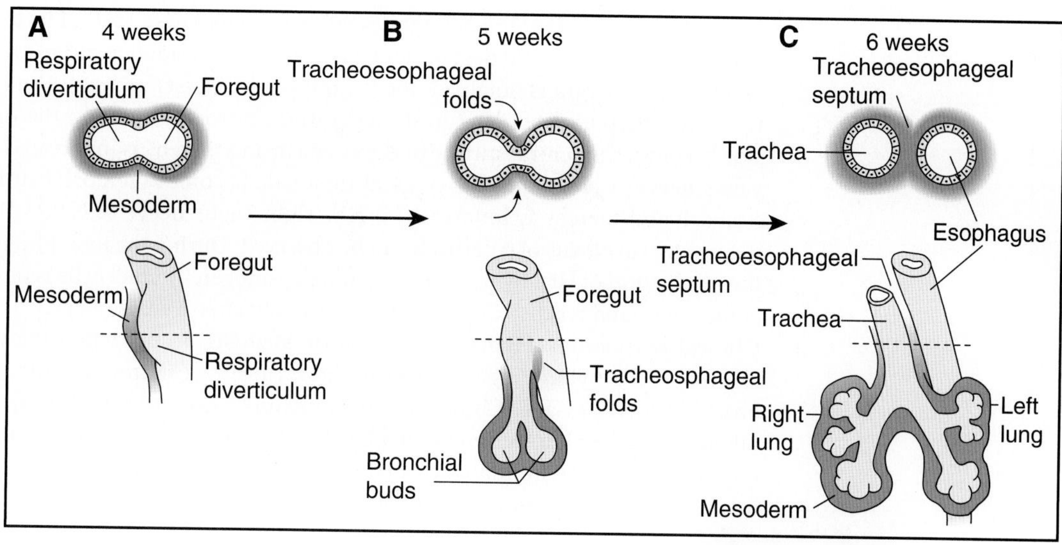

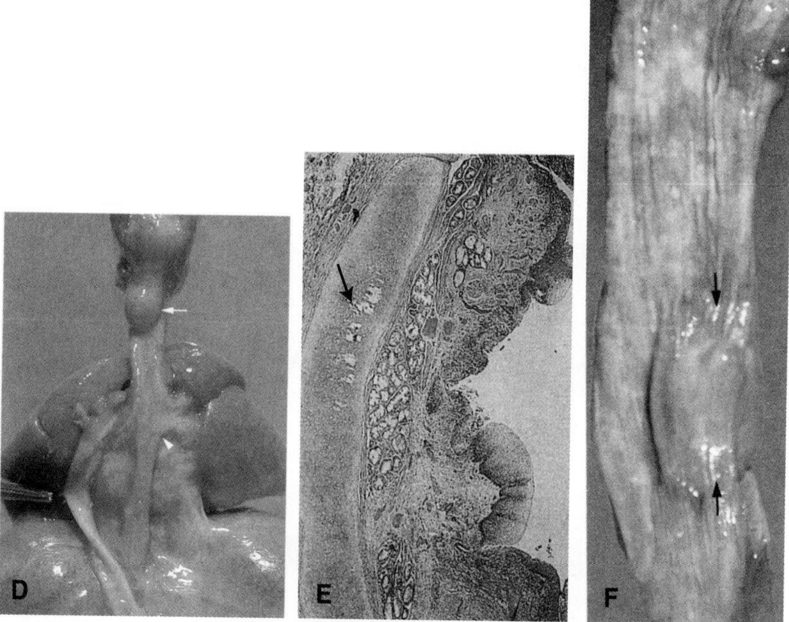

FIGURE 1-2. **Esophagus. (A–C)** Development of esophagus at **(A)** 4 weeks, **(B)** 5 weeks, and **(C)** 6 weeks. Both lateral views and cross-sectional views are shown. Note the relationship of the respiratory diverticulum and foregut. Curved arrows indicate the movement of the tracheoesophageal folds as the tracheoesophageal septum consisting of visceral mesoderm forms between the trachea and esophagus and splits the foregut into two separate tubes. **(D) Esophageal Atresia.** A posterior view shows that the esophagus terminates blindly in a blunted esophageal pouch (arrow). There is a distal esophageal connection with the trachea at the carina (arrowhead). **(E) Esophageal Stenosis.** This micrograph shows the stratified squamous epithelial lining of the esophagus and submucosal glands. Note that a portion of the muscular wall contains remnants of cartilage (arrow), which contributes to a stenosis. **(F) Gross Anatomy Photograph of the Esophagus.** This photograph shows a large intramural duplication cyst (arrows).

ity to pass a catheter into the stomach and radiographs demonstrating air in the infant's stomach.

B. Stomach *(Figure 1-3)*

1. **Formation**. A fusiform dilatation forms in the foregut in week 4, which gives rise to the **primitive stomach**. The primitive stomach is suspended from the posterior body wall by a dorsal mesentery called the **dorsal mesogastrium**. The primitive stomach is also suspended from the anterior body wall by a ventral mesentery called the **ventral mesogastrium**. The dorsal part of the primitive stomach grows faster than the ventral part, thereby resulting in the greater and lesser curvatures, respectively. At

≈week 6, the primitive stomach rotates **90 degree clockwise** around its longitudinal axis. As a result of this 90 degree clockwise rotation, the adult anatomic relationship of all foregut viscera is obtained; the ventral border (lesser curvature) moves to the right and the dorsal border (greater curvature) moves to the left; the original left side becomes the ventral surface of the stomach and thereby is innervated by the **left vagus nerve** (CN X); and the original right side becomes the dorsal surface of the stomach and thereby is innervated by the **right vagus nerve** (CN X). At week 13, the myenteric plexus of Auerbach can be observed. During the first 3 months of life, the production of HCl by parietal cells and pepsinogen by chief cells is only <50% of adult values and reaches mature adult levels only after 2 years of age.

2. **Clinical correlation. Hypertrophic pyloric stenosis** occurs when the muscularis externa in the pyloric region hypertrophies, causing a narrow pyloric lumen that obstructs food passage. Clinical findings include association with projectile, non-bilious vomiting after feeding; a small, palpable mass at the right costal margin; and increased incidence in infants treated with the antibiotic, erythromycin. Treatment involves surgical incision of the hypertrophic muscle.

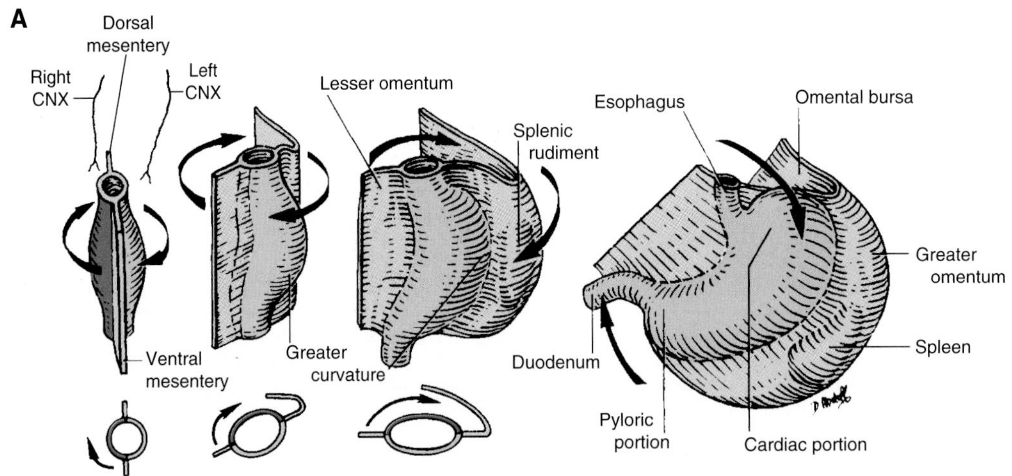

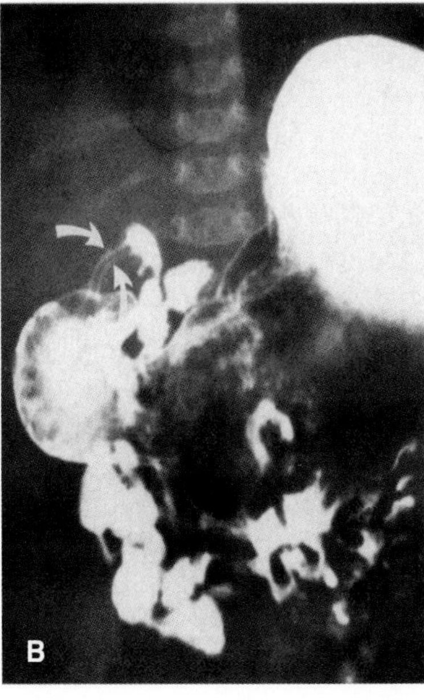

FIGURE 1-3. **Stomach. (A)** Diagram depicting the development and 90 degree clockwise rotation of the stomach from week 4 through week 6. **(B) Hypertrophic Pyloric Stenosis.** Barium contrast radiograph show the long, narrow, double channel of the pylorus (arrows) in a patient with hypertrophic pyloric stenosis.

C. Liver *(Figure 1-4A)*

1. **Formation.** The endodermal lining of the foregut forms an outgrowth called the **hepatic diverticulum**, which pushes into the surrounding mesoderm of the **septum transversum**. Cords of endodermal cells (called **hepatic cords**) from the hepatic diverticulum begin to grow into the mesoderm of the septum transversum. Eventually, the hepatic cords arrange themselves around the **vitelline veins and umbilical veins**, which are coursing through the septum transversum, and form the definitive adult **hepatic sinusoids**. In addition, the mesoderm of the septum transversum is involved in the formation of the **diaphragm**, which explains the intimate gross anatomic relationship between the liver and diaphragm.

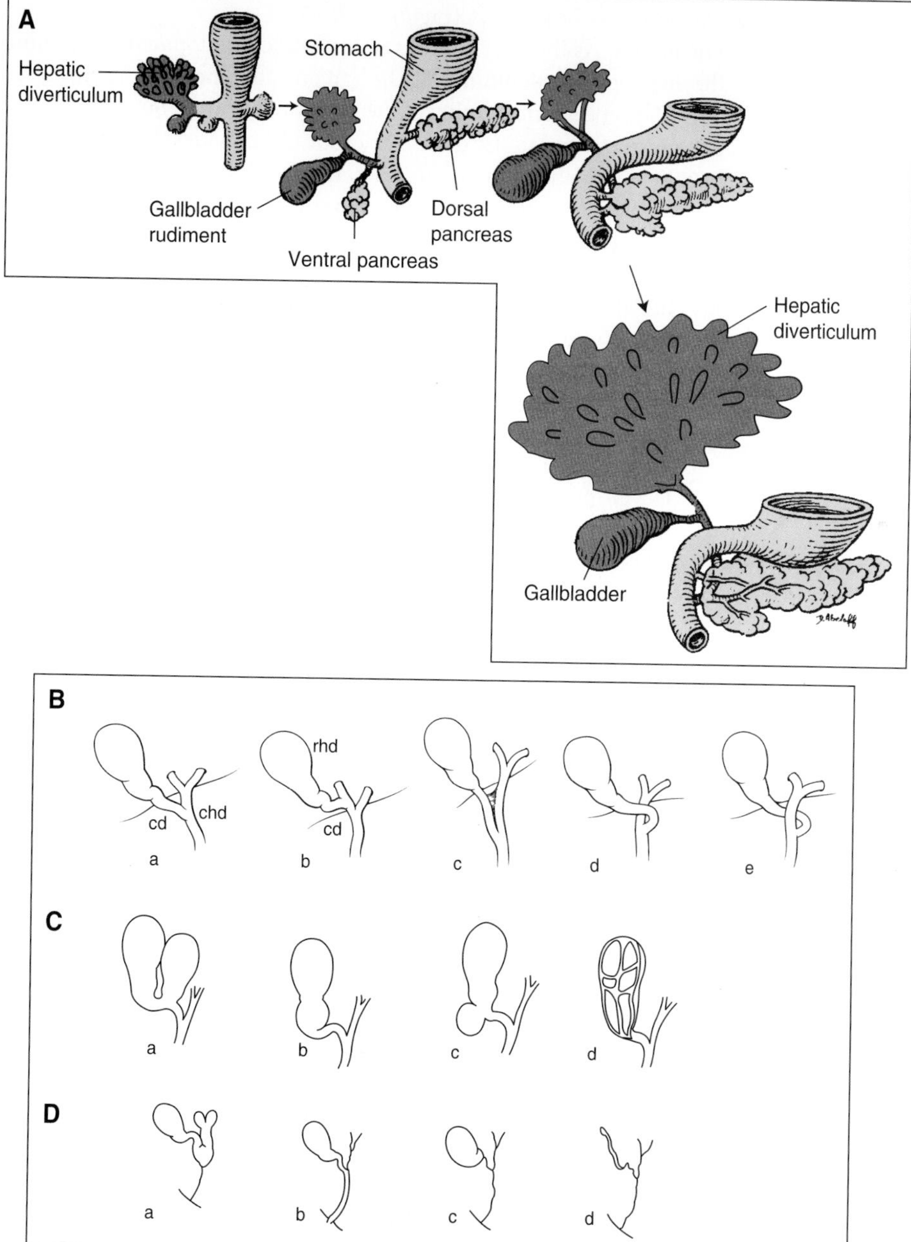

FIGURE 1-4. **Liver and Gallbladder. (A)** Sequence of events in the development of the hepatic diverticulum and gallbladder rudiment from week 4 through week 7. **(B) Developmental Anomalies of the Cystic Duct. (a)** Cystic duct (cd) joins the common hepatic duct (chd) directly (most common anatomical arrangement). **(b)** Cystic duct joins the right hepatic duct (rhd). **(c)** Low junction of cystic duct with the common hepatic duct. **(d)**Anterior spiral of cystic duct. **(e)** Posterior spiral of cystic duct. **(C) Developmental Anomalies of the Gallbladder. (a)** Two gallbladders. **(b)** Bilobed gallbladder. **(c)** Diverticulum of the gallbladder. **(d)** Septated gallbladder is most likely due to incomplete recanalization of the lumen. **(D) Different Forms of Extrahepatic Biliary Atresia. (a–c)** Partial. **(d)** Complete.

At week 6, the liver begins **hematopoiesis** whereby large nests of mesodermally derived cells that produce red and white blood cells are found between the hepatocytes and the hepatic sinusoids.

At week 12, the liver begins **bile production** by the hepatocytes. Since the gallbladder and bile ducts have already developed by week 12, bile can enter the gastrointestinal tract and take on a dark, green color. The bile duct initially opens into the duodenum on the anterior surface. However, because of the 90 degree clockwise rotation, the opening of the bile duct gradually shifts from an initial anterior position to the definitive adult posterior position.

2. **Clinical correlation**. Congenital malformations of the liver are rare.

D. Gallbladder and Bile Ducts *(Figure 1-4B–D)*

1. **Formation**. As the liver continues its prolific development, the connection between the hepatic diverticulum and the foregut stretches and narrows to form the **bile duct**. The endodermal lining of the bile duct forms an outgrowth called the **gallbladder rudiment** and **cystic duct**. The cystic duct divides the bile duct into the common hepatic duct and common bile duct. During development, the endodermal lining of the gallbladder and extrahepatic bile ducts proliferates rapidly and obliterates the lumen; later recanalization occurs.
2. **Clinical correlations**
   a. **Intrahepatic gallbladder** occurs when the gallbladder rudiment advances beyond the hepatic diverticulum and becomes buried within the substance of the liver.
   b. **Floating gallbladder** occurs when the gallbladder rudiment lags behind the hepatic diverticulum and thereby becomes suspended from the liver by a mesentery. A floating gallbladder is at risk for **torsion**.
   c. **Developmental anomalies of the cystic duct** anatomy are fairly common.
   d. **Developmental anomalies of the gallbladder** anatomy are fairly common wherein two, bilobed diverticula and septated gallbladders are found.
   e. **Biliary atresia** is defined as the obliteration of extrahepatic and/or intrahepatic ducts. The ducts are replaced by fibrotic tissue because of acute and chronic inflammation. It is associated clinically with progressive neonatal jaundice with onset soon after birth, white clay-colored stool, and dark-colored urine. The average survival time is 12 to 19 months with a 100% mortality rate.

E. Pancreas *(Figure 1-5)*

1. **Formation.** At week 4, the endodermal lining of the foregut first forms an outgrowth called the **dorsal pancreatic bud** whose formation seems to be induced by the notochord. Shortly afterward, the endodermal lining of the foregut forms another outgrowth called the **ventral pancreatic bud** whose formation seems to be induced by cardiac mesoderm. Within both pancreatic buds, endodermal tubules surrounded by mesoderm branch repeatedly to form **acinar cells** and **ducts** (i.e., exocrine pancreas). At the same time, isolated clumps of endodermal cells bud from the tubules and accumulate within the mesoderm to form **islet cells** (i.e., endocrine pancreas) in the following sequence (first→last): **alpha cells** (glucagon)→ **beta cells** (insulin)→ **delta cells** (somatostatin) and **PP cells** (pancreatic polypeptide). By ≈week 19, typical mature acinar cells, ducts, and islets cells are present along with their differentiated cell secretory products.

   The **dorsal pancreatic bud** forms as an endodermal proliferation between the layers of the dorsal mesentery. The **ventral pancreatic bud** forms as an endodermal proliferation between the layers of the ventral mesentery.

   At ≈week 5, the ventral bud rotates dorsally and fuses with the dorsal bud to form the definitive adult pancreas because of the 90 degree clockwise rotation of the duodenum. The ventral bud forms the **uncinate process** and a **portion of the head**

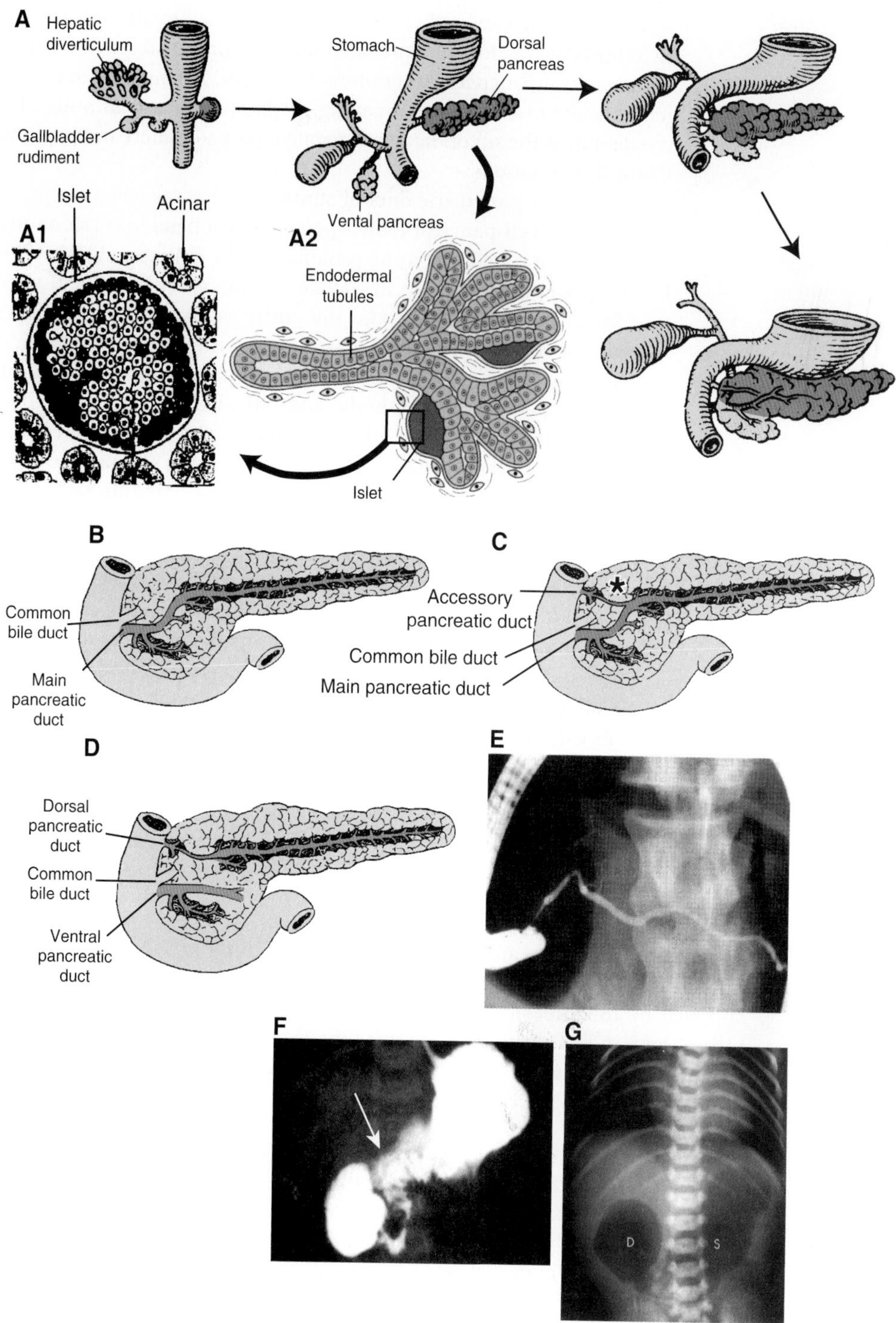

FIGURE 1-5. **Pancreas. (A) Sequence of Events in the Development of the Pancreatic Buds from Week 4 through Week 7.** Note that within the pancreatic buds endodermal tubules branch repeatedly to form the exocrine (acinar) pancreas (see **A2**). Subsequently, endodermal cells bud from the endodermal tubules to form the endocrine (islet) pancreas (see **A1**). **(B)** Normal pattern of the main pancreatic duct (48% incidence in the population). **(C) Accessory Pancreatic Duct (33% Incidence in the Population).** Note that the proximal one third of the dorsal pancreatic duct persists (*). **(D,E) Pancreas Divisum.** Note that distal two thirds of the dorsal pancreatic duct and the ventral pancreatic duct fail to anastomose, thereby forming two separate duct systems. An endoscopic retrograde pancreatogram performed through the accessory minor papillae shows the dorsal pancreatic duct in pancreatic divisum. **(F,G) Annular Pancreas. (F)** Barium contrast radiograph shows a partial duodenal obstruction (arrow) consistent with an annular pancreas. **(G)** Radiograph shows that both the stomach (S) and duodenum (D) are distended with air leading to the "double bubble" sign.

of the pancreas. The dorsal bud forms the **remaining portion of the head, body,** and **tail of the pancreas**.

The main pancreatic duct of Wirsung is formed by the anastomosis of the **distal two thirds of the dorsal pancreatic duct** (the proximal one third regresses) and the **entire ventral pancreatic duct** (48% incidence). The main pancreatic duct and common bile duct form a single opening (**hepatopancreatic ampulla of Vater**) into the duodenum at the tip of the major papillae (**hepatopancreatic papillae**).

2. **Clinical correlations**
   a. **Accessory pancreatic duct of Santorini** develops when the proximal one third of the dorsal pancreatic duct persists and opens into the duodenum through the minor papillae at a site proximal to the ampulla of Vater (33% incidence).
   b. **Pancreas divisum** (4% incidence) occurs when the **distal two thirds of the dorsal pancreatic duct** and the **entire ventral pancreatic duct** fail to anastomose and the proximal one third of the dorsal pancreatic duct persists, thereby forming two separate duct systems. The dorsal pancreatic duct drains a **portion of the head, body,** and **tail of the pancreas** by opening into the duodenum through the minor papillae. The ventral pancreatic duct drains the **uncinate process** and a **portion of the head of the pancreas** by opening into the duodenum through the major papillae. Patients with pancreas divisum are prone to pancreatitis especially if the opening of the dorsal pancreatic duct at the minor papillae is small.
   c. **Annular pancreas** occurs when the ventral pancreatic bud fuses with the dorsal bud both dorsally and ventrally, thereby forming a **ring of pancreatic tissue** around the duodenum causing severe **duodenal obstruction**. Newborns and infants are intolerant of oral feeding and often have bilious vomiting. Radiographic evidence of an annular pancreas is indicated by a duodenal obstruction where a "double bubble" sign is often seen because of dilation of the stomach and distal duodenum.

F. Upper Duodenum

The upper duodenum develops from the caudal portion of the foregut.

III Midgut Derivatives

The midgut derivatives are the lower duodenum, jejunum, ileum, cecum, appendix, ascending colon, and the proximal two thirds of the transverse colon. The midgut derivatives are supplied by the **superior mesenteric artery**. The development of the midgut is characterized by rapid elongation of the gut tube that results in the formation of the U-shaped **midgut loop**. At its apex, the midgut loop remains in open connection with the yolk sac by way of the **vitelline duct**.

A. Lower Duodenum

1. **Formation.** The **lower duodenum** develops from the cranial portion of the midgut. The junction of the upper and lower duodenum is just distal to the opening of the common bile duct. The entire developing duodenum grows rapidly and forms a C-shaped loop that initially projects ventrally. Because of the 90 degree clockwise rotation, the C-shaped duodenum rotates to the right and eventually comes to rest in a retroperitoneal position (except for the first 2 cm of the superior part of the duodenum, which is intraperitoneal and is referred to as the **duodenal cap** or **duodenal bulb**). During development, the endodermal lining of the duodenum proliferates rapidly and obliterates the lumen; later recanalization occurs.
2. **Clinical considerations**
   a. **Duodenal stenosis** occurs when the lumen of the duodenum is narrowed as a result of incomplete recanalization.
   b. **Duodenal atresia** occurs when the lumen of the duodenum is occluded as a result of failed recanalization. Clinical findings include polyhydramnios, bile-containing vomitus, and a distended stomach.

B. Jejunum, Ileum, Cecum, Appendix, Ascending Colon, and Proximal Two Thirds of Transverse Colon (*Figure 1-6*)

1. **Formation**. At week 5, the midgut forms a U-shaped loop (**midgut loop**). During weeks 5 to 10, the midgut loop continues its rapid elongation and herniates through the primitive umbilical ring into the extraembryonic coelom (i.e., **physiological umbilical herniation**). During this period of rapid elongation, the midgut loop rotates **90 degree** around the superior mesenteric artery, which directs the proximal midgut to the right side and the distal midgut to the left side. At ≈week 10, the midgut loop rotates an additional **180 degree** as it returns to the abdominal cavity that directs the proximal jejunum to the left side and the ileum to the right side. When the midgut loop returns to the abdominal cavity, the cecal diverticulum enters last and locates temporarily in the right upper quadrant, just caudal to the liver.

   The midgut loop consists of a **cranial limb** and a **caudal limb**. The cranial limb forms the **jejunum** and **upper part of the ileum**. The caudal limb forms the **cecal diverticulum** from which the **cecum** and **appendix** develop. The rest of the caudal limb forms the **lower part of the ileum, ascending colon**, and **proximal two thirds of the transverse colon**.

2. **Clinical correlations**
   a. **Omphalocele** occurs when abdominal contents herniate through the umbilical ring and persist outside the body covered variably by a translucent peritoneal membrane sac (a light gray, shiny sac) protruding from the base of the umbilical cord. Large omphaloceles may contain stomach, liver, and intestines. Small omphaloceles contain only intestines. Omphaloceles are usually associated with other congenital anomalies (e.g., trisomy 13, trisomy 18, or Beckwith–Wiedemann syndrome).
   b. **Gastroschisis** occurs when there is a defect in the ventral abdominal wall usually to the right of the umbilical ring through which there is a massive evisceration of intestines (other organs may also be involved). The intestines are not covered by a peritoneal membrane, are directly exposed to amniotic fluid, and are thickened and covered with adhesions.
   c. **Nonrotation of the midgut loop** occurs when the midgut loop rotates only 90 degree counterclockwise, thereby positioning the small intestine entirely on the right side and the large intestine entirely on the left side with the cecum located either in the left upper quadrant or in the left iliac fossa.
   d. **Malrotation of the midgut loop** occurs when the midgut loop undergoes only partial counterclockwise rotation. This results in the cecum and appendix lying in a subpyloric or subhepatic location and the small intestine suspended by only a vascular pedicle (i.e., not a broad mesentery). A major clinical complication of malrotation is volvulus (twisting of the small intestines around the vascular pedicle), which may cause necrosis because of compromised blood supply. (Note: The abnormal position of the appendix due to malrotation of the midgut should be considered when diagnosing appendicitis.)
   e. **Reversed rotation of the midgut loop** occurs when the midgut loop rotates clockwise instead of counterclockwise, causing the large intestine to enter the abdominal cavity first. This results in the large intestine being anatomically located posterior to the duodenum and superior mesenteric artery.
   f. **Ileal diverticulum (Meckel diverticulum)** occurs when a remnant of the vitelline duct persists, thereby forming an outpouching located on the antimesenteric border of the ileum. The outpouching may connect to the umbilicus via a fibrous cord or fistula. A Meckel diverticulum is usually located about 30 cm proximal to the ileocecal valve in infants and varies in length from 2 to 15 cm. Heterotopic gastric mucosa may be present, which leads to ulceration, perforation, or gastrointestinal bleeding especially if a large number of parietal cells are present. Clinical findings include symptoms resembling appendicitis and bright-red or dark-red stools (i.e., bloody).

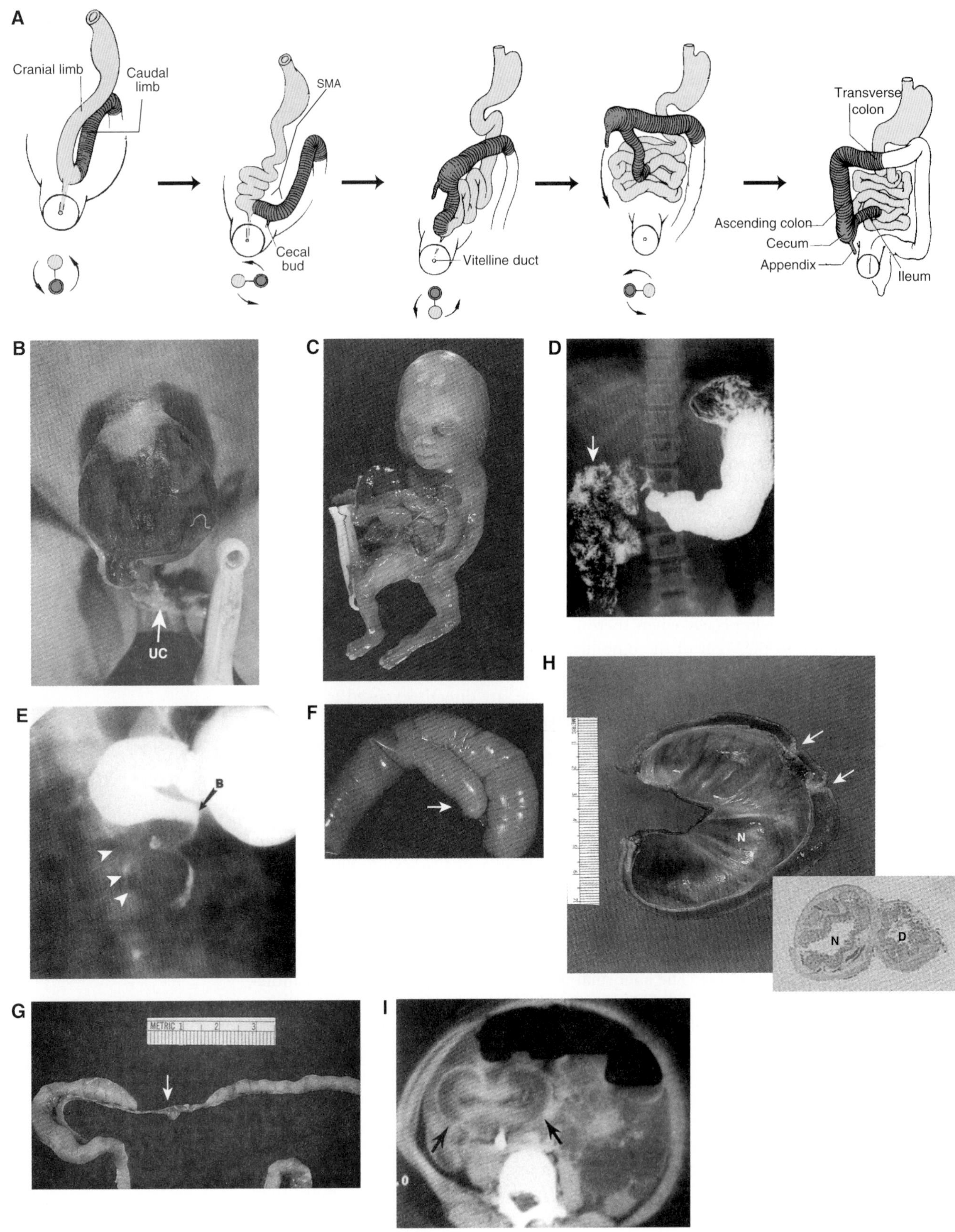
A
Cranial limb
Caudal limb
SMA
Cecal bud
Vitelline duct
Transverse colon
Ascending colon
Cecum
Appendix
Ileum
B
UC
C
D
E
B
F
G
METRIC 1 2 3
H
N
N
D
I

g. **Intestinal atresia and stenosis.** Atresia occurs when the lumen of the intestines is completely occluded; whereas, stenosis occurs when the lumen of the intestines is narrowed. The causes of these conditions seem to be both failed recanalization and an ischemic intrauterine event ("vascular accident").

h. **Duplication of the intestines** occurs when a segment of the intestines is duplicated as a result of abnormal recanalization (most commonly near the ileocecal valve). The duplication is found on the mesenteric border; its lumen generally communicates with the normal bowel, shares the same blood supply as the normal bowel, and is lined by normal intestinal epithelium but heterotopic gastric and pancreatic tissues have also been identified. Clinical findings include an abdominal mass, bouts of abdominal pain, vomiting, chronic rectal bleeding, intussusception, and perforation.

i. **Intussusception occurs** when a segment of bowel invaginates or telescopes into an adjacent bowel segment leading to obstruction or ischemia. This is one of the most common causes of obstruction in children that are 2 years of age, is most often idiopathic, and most commonly involves the ileum and colon (i.e., ileocolic). Clinical findings include acute onset of intermittent abdominal pain, vomiting, bloody stools, diarrhea, and somnolence.

j. **Retrocecal and retrocolic appendix** occurs when the appendix is located on the posterior side of the cecum or colon, respectively. These anomalies are very common and important to remember during appendectomies. (Note: The appendix is normally found on the medial side of the cecum.)

IV Hindgut Derivatives *(Figure 1-7)*

The hindgut derivatives are the distal one third of the transverse colon, descending colon, sigmoid colon, rectum, and the upper anal canal. The hindgut derivatives are supplied by the **inferior mesenteric artery**.

A. Formation. The cranial end of the hindgut develops into the distal one third of the transverse colon, descending colon, and sigmoid colon. The terminal end of the hindgut is an endoderm-lined pouch called the **cloaca**, which contacts the surface ectoderm of the **proctodeum** to form the **cloacal membrane**. As development proceeds, the cloaca is partitioned by the **urorectal septum** into a posterior portion, which develops into the rectum and upper anal canal, and an anterior portion, which develops into the **urogenital sinus.** By week 7, the urorectal septum has fused with the cloacal membrane, thereby partitioning the **cloacal membrane** into the posterior **anal membrane** and anterior **urogenital membrane**. The urorectal septum fuses with the cloacal membrane at the future site of the gross anatomical structure called the **perineal body**. At the end of week 7, the cloacal membrane ruptures thereby creating a posterior opening for the hindgut and an anterior opening for the urogenital sinus.

B. Clinical Correlation. Colonic aganglionosis (Hirschsprung disease) is caused by the arrest of the caudal migration of neural crest cells. The hallmark is the absence of ganglionic cells in the myenteric and submucosal plexuses most commonly in the sigmoid colon and rectum resulting in a narrow segment of colon (i.e., the colon fails to relax). The most characteristic functional finding is the failure of internal anal

FIGURE 1-6. **Midgut Derivatives. (A) Diagram Depicting the 270 Degree Counterclockwise Rotation of the Midgut Loop.** Note the orientation of the cranial limb and caudal limb. After the 270 degree rotation, the cecum and appendix are located in the upper abdominal cavity. Later in development, there is growth in the direction indicated by the arrow so that the cecum and appendix end up in the lower right quadrant. **(B) Omphalocele.** Note the clamp on the umbilical cord (UC). **(C) Gastroschisis. (D) Nonrotation of Midgut Loop.** Radiograph after barium swallow shows the small intestine lying entirely on the right side (arrow). **(E) Volvulus.** Radiograph after a barium swallow shows the typical "beak sign" (arrow; B) that occurs secondary to the twisting of the intestines (volvulus) and an early spiraling of the small intestine (arrowheads). **(F) Ileal (Meckel) Diverticulum.** Photograph shows an ileal or Meckel diverticulum (arrow) outpouching from the ileum. **(G) Intestinal Atresia and Stenosis.** Photograph shows two blind ends of the small intestine connected by a fibrous cord (arrow) with the mesentery intact. **(H) Duplication.** Note the larger diameter of normal bowel segment (N) and the smaller diameter of the duplicated segment (D). Atretic areas (arrows) are indicated in the duplicated segment. **(I) Intussusception.** CT scan shows two loops of the intussusception (arrows) with fluid present in one loop and a concentric appearance in the other. SMA — superior mesenteric artery.

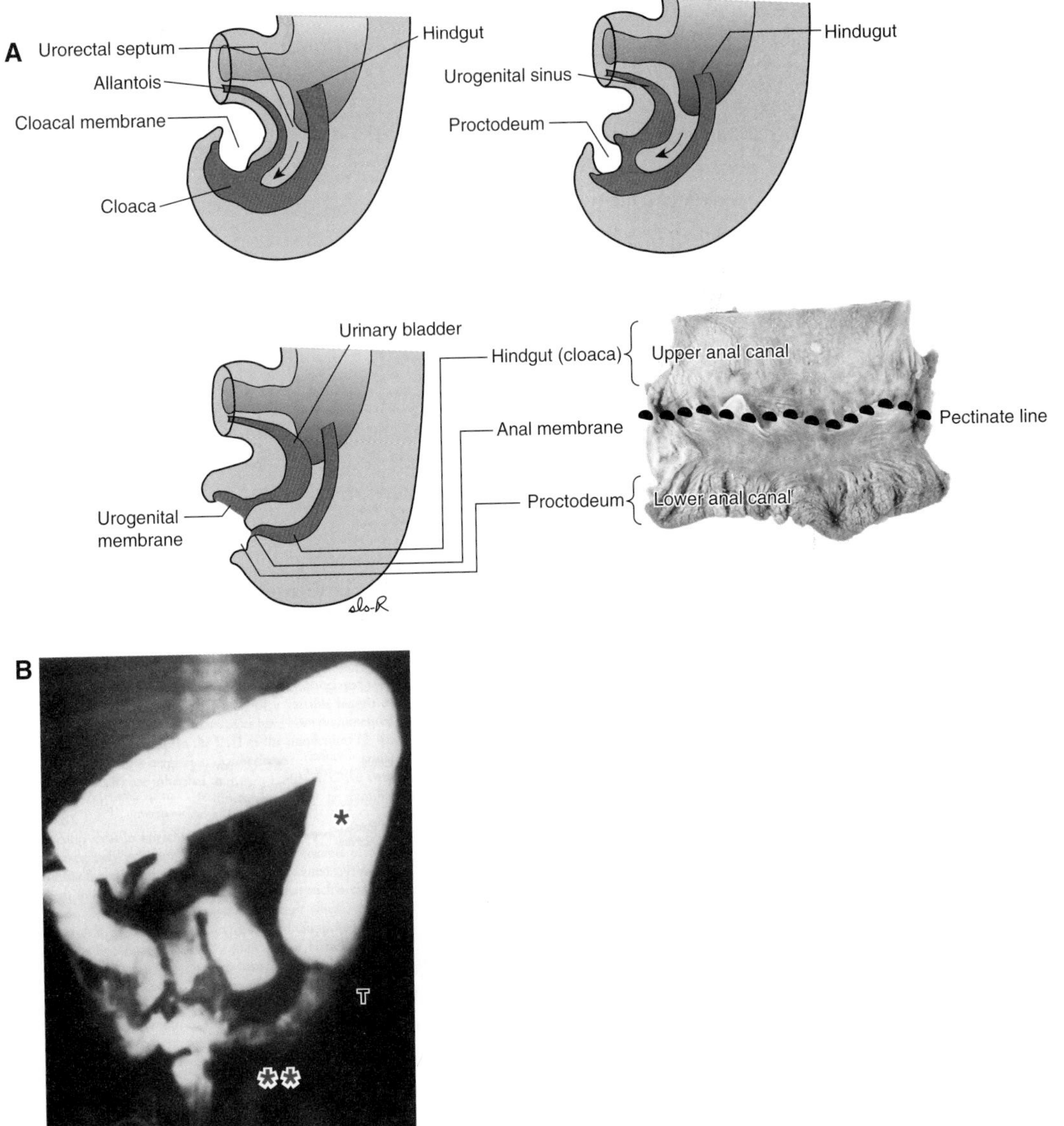

FIGURE 1-7. **Hindgut Derivatives. (A) Diagram Depicting the Partitioning of the Cloaca by Urorectal Septum.** The bold arrow shows the direction of growth of the urorectal septum. **(B) Hirschsprung Disease.** Radiograph after barium enema of a patient with Hirschsprung disease. The upper segment of the normal colon (*) is distended with fecal material. The lower segment of the colon (**) is narrow. The lower segment is the portion of the colon where the ganglionic cells in the myenteric and submucosal plexuses are absent. This case shows a low transition zone (T) between the normal colon and aganglionic colon.

sphincter to relax following rectal distention (i.e., abnormal rectoanal reflex). Clinical findings include a distended abdomen, inability to pass meconium, gushing of fecal material upon a rectal digital exam, and a loss of peristalsis in the colon segment distal to the normal innervated colon.

V The Anal Canal *(Figure 1-8)*

A. **Formation.** The **upper anal canal** develops from the **hindgut**. The **lower anal canal** develops from the **proctodeum**, which is an invagination of surface ectoderm caused by a proliferation of mesoderm surrounding the anal membrane. The dual components (hindgut and proctodeum) involved in the embryological formation of the entire anal canal determine the gross anatomy of this area, which becomes important when considering the characteristics and metastasis of anorectal tumors. The junction between the upper and lower anal canals is indicated by the **pectinate line**, which also marks

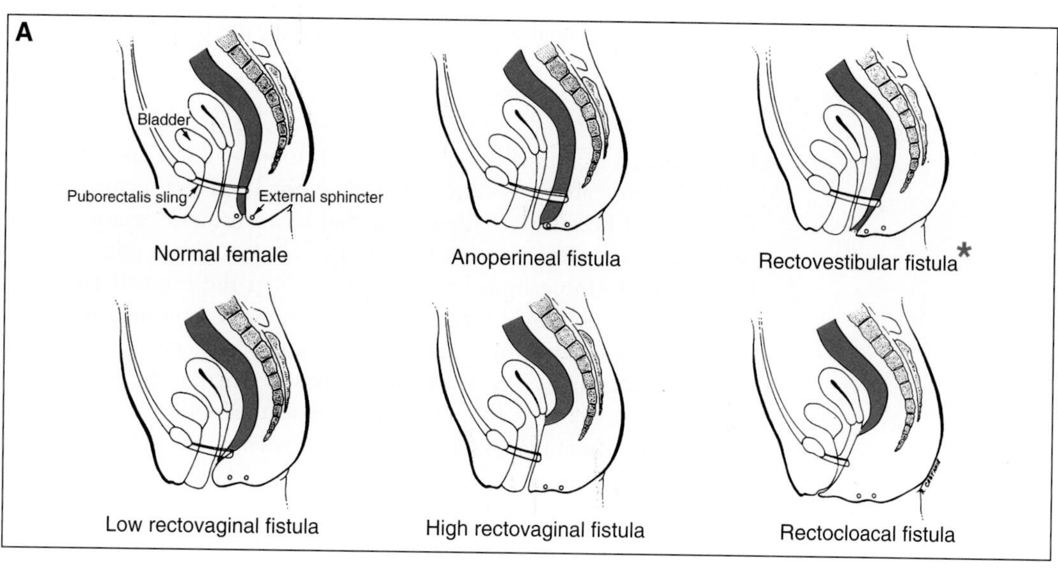

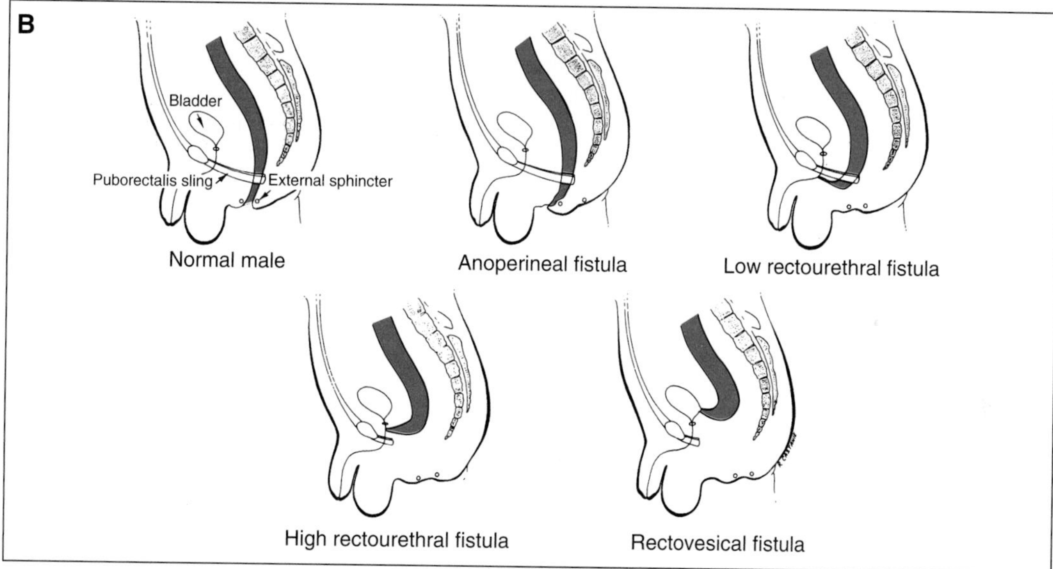

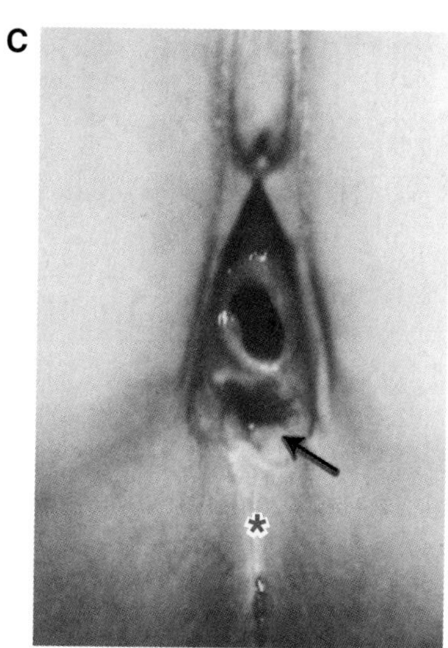

FIGURE 1-8. **Anal Canal. (A) Types of Ectopic Anus in Females.** In ectopic anus, the anus opens ectopically through various types of fistulas. The rectovestibular fistula (*) is the most common type of fistula found associated with ectopic anus. The location of the puborectalis muscle (or sling) is shown. **(B) Types of Ectopic Anus in Males.** Ectopic anus, the anus opens ectopically through various types of fistulas. The location of the puborectalis muscle (or sling) is shown. **(C) Photograph of a Female Infant with Ectopic Anus.** The * indicates the normal site of the anus. This case of ectopic anus is associated with a rectovestibular fistula (arrow) located immediately below the hymenal ring.

the site of the former **anal membrane**. In the adult, the pectinate line is located at the lower border of the anal columns.

B. Clinical Correlations

1. **Rectal atresia** occurs when the anus is both present and open, but a variable segment of rectum above it is atretic. The anal canal and rectum are present but remain unconnected because of either abnormal recanalization or a compromised blood supply (i.e., ischemia) causing focal atresia. No fistulas are present in rectal atresia.
2. **Ectopic anus (Imperforate anus)** occurs when the hindgut ends as a blind sac because of the abnormal formation of the urorectal septum. There are two general types of ectopic anus. In the first type, the hindgut ends **above the puborectalis muscle** (sometimes called **anorectal agenesis**) wherein the puborectalis muscle is hypoplastic or even absent. In the second type, the hindgut ends below the puborectalis muscle (sometime called **anal agenesis**) wherein the puborectalis muscle is well developed and functional. The most important consideration in the surgical correction of ectopic anus so that anal continence is established is the integrity of the puborectalis muscle since the internal and external anal sphincters are usually underdeveloped and functionally inadequate. In ectopic anus, the anus opens ectopically through various types of fistulas. In the female, **anoperineal fistulas, rectovestibular fistulas** (most common), **low rectovaginal fistulas, high rectovaginal fistulas**, and **rectocloacal fistulas** have been reported. In the male, **anoperineal fistulas, low rectourethral fistulas, high rectourethral fistulas**, and **rectovesical fistulas** have been reported.

VI Mesenteries *(Table 1-1)*

The primitive gut tube is suspended within the peritoneal cavity of the embryo by the **septum transversum** and **dorsal mesentery** from which all adult mesenteries are derived. The septum transversum is present only in the region of the lower esophagus, stomach, liver, and upper duodenum. When the hepatic cords grow into the septum transversum, the septum transversum is stretched and divided into the **lesser omentum** and the **falciform ligament**. The dorsal mesentery is present in the region of the lower esophagus and extends all the way down to the cloacal region of the hindgut. The dorsal mesentery is called the **dorsal mesogastrium** in the region of the stomach, **dorsal mesoduodenum** in the region of the duodenum, **mesentery proper** in the region of the jejunum and ileum, and **dorsal mesocolon** in the region of the colon.

TABLE 1-1 DERIVATION OF ADULT MESENTERIES

Embryonic Mesentery	Adult Mesentery
Ventral mesogastrium	Lesser omentum (hepatogastric and hepatoduodenal ligaments), falciform ligament, coronary ligament of the liver, and triangular ligaments of the liver
Dorsal mesentery	Greater omentum (gastrorenal, gastrosplenic, gastrocolic, and splenorenal ligaments), mesentery of small intestine, mesoappendix, transverse mesocolon, sigmoid mesocolon

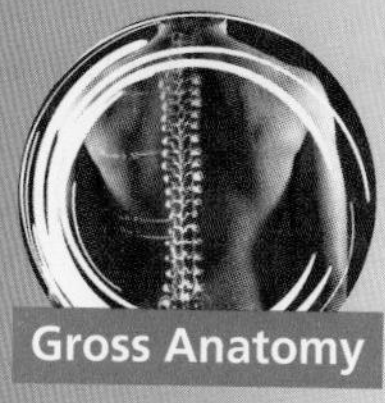

Chapter **2**

Gross Anatomy

Vasculature of the Gastrointestinal Tract

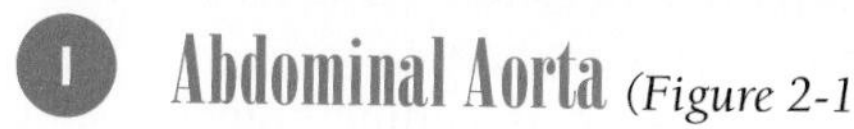

I Abdominal Aorta *(Figure 2-1)*

A. Major Branches

1. **Celiac trunk** is located at **T12** vertebral level and supplies viscera that derive embryologically from the **foregut** (i.e., intra-abdominal portion of esophagus, stomach, upper part of duodenum, liver, gallbladder, and pancreas). It further branches into the following arteries:
   a. **Left gastric artery.** The left gastric artery runs along the lesser curvature of the stomach, anastomoses with the right gastric artery, and gives rise to esophageal and hepatic branches
   b. **Splenic artery.** The splenic artery runs along the superior border of the pancreas. The splenic artery gives rise to the
      i. **Dorsal pancreatic artery**
      ii. **Short gastric arteries**
      iii. **Left gastroepiploic artery**
   c. **Common hepatic artery.** The common hepatic artery runs along the superior border of the pancreas. The common hepatic artery gives rise to the
      i. **Proper hepatic artery.** The proper hepatic artery gives rise to the **right hepatic artery** and **left hepatic artery.** The right hepatic artery gives rise to the **cystic artery** (in 70% of cases) that supplies the gallbladder. The right hepatic artery originates from the common hepatic artery (in 85% of cases) and can be commonly found arising from the superior mesenteric artery.
      ii. **Right gastric artery.** The right gastric artery runs along the lesser curvature of the stomach and anastomoses with the left gastric artery.
      iii. **Gastroduodenal artery.** The gastroduodenal artery runs posterior to the first part of the duodenum. The gastroduodenal artery gives rise to the **right gastroepiploic artery** and the **superior pancreaticoduodenal artery** that further divides into the **anterior superior pancreaticoduodenal artery** and the **posterior superior pancreaticoduodenal artery**.
2. **Superior mesenteric artery** is located at **L1** vertebral level and supplies viscera that derive embryologically from the **midgut** (i.e., lower part of duodenum, jejunum, ileum, cecum, appendix, ascending colon, and proximal two thirds of transverse colon). The superior mesenteric artery gives rise to the following arteries:
   a. **Inferior pancreaticoduodenal artery.** The inferior pancreaticoduodenal artery further divides into the **anterior inferior pancreaticoduodenal artery** and **posterior inferior pancreaticoduodenal artery** which anastomose with the corresponding branches of the superior pancreaticoduodenal artery.
   b. **Middle colic artery.** The middle colic artery runs within the transverse mesocolon. The middle colic artery gives rise to a **right branch** that anastomoses with the right colic artery and a **left branch** that anastomoses with the left colic artery. This forms an anastomotic channel along the margin of the large intestine called the **marginal artery**.

c. **Right colic artery**. The right colic artery gives rise to **ascending branches** and **descending branches** that supply the ascending colon.
d. **Ileocolic artery.** The ileocolic artery gives rise to **ascending colic artery** that anastomoses with the right colic artery, **anterior and posterior cecal arteries**, and the **appendicular artery**.
e. **Intestinal arteries.** The 12 to 15 intestinal arteries supply the jejunum and ileum as they branch and anastomose to form a series of arcades within the mesentery.

3. **Renal arteries** supply the kidneys.
4. **Gonadal arteries** supply the testes or ovaries.
5. **Inferior mesenteric artery** is located at **L3** vertebral level and supplies viscera that derive embryologically from the **hindgut** (i.e., distal one third of transverse colon, descending colon, sigmoid colon, and upper portion of rectum). The inferior mesenteric artery gives rise to the following arteries:
   a. **Left colic artery.** The left colic artery gives rise to **ascending branches** and **descending branches** that supply the descending colon.
   b. **Sigmoid arteries.** The 2 to 3 sigmoid arteries supply the sigmoid colon.
   c. **Superior rectal artery.** The superior rectal artery is the termination of the inferior mesenteric artery. The superior rectal artery anastomoses with the middle and inferior rectal arteries.
6. **Common iliac arteries** are the terminal branches of the abdominal aorta.

B. Clinical Considerations. **Abdominal aortic aneurysm (AAA)** is most commonly seen in atherosclerotic elderly males below the L1 vertebral level (i.e., below the renal arteries and superior mesenteric artery). The most common site of a ruptured AAA is below the renal arteries in the **left posterolateral wall (i.e., retroperitoneal)**. In a patient with a ruptured AAA, the first step is immediate compression of the aorta against the vertebral bodies **above the celiac trunk**. During a transabdominal surgical approach to correct a ruptured AAA, the **left renal vein** is put in jeopardy; however, ligation and isolation of the left renal vein to remove it from the operating field to avoid laceration has no effect on overall long-term postoperative renal function. The **inferior mesenteric artery** generally lies in the middle of an AAA. Clinical findings include sudden onset of severe, central abdominal pain that may radiate to the back, a pulsatile tender abdominal mass; if rupture occurs, hypotension and delirium may occur. Surgical complications include **ischemic colitis** due to ligation of the inferior mesenteric artery or **spinal cord ischemia** due to ligation of the great radicular artery.

II Venous Drainage of Abdomen *(Figure 2-2A)*

A. Azygos Venous System. The **azygos vein** ascends on the right side of the vertebral column and drains blood from the inferior vena cava (IVC) to the superior vena cava (SVC). The **hemiazygos vein** ascends on the left side of the vertebral column and drains blood from the left renal vein to the azygos vein.

B. Inferior Vena Cava is formed by the union of the right and left common iliac veins at vertebral level L5. The IVC drains all the blood from below the diaphragm (even portal blood from the gastrointestinal (GI) tract after it percolates through the liver) to the right atrium. It is in jeopardy during surgical repair of a herniated intervertebral disc. The IVC above the kidneys (suprarenal) should never be ligated (there is a 100% mortality rate); the IVC below the kidneys (infrarenal) may be ligated (there is a 50% mortality rate).

1. The **right gonadal vein** drains directly into the IVC, whereas the **left gonadal vein** drains into the left renal vein. This is important in females where the appearance of a **right side hydronephrosis** may indicate thrombosis of the right ovarian vein that constricts the ureter since the right ovarian vein crossed the ureter to drain into the

IVC. This is also important in males where the appearance of a **left side testicular varicocele** may indicate occlusion of the **left testicular vein** and/or **left renal vein** due to a malignant tumor of the kidney.

2. **Routes of collateral venous return** exist in case the IVC is blocked by either a malignant retroperitoneal tumor or a large blood clot (thrombus). These include:
   a. Azygous vein → superior vena cava→ right atrium
   b. Lumbar veins→ external and internal vertebral venous plexuses→ cranial dural sinuses→ internal jugular vein → right atrium

III Hepatic Portal System *(Figure 2-2B–D)*

In general, the term "portal" refers to a vein interposed between two capillary beds, i.e., capillary bed → vein → capillary bed. The hepatic portal system consists specifically of the following vascular structures: capillaries of GI tract → portal vein → hepatic sinusoids. The **portal vein** is formed posterior to the neck of pancreas by the union of the **splenic vein** and **superior mesenteric vein**. The **inferior mesenteric vein** usually ends by joining the splenic vein. The blood within the portal vein carries high levels of nutrients from the GI tract and

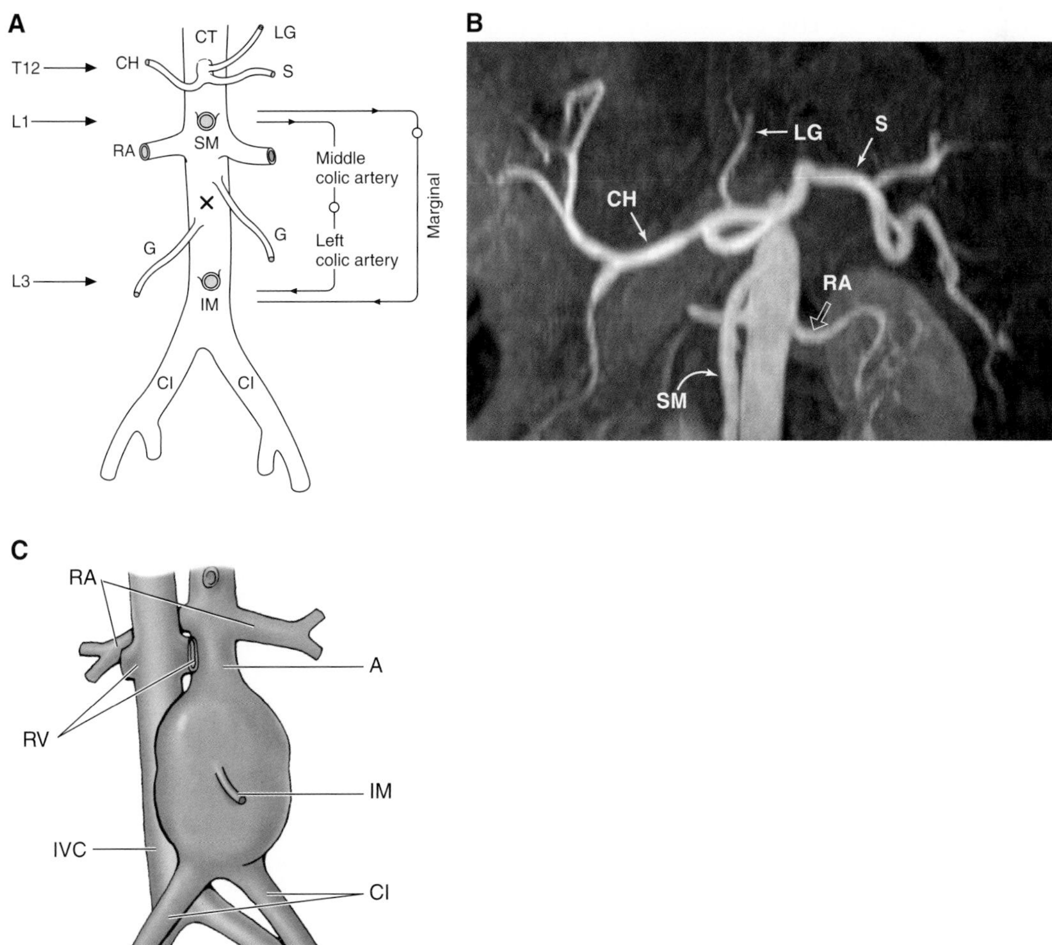

FIGURE 2-1. **Abdominal Aorta. (A) Diagram of the Abdominal Aorta.** The major branches are indicated. The abdominal vasculature has a fairly robust collateral circulation. Any blockage (see X) between the superior mesenteric artery (SM; at L1 vertebral level) and inferior mesenteric artery (IM; at L3 vertebral level) will cause the blood to be diverted along two routes of collateral circulation. The first route uses the middle colic artery (a branch of SM) that anastomoses with the left colic artery (a branch of IM). The second route uses the marginal artery. **(B)** An arteriogram showing the branches of the celiac trunk and other arteries in the vicinity. **(C)** Diagram of an abdominal aortic aneurysm. A — aorta; CH — common hepatic artery; CI — common iliac artery; CT — celiac trunk; G — gonadal artery; LG — left gastric artery; RA — renal artery; RV — renal vein; S — splenic artery; T12, L1, and L3 indicate the vertebral level of the various branches.

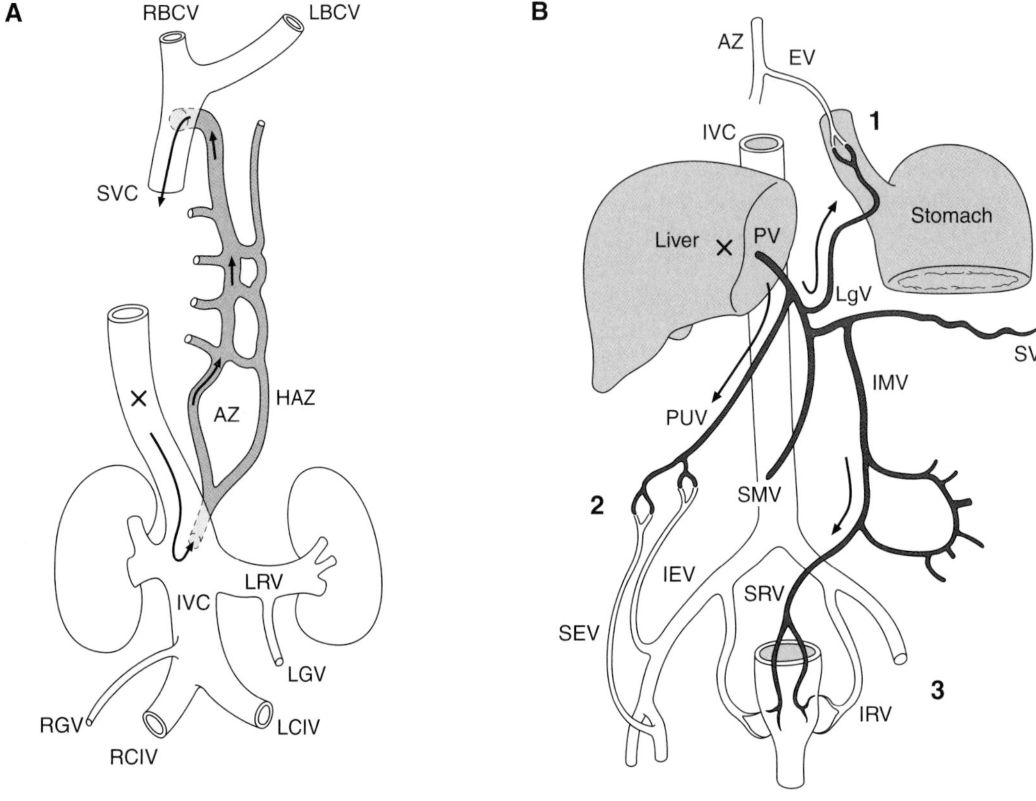

C

Site of Anastomosis	Clinical Sign	Veins Involved in Portal ↔ Inferior Venal Caval Anastomosis
1. Esophagus	Esophageal varices	Left gastric vein ↔ esophageal vein
2. Umbilicus	Caput medusa	Paraumbilical vein ↔ superficial and inferior epigastric veins
3. Rectum	Anorectal varices	Superior rectal vein ↔ middle and inferior rectal veins

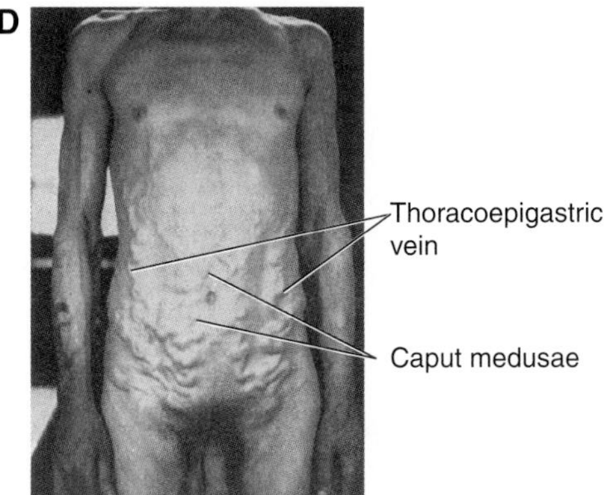

FIGURE 2-2. **Venous Drainage of GI Tract. (A) Diagram of the Azygos Venous System and the IVC.** Note that the left gonadal vein (LGV) drains into the left renal vein (LRV) which has clinical implications in the case of males (e.g., left testicular varicocele). Note how the azygos vein provides a route of collateral venous (arrows) return in cases where the IVC is blocked (X). **(B–D) Hepatic Portal System. (B)** Diagram of the hepatic portal system. Note the three main sites (1,2,3) of portal–IVC (caval) anastomosis. In case of portal hypertension where blood flow through the liver is severely reduced (X), these anastomoses provide collateral circulation (arrows) through the IVC back to the heart. **(C)** Table showing the clinical signs of portal hypertension. **(D)** Photograph of a patient with portal hypertension and caput medusae. AZ — azygos vein; EV — esophageal vein; HAZ — hemiazygos vein; IEV — inferior epigastric vein; IMV — inferior mesenteric vein; IRV — inferior rectal vein; LBCV — left brachiocephalic vein; LCIV — left common iliac vein; LgV — left gastric vein; PUV — paraumbilical vein; PV — portal vein; RBCV — right brachiocephalic vein; RCIV — right common iliac vein; RGV — right gonadal vein; SEV — superior epigastric vein; SMV — superior mesenteric vein; SRV — superior rectal vein; SV — splenic vein; SVC — superior vena cava.

products of red blood cell destruction from the spleen. **Portal–IVC (caval) anastomosis** becomes clinically relevant when **portal hypertension** occurs. Portal hypertension will cause blood within the portal vein to reverse its flow and enter the IVC in order to return to the heart. There are three main sites of portal–IVC anastomosis: esophagus, umbilicus, and rectum. Other sites of portal–caval anastomosis are the hepatic capsule/bare area of the liver → IVC and a patent ductus venous → IVC. Clinical findings of portal hypertension include vomiting copious amounts of blood, alcoholism, liver cirrhosis, schistosomiasis, enlarged abdomen due to ascites fluid, and splenomegaly.

Innervation of the Gastrointestinal Tract

The GI tract is innervated by the autonomic nervous system that consists of two components: the **intrinsic component (or enteric nervous system)** and the **extrinsic component** (*Figure 2-3*).

I Intrinsic Component (or Enteric Nervous System)

The phylogenetically primitive enteric nervous system is an entirely separate nervous system in the body since most functions of the GI tract are controlled by the enteric nervous system even in the absence of the extrinsic component, i.e., the enteric nervous system can function autonomously. Many different neurotransmitters have been localized in the enteric nervous system: **acetylcholine** (ACh; released from the "traditional" postganglionic parasympathetic neuron), **nitric oxide** (NO), **vasoactive intestinal polypeptide, adenosine 5'-triphosphate** (ATP), **serotonin, and somatostatin.** The enteric nervous system is composed of **two distinct** interconnected neuronal circuits as indicated below:

A. **Submucosal Plexus of Meissner.** The neuronal cell bodies of the submucosal plexus are found in the submucosa. This plexus extends from the small intestine to the upper anal canal.
   1. **Motor component.** The motor component of this plexus controls primarily **mucosal and submucosal gland secretion and blood flow.**
   2. **Sensory component.** The sensory component of this plexus consists of **mucosal mechanosensitive neurons.**

B. **Myenteric Plexus of Auerbach.** The neuronal cell bodies of the myenteric plexus are found between the inner circular and outer longitudinal layer of the muscularis externa. This plexus extends from the esophagus to the upper anal canal.
   1. **Motor component.** The motor component of this plexus controls primarily **GI motility (contraction/relaxation of GI smooth muscle).**
   2. **Sensory component.** The sensory component of this plexus consists of **tension-sensitive neurons** and **chemo-sensitive neurons.**

II Extrinsic Component (Parasympathetic and Sympathetic Nervous Systems)

The extrinsic component **modulates** the activity of the enteric nervous system, although specific functions are hard to detail. The extrinsic component is composed of two distinct pathways:

A. **Parasympathetic Nervous System**
   1. **Motor component.** Preganglionic neuronal cell bodies are located in the **dorsal nucleus of the vagus** and the **nucleus ambiguus** in the medulla or in the **gray matter**

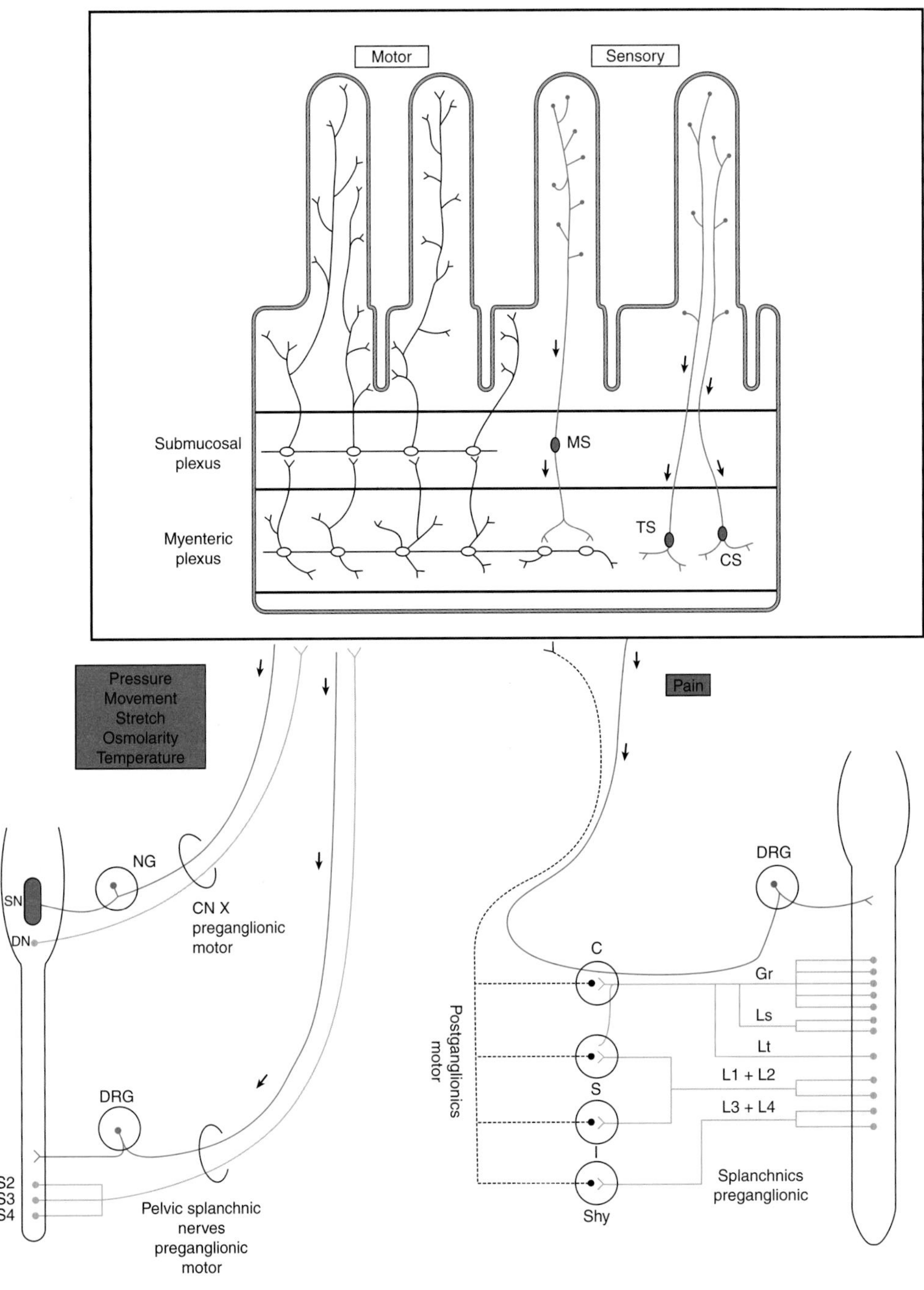

FIGURE 2-3. **Innervation of the GI Tract.** The enteric nervous system consists of both motor and sensory neuronal cell bodies located in the GI wall. The neuronal cell bodies are grouped in small aggregates called the enteric ganglia that are connected by bundles of neuronal cell processes to form the submucosal plexus of Meissner and myenteric plexus of Auerbach. The parasympathetic system provides preganglionic motor axons that run with CN X and pelvic splanchnic nerves and synapse in the complex neuronal circuitry of the enteric nervous system. The parasympathetic system also carries sensory information (e.g., pressure, movement, stretch, osmolarity, and temperature) from the GI tract back to the central nervous system via pseudounipolar neurons that run with CN X and pelvic splanchnic nerves. The sympathetic system provides postganglionic motor axons that run with blood vessels and synapse in the complex neuronal circuitry of the enteric nervous system. The sympathetic system also carries sensory information (predominately pain) from the GI tract back to the central nervous system via pseudounipolar neurons that run with the splanchnic nerves. MS — mucosal mechanosensitive sensory neuron; TS — tension-sensitive sensory neuron; CS — chemo-sensitive sensory neuron; NG — nodose (inferior) ganglion of CN X; SN, solitary nucleus; DN — dorsal nucleus of CN X; DRG — dorsal root ganglion; Gr — greater splanchnic nerve; Ls — lesser splanchnic nerve; Lt — least splanchnic; L1 and L2 — lumbar 1 and lumbar 2 splanchnic nerves; L3 and L4 — lumbar 3 and lumbar 4 splanchnic nerves; C — celiac ganglion; S — superior mesenteric ganglion; I — inferior mesenteric ganglion; Shy — superior hypogastric plexus.

of the S2–S4 spinal cord.** Preganglionic axons travel in **CN X (vagus nerve)** and **pelvic splanchnic nerves (S2–S4)** and synapse on postganglionic neurons in the complex circuitry of the enteric nervous system. Some of these postganglionic neurons release ACh as a neurotransmitter and, therefore, can be considered the "traditional" postganglionic parasympathetic neuron. Hence, it is difficult to detail specific parasympathetic motor functions although they are usually considered excitatory in nature.

2. **Sensory component.** The neuronal cell bodies are located in the **nodose (inferior) ganglion of CN X** and the **dorsal root ganglion of S2–S4 spinal nerves.** These neurons send a peripheral process to the viscera and a central process to either the solitary nucleus in the brainstem or the spinal cord. These neurons transmit the sensations of **visceral pressure, visceral movement, visceral stretch, visceral osmolarity, and visceral temperature.** Reflexes in which the sensory and motor components travel in CN X are called **vagovagal reflexes.**

B. Sympathetic Nervous System

1. **Motor component.** Preganglionic neuronal cell bodies are located in the **intermediolateral cell column** of the T5–L2/L3 spinal cord. Preganglionic axons travel in the **greater splanchnic nerve, lesser splanchnic nerve, least splanchnic nerve**, and **lumbar splanchnic nerves** and synapse on postganglionic neuronal cell bodies located in the **celiac ganglion, superior mesenteric ganglion, inferior mesenteric ganglion** (also called prevertebral ganglia), and the **superior hypogastric plexus.** Postganglionic axons synapse in the complex circuitry of the enteric nervous system. Hence, it is difficult to detail the specific sympathetic motor functions although they are usually considered inhibitory in nature. However, one motor function that is fairly well established is the **regulation of GI blood flow.**
2. **Sensory component.** The neuronal cell bodies are located in the dorsal root ganglia at T5–L2/L3 spinal cord levels. These neurons send a peripheral process to the viscera via splanchnic nerves and a central process to the spinal cord. These neurons transmit the sensation of **visceral pain.**

Esophagus

I General Features *(Figure 2-4A)*

The esophagus is a muscular tube that is continuous with the pharynx and runs in the thorax through the superior and posterior mediastinum. The esophagus begins at the **cricoid cartilage** (at vertebral level C6) and ends at the **gastroesophageal junction.** The esophagus pierces the diaphragm to form the esophageal hiatus (at vertebral level T10). The muscular wall of the esophagus (i.e., the muscularis externa histologically) changes from cephalad to caudad. The **upper** 5% of the esophagus consists of **skeletal muscle** only. The **middle** 45% of the esophagus consists of both **skeletal muscle and smooth muscle** interwoven together. The **distal 50%** of the esophagus consists of **smooth** muscle only. The overall length of the esophagus obviously varies with trunk length but the average adult length of the esophagus is **23 to 25 cm.** In clinical practice, endoscopic distances are measured from the incisor teeth and in the average male, the gastroesophageal junction is 38 to 43 cm away from the incisor teeth. For purposes of classification, staging, and reporting of esophageal malignancies, the esophagus is divided into four segments based on the distance from the incisor teeth: cervical segment, upper thoracic segment, midthoracic segment, and lower thoracic segment.

II Constrictions

Along the course of the esophagus, there are five main sites where the esophagus is constricted: (a) at the junction of pharynx and esophagus (cricoid origin), (b) at the aortic arch, (c) at the tracheal bifurcation (vertebral level T4) where the left main bronchus crosses the esophagus, (d) at the left atrium, and (e) at the esophageal hiatus.

III Sphincters

A. **The Upper Esophageal Sphincter (UES)** separates the pharynx from the esophagus. The UES is composed of **opening muscles** (i.e., thyrohyoid and geniohyoid muscles) and **closing muscles** (i.e., inferior pharyngeal constrictor and **cricopharyngeus** [main player]). The UES is a **skeletal muscle.**

B. **The Lower Esophageal Sphincter (LES)** separates the esophagus from the stomach. The LES is composed of **smooth muscle** and it is difficult to identify anatomically. Human autopsies have found an asymmetric, thickened, ringlike area in the area of the gastroesophageal junction, which may aid the muscularis externa in the physiological role as a sphincter. The LES **prevents gastroesophageal reflux.**

IV Vasculature of the Esophagus *(Figure 2-4B)*

A. **Arterial Supply.** The arterial supply of the cervical esophagus is from the **inferior thyroid arteries** (subclavian artery → thyrocervical trunk → inferior thyroid artery) that give off ascending and descending branches that anastomose with each other across the midline. The arterial supply of the thoracic esophagus is from **four to five branches from the descending thoracic aorta**. The arterial supply of the abdominal esophagus is from the **left gastric artery** (abdominal aorta → celiac trunk → left gastric artery).

B. **Venous Drainage.** The venous drainage of the cervical esophagus is to the **inferior thyroid veins** (inferior thyroid veins → brachiocephalic veins → superior vena cava). The venous drainage of the thoracic esophagus is to the **esophageal plexus of veins** (esophageal plexus of veins → azygous veins → superior vena cava). The venous drainage of the abdominal esophagus is to the **left gastric vein** (left gastric vein → portal vein → hepatic sinusoids → central veins → hepatic veins → IVC).

V Innervation of the Esophagus *(Figure 2-4C)*

The innervation of the esophagus is done by the **somatic nervous system** (upper portion only) and the **enteric nervous system** which, in the esophagus, consists of the myenteric plexus of Auerbach only. The enteric nervous system is modulated by the parasympathetic and sympathetic nervous systems.

A. **Somatic Innervation.** Somatic neuronal cell bodies are located in the ventral horn of the spinal cord at **cervical level 1 (C1)** and travel with the **hypoglossal nerve (CN XII)** to innervate the opening muscles (i.e., thyrohyoid and geniohyoid muscles) of the UES.

B. **Parasympathetic**

1. Preganglionic neuronal cell bodies are located in the **dorsal nucleus of the vagus**. Preganglionic axons run in **CN X** and enter the **esophageal plexus.** Postganglionic neuronal cell bodies are located in the **enteric nervous system**, some of which are the "traditional" postganglionic parasympathetic neurons that release ACh as a neurotransmitter. The postganglionic axons terminate on mucosal glands, submucosal glands, and smooth muscle.

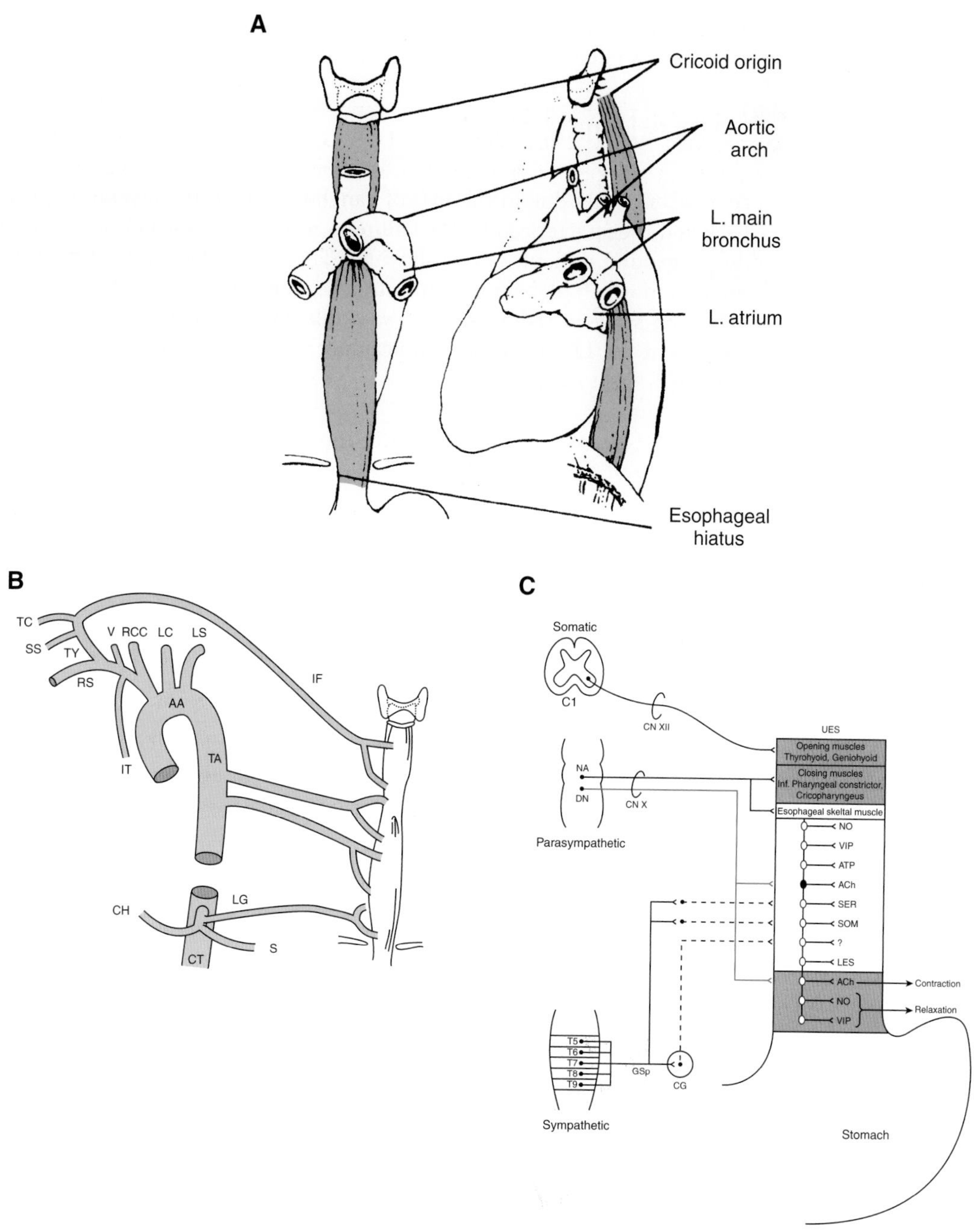

FIGURE 2-4. **Esophagus. (A) Diagram of the Esophagus (Anterior and Lateral Views).** Note the various anatomic relationships of the esophagus. **(B)** Arterial supply of the esophagus. **(C)** Innervation of the esophagus. TC — transverse cervical artery; SS — suprascapular artery; V — vertebral artery; RCC — right common carotid artery; LC — left common carotid artery; LS — left subclavian artery; IT, internal thoracic artery; IF — inferior thyroid artery; LG — left gastric artery; S — splenic artery; CH — common hepatic artery; AA — aortic arch; TA — thoracic artery; RS — right subclavian artery; TY — thyrocervical trunk; CT — celiac trunk; NA — nucleus ambiguus; DN — dorsal nucleus of the vagus; CN X — cranial nerve X (vagus nerve); CN XII — cranial nerve XII (hypoglossal nerve); C1 — spinal cord level cervical 1; GSp — greater splanchnic nerve; CG — celiac ganglion; LES — lower esophageal sphincter; NO — nitric oxide; SER — serotonin; SOM — somatostatin;?, other neurotransmitters.

2. Neuronal cell bodies located in the **nucleus ambiguus** send axons that run in **CN X (recurrent laryngeal nerves)** and enter the **esophageal plexus**. These axons terminate on the **closing muscles of the upper esophageal sphincter (UES; inferior pharyngeal constrictor and the cricopharyngeus muscle)** and the **esophageal skeletal muscle**.

C. **Sympathetic.** Preganglionic neuronal cell bodies are located in the **intermediolateral cell column** of the spinal cord (T5 to T9). Preganglionic axons form the **greater splanchnic nerve**. Postganglionic neuronal cell bodies are located in the **diffuse**

ganglia along the esophagus and the **celiac ganglion**. Postganglionic axons synapse in the complex circuitry of the enteric nervous system.

VI Clinical Considerations

A. **Achalasia** occurs due to the loss of ganglion cells in the myenteric plexus of Auerbach and is characterized by the failure to relax the LES which will cause progressive dysphagia and difficulty in swallowing. The most effective treatment is **pneumatic dilation** in which high air pressure stretches the constricted LES to induce relaxation. A barium swallow radiograph shows a dilated esophagus above the LES and distal stenosis at the LES (bird beak appearance). Chagas disease caused by *Trypanosoma cruzi* may lead to achalasia.

B. **Enlarged Left Atrium** may constrict the esophagus due to their close anatomical relationship.

C. **Bronchogenic Carcinoma** may indent the esophagus due to the enlargement of mediastinal lymph nodes. This indentation can be observed radiologically during a barium swallow.

D. **Malignant Tumors of the Esophagus** most commonly occur in the lower one third of the esophagus and metastasize below the diaphragm to the **celiac lymph nodes**.

E. **Sliding Hiatal Hernia** occurs when the stomach along with the gastroesophageal junction herniates through the diaphragm into the thorax. Clinical findings include deep burning retrosternal pain and reflux of gastric contents into the mouth (i.e., heartburn) which are accentuated in the supine position.

F. **Paraesophageal Hiatal Hernia** occurs when only the stomach herniates through the diaphragm into the thorax. Clinical findings include no reflux of gastric contents but strangulation or obstruction may occur.

G. **Esophageal Varices** refer to the dilated subepithelial and submucosal venous plexuses of the esophagus that drain into the **left gastric (coronary) vein**. The left gastric vein empties into the portal vein from the distal esophagus and proximal stomach. Esophageal varices are caused by **portal hypertension.** Portal hypertension may be caused by **intrahepatic events** (e.g., cirrhosis, schistosomiasis, and sarcoidosis), **prehepatic events** (e.g., portal vein thrombosis and increased splenic flow), and **posthepatic events** (e.g., vena cava obstruction, Budd–Chiari syndrome, and veno-occlusive disease).

Stomach

I General Features *(Figure 2-5A)*

The stomach is a J-shaped muscular organ that macerates, homogenizes, and partially digests the swallowed food to produce a semisolid paste called **chyme**. The stomach is also a reservoir for food capable of holding 2 to 3 L of food. The stomach receives food from the esophagus and releases its contents into the duodenum. The stomach has two openings: the **cardiac orifice** (where the esophagus opens into the stomach) and the **pyloric orifice** (where the stomach opens into the duodenum). The stomach has two curvatures: the **lesser curvature** that forms the right border of the stomach and is connected to the liver by the lesser omentum and the **greater curvature** that forms the left border of the stomach and from which, the greater omentum hangs. The stomach is divided into four parts:

1. **Cardia** is near the gastroesophageal junction.
2. **Fundus** is above the gastroesophageal junction.
3. **Body** is between the fundus and antrum.
4. **Pylorus** is the distal part of the stomach and is divided into the **pyloric antrum** (wide part) and the **pyloric canal** (narrow part). The pyloric orifice is surrounded by the **pyloric sphincter** that is a well-defined muscular sphincter that controls the movement of food out of the stomach and prevents reflux of duodenal contents into the stomach.

II Vasculature of the Stomach *(Figure 2-5B)*

A. **Arterial Supply.** The arterial supply of the stomach is from the **right and left gastric arteries** that supply the lesser curvature (abdominal aorta → celiac trunk → common hepatic artery → right gastric artery; abdominal aorta → celiac trunk → left gastric artery); **right and left gastroepiploic arteries** that supply the greater curvature (abdominal aorta → celiac trunk → common hepatic artery → gastroduodenal artery → right gastroepiploic artery; abdominal aorta → celiac trunk → splenic artery → left gastroepiploic artery); and **short gastric arteries** that supply the fundus (abdominal aorta → celiac trunk → splenic artery → short gastric arteries).

B. **Venous Drainage.** The venous drainage of the stomach is to the **right and left gastric veins** (right and left gastric veins → portal vein → hepatic sinusoids → central veins

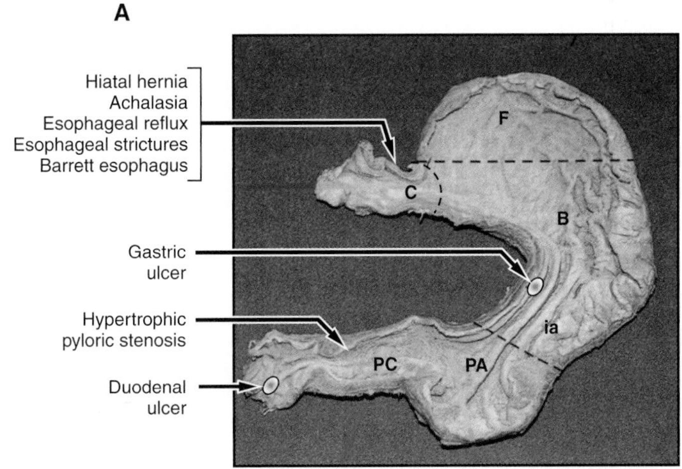

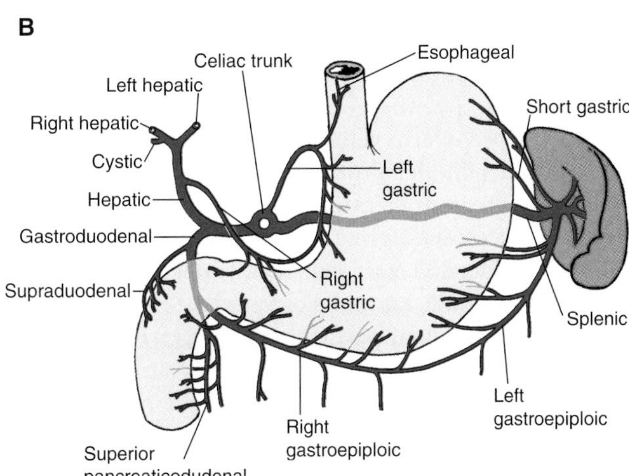

FIGURE 2-5. Stomach. (A) Photograph of the Inner Luminal Surface of the Stomach. Note the various parts of the stomach. High-yield clinical considerations associated with the esophagus, stomach, and duodenum are indicated. **(B)** Arterial supply of the stomach. C — cardia; F — fundus; B — body; ia — incisura angularis; PA — pyloric antrum; PC — pyloric canal.

→ hepatic veins → IVC); **left gastroepiploic vein** and **short gastric veins** (left gastroepiploic vein and short gastric veins → splenic vein → portal vein → hepatic sinusoids → central veins → hepatic veins → IVC); and **right gastroepiploic vein** (right gastroepiploic vein → superior mesenteric vein → portal vein → hepatic sinusoids → central veins → hepatic veins → IVC).

III Clinical Consideration

Carcinomas of the stomach are most commonly found in the **pylorus** of the stomach and may metastasize to the **supraclavicular lymph nodes (Virchow node)** on the left side which can be palpated within the posterior triangle of the neck (**Troisier sign**). Virchow node is a single node in the supraclavicular region most commonly referred to as the node found between the heads of the sternocleidomastoid muscle. Carcinoma of the stomach may also metastasize to the ovaries where it is called **Krukenberg tumor**.

Small Intestine

General Features *(Figure 2-6A)*

The function of the small intestine is to continue digestion of chyme received from the stomach using enzymes of the glycocalyx, pancreatic enzymes, and liver bile and absorb nutrients derived from the digestive process, H_2O, electrolytes, and minerals. The small intestine extends from the stomach (pyloric sphincter) to the colon (ileocecal valve) and is ≈6 to 7 m long. The inner luminal surface of the small intestine contains semilunar folds of mucosa and submucosa called **plicae circularis (valves of Kerckring)** and fingerlike projections of epithelium and lamina propria called **villi**. The small intestine is divided into the **duodenum**, **jejunum**, and **ileum**.

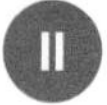

Duodenum

A. **General Features.** The duodenum is an ≈25 cm long portion of the small intestine that extends from the pyloric sphincter to the duodenojejunal flexure. The duodenum pursues a C-shaped course around the head of the pancreas. The villi of the duodenum are broad, leaf shaped. The duodenum is divided into four parts:
    1. **Superior part (first part).** The first 2 cm of the superior part is intraperitoneal and, therefore, has a mesentery and is mobile; the remaining distal 3 cm of the superior part is retroperitoneal. Radiologists refer to the first 2 cm of the superior part of the duodenum as the **duodenal cap** or **bulb**. The superior part begins at the pylorus of the stomach (**gastroduodenal junction**) which is marked by the **prepyloric vein**. Posterior relationships include the **common bile duct** and **gastroduodenal artery**. The **hepatoduodenal ligament** attaches superiorly and the **greater omentum** attaches inferiorly.
    2. **Descending part (second part)** is retroperitoneal and receives the **common bile duct** and **main pancreatic duct** on its posterior/medial wall at the **hepatopancreatic ampulla (ampulla of Vater)**.
    3. **Horizontal part (third part)** is retroperitoneal and runs horizontally across the L3 vertebra between the superior mesenteric artery anteriorly and the aorta and IVC posteriorly. In severe abdominal injuries, this part of the duodenum may be crushed against the L3 vertebra.
    4. **Ascending part (fourth part)** is intraperitoneal and ascends to meet the jejunum at the **duodenojejunal junction**, which occurs approximately at L2 vertebral level about 2 to 3 cm to the left of the midline. This junction usually forms an acute angle that is called the **duodenojejunal flexure** which is supported by the **ligament**

of Treitz (also called the **suspensory muscle of the duodenum** and represents the cranial end of the dorsal mesentery).

B **Vasculature of the Duodenum** (*Figure 2-6B*)

1. **Arterial supply.** The arterial supply of the duodenum is from the **supraduodenal artery** that supplies the upper portion of the duodenum (abdominal aorta → celiac trunk → common hepatic artery → gastroduodenal artery → supraduodenal artery); **anterior and posterior superior pancreaticoduodenal arteries** (abdominal aorta → celiac trunk → common hepatic artery → gastroduodenal artery → anterior and posterior superior pancreaticoduodenal arteries); and **anterior and posterior inferior pancreaticoduodenal arteries** (abdominal aorta → superior mesenteric artery → anterior and posterior inferior pancreaticoduodenal arteries).
2. **Venous drainage.** The venous drainage of the duodenum is to the **anterior and posterior superior pancreaticoduodenal veins** (anterior and posterior superior pancreaticoduodenal veins → portal vein → hepatic sinusoids → central veins → hepatic veins → IVC) and **anterior and posterior inferior pancreaticoduodenal veins** (anterior and posterior inferior pancreaticoduodenal veins → superior mesenteric vein → portal vein → hepatic sinusoids → central veins → hepatic veins → IVC).

III Jejunum

A. **General Features** ***(see Table 2-1).*** The jejunum is an ≈2.5 m long portion of the small intestine that extends from the duodenojejunal flexure to the beginning of the ileum (i.e., the initial two thirds of the small intestine). The jejunum has long, finger-shaped villi; is >3 cm in diameter; has large, numerous, palpable plicae circularis; is located in the umbilical region on the left side of the abdomen; has long vasa recta with one to two arterial arcades; is often empty with no fecal contents; is the main site of nutrient absorption; and has no Peyer patches. In general, the jejunum is thicker walled, more vascular, and redder in the living person than the ileum.

B. **Vasculature**

1. **Arterial supply.** The arterial supply of the jejunum is from the **vasa rectae** (abdominal aorta → superior mesenteric artery → jejunal arteries → 1 to 2 arterial arcades → vasa rectae).
2. **Venous drainage.** The venous drainage of the jejunum is to the **veins associated with the arcades** (veins associated with the arcades → jejunal veins → superior mesenteric vein → portal vein → hepatic sinusoids → central veins → hepatic veins → IVC).

IV Ileum

A. **General Features** ***(see Table 2-1).*** The ileum is an ≈3.6 m long portion of the small intestine that extends from the beginning of the ileum to the ileocecal valve located just above the cecal tip (i.e., the terminal three fifth of the small intestine). The ileum has short, club-shaped villi; is <3 cm in diameter; has small and few plicae circularis; is located in the hypogastric and inguinal regions on the right side of the abdomen; has short vasa recta with three to four arterial arcades; is the main site of vitamin B_{12} and H_2O/electrolyte absorption; is the site of bile recirculation; has Peyer patches that are prominent.

B. **Vasculature**

1. **Arterial supply.** The arterial supply of the ileum is from the **vasa rectae** (abdominal aorta → superior mesenteric artery → ileal arteries → three to four arterial arcades → vasa rectae).
2. **Venous drainage.** The venous drainage of the ileum is to the **veins associated with the arcades** (veins associated with the arcades → ileal veins → superior mesenteric vein → portal vein → hepatic sinusoids → central veins → hepatic veins → IVC).

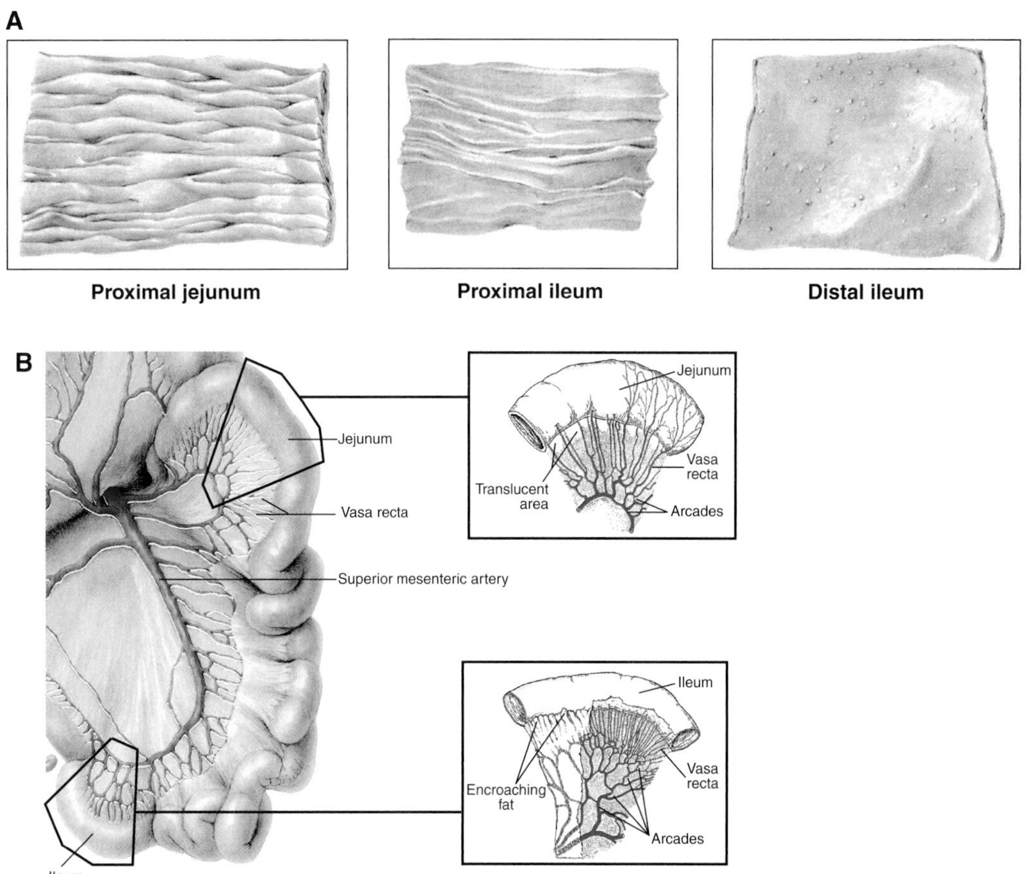

FIGURE 2-6. **Small Intestine. (A) Photograph of the Inner Luminal Surface of Various Portions of the Small Intestine.** The proximal jejunum has large, numerous, and palpable plicae circularis. The proximal ileum has small and few plicae circularis. The distal ileum has no plicae circularis, instead Peyer patches are prominent. **(B)** Arterial supply of the small intestine.

TABLE 2-1 CHARACTERISTICS OF THE JEJUNUM AND ILEUM

Jejunum	Ileum
Villi present (long, finger shaped)	Villi present (short, club shaped)
Intestinal glands (crypts) present	Intestinal glands (crypts) present
>3 cm in diameter	<3 cm in diameter
Large, numerous, and palpable plicae circulares *	Small and few plicae circulares that disappear distally
Initial two fifths of small intestine	Terminal three fifths of small intestine
Located in the umbilical region on left side of abdomen	Located in the hypogastric and inguinal regions on the right side of abdomen
Long vasa recta	Short vasa recta
Peyer patches (GALT) are present	Peyer patches (GALT) are prominent
Main site of NaCl absorption	Main site of Vitamin B_{12} absorption
Often empty (no fecal contents)	Main site of $NaHCO_3^-$ absorption site of bile recirculation
Thicker wall, more vascular, and redder in the living person than ileum	Terminal ileum ends several centimeters above the cecal tip

*These are folds of the mucosa and submucosa
GALT, gut-associated lymphatic tissue.

Large Intestine

 General Features *(Figure 2-7A,B)*

The function of the large intestine is to absorb Na^+, Cl^-, and H_2O from the lumen; soften the fecal mass by addition of mucus; and store, support, and eliminate the fecal mass. The large intestine extends from the ileocecal junction to the upper anal canal and is ≈1.5 m long. The inner luminal surface of the large intestine is relatively smooth with some semilunar folds of mucosa and submucosa called **plicae semilunares**. The large intestine is divided into the **cecum**, **appendix**, **ascending colon**, **transverse colon**, **descending colon**, **sigmoid colon**, **rectum**, and **upper anal canal**.

 Cecum

A. **General Features.** The cecum is the intraperitoneal blind-ended pouch of the large intestine which lies in the right iliac fossa. At the junction of the cecum and ascending colon, the terminal part of the ileum joins. From the posteromedial surface of the cecum, the appendix extends.

B. **Anatomic Relationships.** The anterior relationships include the right inguinal region of the anterior abdominal wall and coils of ileum. The posterior relationship includes the iliopsoas muscle.

C. **Vasculature of the Cecum**

1. **Arterial supply.** The arterial supply of the cecum is from the **anterior and posterior cecal arteries** (abdominal aorta → superior mesenteric artery → ileocolic artery → anterior and posterior cecal arteries).
2. **Venous drainage.** The venous drainage of the cecum is to the **anterior and posterior cecal veins** (anterior and posterior cecal veins → superior mesenteric vein → portal vein → central veins → hepatic veins → IVC).

III Appendix

A. **General Features.** The appendix is an intraperitoneal (**mesoappendix**), narrow, muscular tube attached to the posteromedial surface of the cecum. The appendix is located ≈2.5 cm below the ileocecal valve. The appendix may lie in the following positions: **retrocecal** (65%), **pelvis** (32%), **subcecal** (2%), **anterior juxta-ileal** (1%), **and posterior juxta-ileal** (0.5%).

B. **Anatomic Relationships.** The anterior relationships include the **right inguinal region** of the anterior abdominal wall. **McBurney point** is located by drawing a line from the right anterior superior iliac spine to the umbilicus. Two thirds of the distance from the umbilicus along this line locates the root of the appendix at the junction of the right inguinal region and the umbilical region of the anterior abdominal wall.

C. **Vasculature of the Appendix**

1. **Arterial supply.** The arterial supply of the appendix is from the **appendicular artery** (abdominal aorta → superior mesenteric artery → ileocolic artery → posterior cecal artery → appendicular artery).
2. **Venous drainage.** The venous drainage of the appendix is to the **posterior cecal vein** (posterior cecal vein → superior mesenteric vein → portal vein → hepatic sinusoids → central veins → hepatic veins → IVC).

D. **Appendicitis** begins with the obstruction of the appendix lumen with a fecal concretion (fecalith) and lymphoid hyperplasia followed by distention of the appendix. Clinical findings include initial pain in the umbilical or epigastric region, later pain localizing in the right lumbar region, nausea, vomiting, anorexia, tenderness to palpation, and percussion in the right lumbar region. Complications may include peritonitis due to rupture of the appendix.

IV Ascending Colon

A. **General Features.** The ascending colon is an ≈13 cm long retroperitoneal portion of the large intestine that extends on the right side from the cecum to the inferior lobe of the liver at the **right colic flexure**. The ascending colon is characterized by the **teniae coli** (three narrow bands of smooth muscle), **haustra** (sacculations formed by the contraction of the teniae coli), and **epiploic appendages** (fatty tags attached in rows along the teniae coli).

B. **Vasculature of the Ascending Colon**

1. **Arterial supply.** The arterial supply of the ascending colon is from the **ileocolic artery** and **right colic artery** (abdominal aorta → superior mesenteric artery → ileocolic artery and right colic artery). The **marginal artery** is formed by an anastomotic connection between the superior mesenteric artery and inferior mesenteric artery.
2. **Venous drainage.** The venous drainage of the ascending colon is to the **ileocolic vein** and **right colic vein** (ileocolic vein and right colic vein → superior mesenteric vein → portal vein → hepatic sinusoids → central veins → hepatic veins → IVC).

V Transverse Colon

A. **General Features.** The transverse colon is an ≈38 cm long intraperitoneal (suspending by the **transverse mesocolon**) portion of the large intestine that extends from the right colic flexure to the spleen at the **left colic flexure**. The transverse colon is also characterized by the **teniae coli** (three narrow bands of smooth muscle), **haustra** (sacculations formed by the contraction of the teniae coli), and **epiploic appendages** (fatty tags attached in rows along the teniae coli).

B. **Vasculature of the Transverse Colon**

1. **Arterial supply.** The arterial supply of the proximal two thirds of the transverse colon is from the **middle colic artery** (abdominal aorta → superior mesenteric artery → middle colic artery). The arterial supply of the distal one third of the transverse colon is from the **left colic artery** (abdominal aorta → inferior mesenteric artery → left colic artery). The **marginal artery** is formed by an anastomotic connection between the superior mesenteric artery and inferior mesenteric artery.
2. **Venous drainage.** The venous drainage of the proximal two thirds of the transverse colon is to the **middle colic vein** (middle colic vein → superior mesenteric vein → portal vein → hepatic sinusoids → central veins → hepatic veins → IVC). The venous drainage of the distal one third of the transverse colon is to the **left colic vein and other unnamed veins** (left colic vein and other unnamed veins → inferior mesenteric vein → portal vein → hepatic sinusoids → central veins → hepatic veins → IVC).

VI Descending Colon

A. **General Features.** The descending colon is an ≈25 cm long retroperitoneal portion of the large intestine that extends from the left colic flexure to vertebral level S1 (sacral promontory; pelvic inlet) where it is continuous with the sigmoid colon. The descending colon is also characterized by the **teniae coli** (three narrow bands of smooth muscle), **haustra** (sacculations formed by the contraction of the teniae coli), and **epiploic appendages** (fatty tags attached in rows along the teniae coli).

B. Vasculature of the Descending Colon

1. **Arterial supply.** The arterial supply of the upper portion of the descending colon is from the **left colic artery** (abdominal aorta → inferior mesenteric artery → left colic artery). The arterial supply of the lower descending colon is from the **sigmoid arteries** (abdominal aorta → inferior mesenteric artery → sigmoid arteries). The **marginal artery** is formed by an anastomotic connection between the superior mesenteric artery and inferior mesenteric artery.
2. **Venous drainage.** The venous drainage of the upper portion of the descending colon is to the **left colic vein** (left colic vein → inferior mesenteric vein → portal vein → hepatic sinusoids → central veins → hepatic veins → IVC). The venous drainage of the lower portion of the descending colon is to the **sigmoid veins** (sigmoid veins → inferior mesenteric vein → portal vein → hepatic sinusoids → central veins → hepatic veins → IVC).

VII Sigmoid Colon

A. General Features. The sigmoid colon is an ≈25 to 38 cm long intraperitoneal (**sigmoid mesocolon**) portion of the large intestine that extends from vertebral level S1 (sacral promontory; pelvic inlet) to vertebral level S3 (rectosigmoid junction) where it is continuous with the rectum. The sigmoid colon is also characterized by the **teniae coli** (three narrow bands of smooth muscle), **haustra** (sacculations formed by the contraction of the teniae coli), and **epiploic appendages** (fatty tags attached in rows along the teniae coli).

B. Vasculature of the Sigmoid Colon

1. **Arterial supply.** The arterial supply of the sigmoid colon is from the **sigmoid arteries** (abdominal aorta → inferior mesenteric artery → sigmoid arteries).
2. **Venous drainage.** The venous drainage of the sigmoid colon is to the **sigmoid veins** (sigmoid veins → inferior mesenteric vein → portal vein → hepatic sinusoids → central veins → hepatic veins → IVC).

C. Clinical Considerations

1. **Flexible sigmoidoscopy** permits examination of the sigmoid colon and rectum. During sigmoidoscopy, the large intestine may be punctured if the angle at the rectosigmoid junction is not negotiated properly. At the rectosigmoid junction, the sigmoid colon bends in an **anterior direction and to the left**. During sigmoidoscopy, the transverse rectal folds (Houston valves) must be negotiated.
2. **Colostomy.** The sigmoid colon is often used in a **colostomy** due to the mobility rendered by the sigmoid mesocolon (mesentery). An ostomy is an intestinal diversion that brings out a portion of the GI tract through the **rectus abdominis muscle**. A colostomy may ablate the pelvic nerve plexus which results in a loss of ejaculation, loss of erection, urinary bladder retention, and decreased peristalsis in the remaining colon.

VIII Rectum

A. General Features. The rectum is an ≈13 cm long retroperitoneal portion of the large intestine that extends from vertebral level S3 (rectosigmoid junction) to the tip of the coccyx at the anorectal junction where the puborectalis muscle forms a U-shaped sling causing a **90 degree perineal flexure**. The **ampulla of the rectum** lies just above the

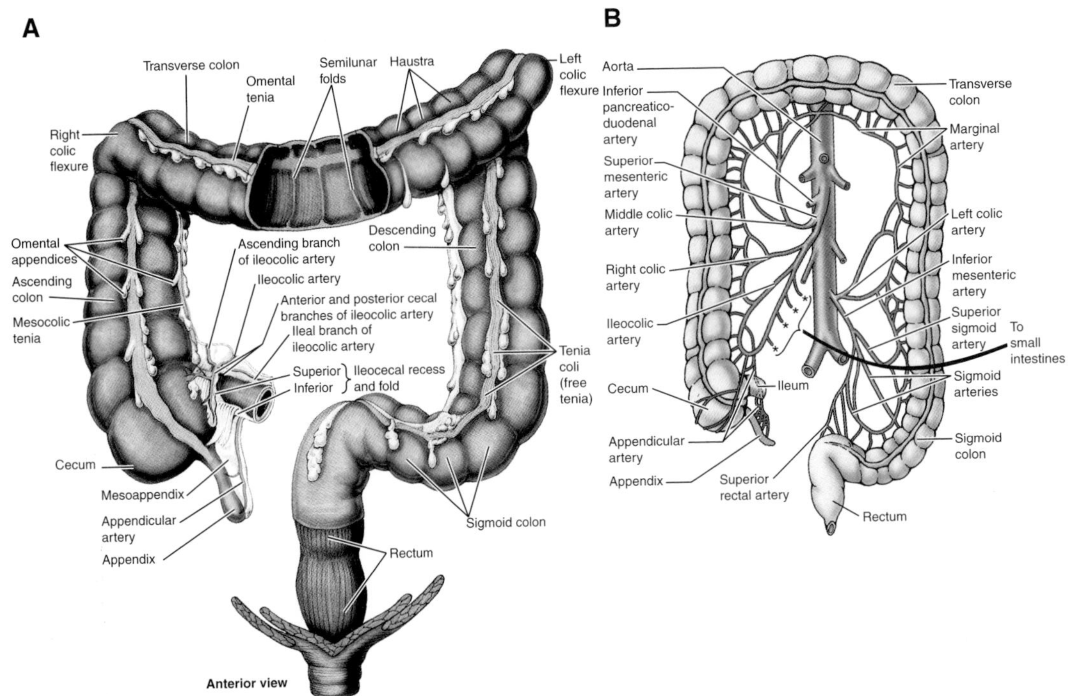

FIGURE 2-7. **Large Intestine. (A)** General features of the large intestine. **(B)** Arterial supply of the large intestine.

pelvic diaphragm. The rectum contains three **transverse rectal folds (Houston valves)** formed by the mucosa, submucosa, and inner circular layer of smooth muscle that permanently extend into the lumen of the rectum to support the fecal mass. The **teniae coli, haustra**, and **epiploic appendages** are not present in the rectum.

B. Vasculature of the Rectum

1. **Arterial supply.** The arterial supply of the rectum is from the **superior rectal artery** (abdominal aorta → inferior mesenteric artery → superior rectal artery), **middle rectal artery** (abdominal aorta → common iliac artery → internal iliac artery → middle rectal artery), and **inferior rectal artery** (abdominal aorta → common iliac artery → internal iliac artery → internal pudendal artery → inferior rectal artery).
2. **Venous drainage.** The venous drainage of the upper portion of the rectum is to the **superior rectal vein** (superior rectal vein → inferior mesenteric vein → portal vein → hepatic sinusoids → central veins → hepatic veins → IVC). The venous drainage of the middle portion of the rectum is to the **middle rectal vein** (middle rectal vein → internal iliac vein → common iliac vein → IVC). The venous drainage of the lower portion of the rectum is to the **inferior rectal vein** (inferior rectal vein → internal pudendal vein → internal iliac vein → common iliac vein → IVC).

D. Clinical Consideration. Rectal prolapse is the protrusion of the **full thickness of the rectum** through the anus (should be distinguished from **mucosal prolapse**, which is the protrusion of only the rectal mucosa through the anus). Clinical findings include bowel protruding through anus, bleeding, anal pain, mucous discharge, and anal incontinence caused by stretching of the **internal and external anal sphincters** or stretch injury to the **pudendal nerve**.

IX Anal Canal *(Figure 2-8)*

A. General Features. The entire anal canal is ≈4 cm long which extends from the rectum at the anorectal junction to the surface of the body at the anus. The anal

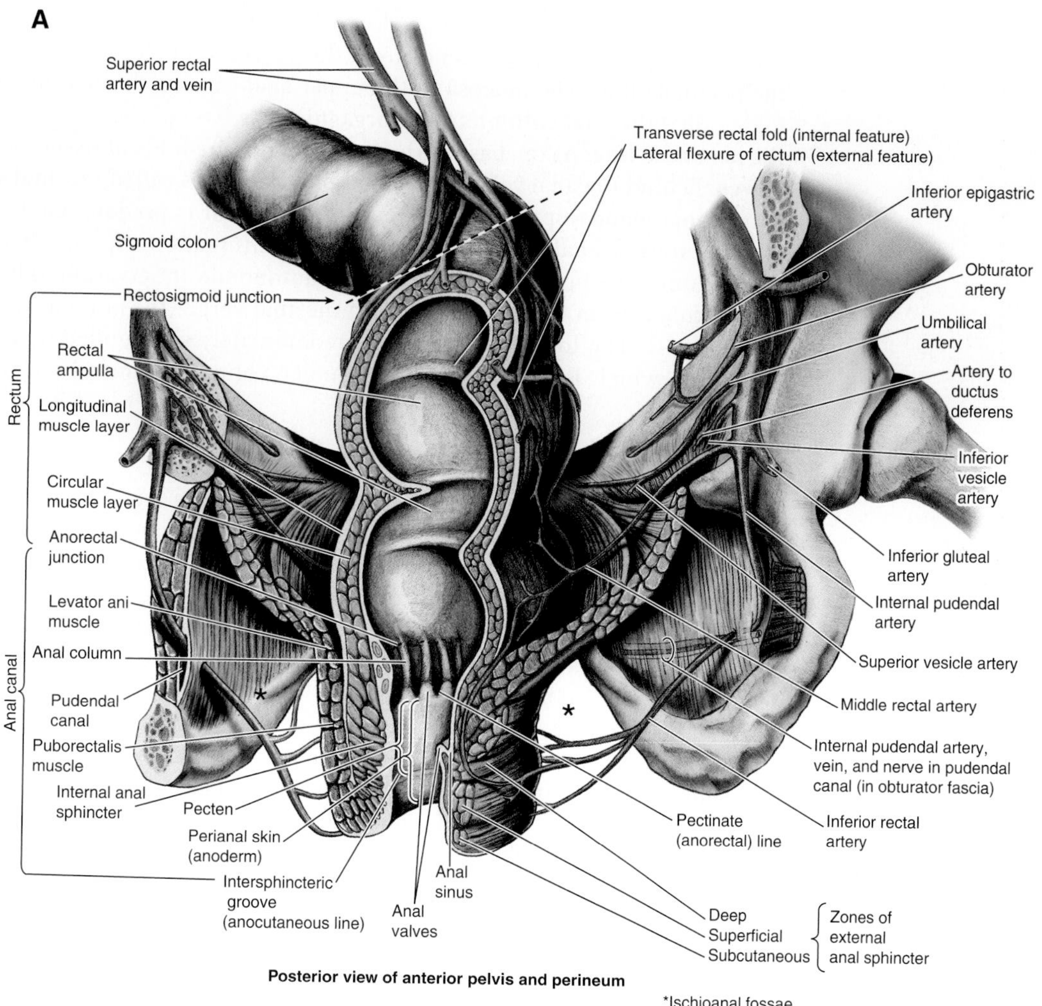

B

Feature	Upper Anal Canal	Lower Anal Canal
Aterial supply	Superior rectal artery (branch of inferior mesenteric artery)	Inferior rectal artery (branch of internal pudendal artery)
Venous drainage	Superior rectal vein → inferior mesenteric vein → hepatic portal system	Inferior rectal vein → internal pudendal vein → internal iliac vein → IVC
Lymphatic drainage	Deep nodes	Superficial inguinal nodes
Innervation	Motor: autonomic innervation of internal anal sphincter (smooth muscle) Sensory: stretch sensation; no pain sensation	Motor: somatic innervation (pudendal nerve) of external anal sphincter (striated muscle) Sensory: pain, temperature, touch sensation
Embryologic derivation	Endoderm (hindgut)	Ectoderm (proctodeum)
Epithelium	Simple columnar	Stratified squamous
Tumors	Palpable enlarged superficial nodes will not be found Patients do not complain of pain	Palpable enlarged superficial nodes will be found Patients do complain of pain
Hemorrhoids	Internal hemorrhoids (varicosities of superior rectal veins) Covered by rectal mucosa Patients do not complain of pain	External hemorrhoids (varicosities of inferior rectal veins) Covered by skin Patients do complain of pain

FIGURE 2-8. **Rectum and Anal Canal. (A)** The wall of the rectum and anal canal has been cut open to reveal the luminal surface. Note the pudendal canal that transmits the pudendal vessels and nerves. **(B)** Table of the anatomic characteristics of the upper and lower anal canal.

canal is divided into the **upper anal canal** and **lower anal canal** by the **pectinate line**. The upper anal canal extends from the anorectal junction (perineal flexure) to the pectinate line. The mucosa of the upper anal canal is thrown into longitudinal folds called the **anal columns (of Morgagni)**. The base of the anal columns defines the **pectinate line**. At the base of the anal columns are folds of tissue called the **anal valves**. Behind the anal valves are small, blind pouches called the **anal sinuses** into which **anal glands** open into. The upper anal canal is predominately surrounded by the **internal anal sphincter** which is a continuation of smooth muscle from the rectum with involuntary control via autonomic innervation. The lower anal canal extends from the pectinate line to the **anal verge** (the point at which perianal skin begins). The lower anal canal is predominately surrounded by **external anal sphincter**, which is a striated muscle under voluntary control via the pudendal nerve.

B. Vasculature of the Anal Canal

1. **Arterial supply.** The arterial supply of the upper anal canal is from the **superior rectal artery** (abdominal aorta → inferior mesenteric artery → superior rectal artery). The arterial supply of the lower anal canal is from the **inferior rectal artery** (abdominal aorta → common iliac artery → internal iliac artery → internal pudendal artery → inferior rectal artery). The **middle rectal artery** (abdominal aorta → common iliac artery → internal iliac artery → middle rectal artery) forms an anastomosis with the superior and inferior rectal arteries.
2. **Venous drainage.** The venous drainage of the upper anal canal is to the **superior rectal vein** (superior rectal vein → inferior mesenteric vein → portal vein → hepatic sinusoids → central veins → hepatic veins → IVC). The venous drainage of the lower anal canal is to the **inferior rectal vein** (inferior rectal vein → internal pudendal vein → internal iliac vein → common iliac vein → IVC).

C. Clinical Considerations

1. **Internal hemorrhoids** are varicosities of the **superior rectal veins** (arterioles and venules are also dilated). They are located above the pectinate line and covered by rectal mucosa. Clinical findings include bleeding, mucus discharge, prolapse, pruritus, and painlessness.
2. **External hemorrhoids** are varicosities of the **inferior rectal veins** (arterioles and venules are also dilated). They are located below the pectinate line near the anal verge and covered by skin. Clinical findings include bleeding, swelling, and pain.

Liver

I General Features *(Figure 2-9)*

The liver is the largest internal gland in the body. The **liver parenchyma** consists of radially arranged plates of **hepatocytes**. The **liver stroma** consists of **reticular fibers (Type III collagen)**. The stroma begins as a thin connective tissue capsule called **Glisson capsule** that extends into the liver around the portal triads, around the periphery of hepatic lobules, extends into the perisinusoidal space of Disse to surround the hepatocytes, and then terminates around the central vein. Gross anatomically, one can identify at the **porta hepatis**, the components of the: (a) **common bile duct**, (b) **portal vein**, (c) **hepatic artery**, and (d) **lymphatics**. The hepatic bile duct, portal vein, and hepatic artery are referred to as the **portal triad** (the lymphatics are forgotten about in this designation). Histologically, branches of these same components can be found within the substance of the liver as they help define a classic hepatic lobule.

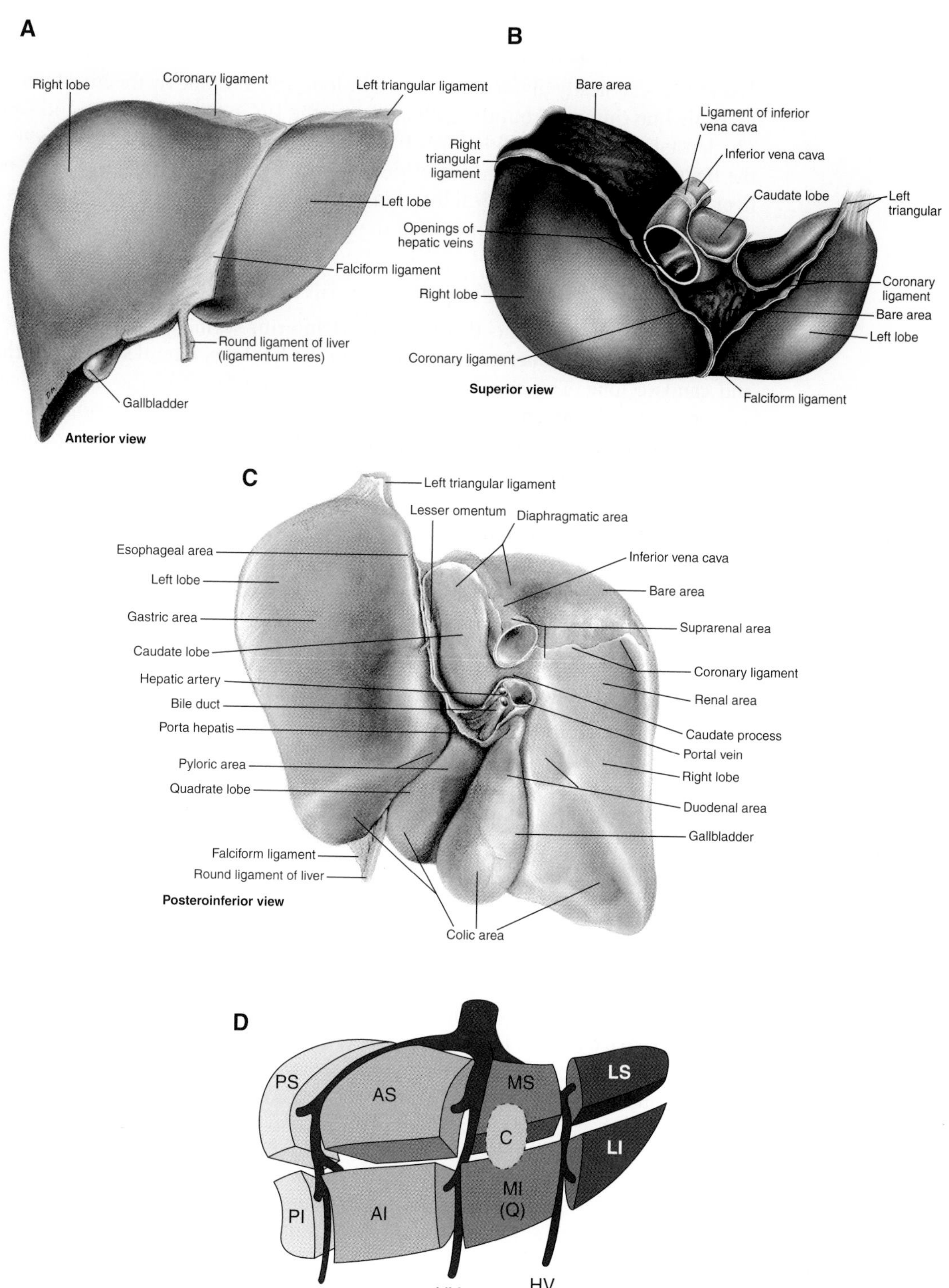

FIGURE 2-9. **Liver. (A)** Diaphragmatic surface of the liver (anterior view). **(B)** Diaphragmatic surface of the liver (superior view). **(C)** Visceral surface of the liver. **(D) Diagram of the Five Liver Segments and Nine Liver Subsegments Used in Liver Resectioning.** The five liver segments include the posterior segment and anterior segment of the right lobe, the medial segment and lateral segment of the left lobe, and the caudate lobe. Note the hepatic veins (HV) at the periphery of the liver segments. The nine liver subsegments include posterior superior (PS), posterior inferior (PI), anterior superior (AS), anterior inferior (AI), medial superior (MS), medial inferior (MI) that corresponds to the classic quadrate lobe (Q), lateral superior (LS), lateral inferior (LI), and the classic caudate lobe (C).

II Lobes of the Liver

The liver is classically divided into the **right lobe** and **left lobe** by the **interlobar fissure** (an invisible line running from the gallbladder to the IVC), **quadrate lobe**, and **caudate lobe**. The left lobe contains the **falciform ligament** (a derivative of the ventral mesentery) with the **ligamentum teres** (a remnant of the left umbilical vein) along its inferior border. The liver is secured in its anatomical location by the attachment of the hepatic veins to the IVC which allows for very little rotation of the liver during surgery.

III Segments and Subsegments of the Liver *(Figure 2-9D)*

There are five liver segments that include the **anterior segment of the right lobe, posterior segment of the right lobe, medial segment of the left lobe, lateral segment of the left lobe**, and **caudate lobe**. The hepatic veins define the boundaries of the liver segments. There are nine liver subsegments that include the **posterior superior, posterior inferior, anterior superior, anterior inferior, medial superior, medial inferior**, which corresponds to the classical quadrate lobe, **lateral superior, lateral inferior**, and the classic **caudate lobe**.

IV Vasculature of the Liver

A. **Arterial Supply.** The arterial supply of the liver is from the **right hepatic artery** and **left hepatic artery** (abdominal aorta → celiac trunk → common hepatic artery → proper hepatic artery → right hepatic artery and left hepatic artery → hepatic sinusoids).

B. **Portal Supply.** The portal supply of the liver is from the **portal vein** (superior mesenteric vein, inferior mesenteric vein, and splenic vein → portal vein → hepatic sinusoids). The portal vein is formed by the union of the splenic vein and superior mesenteric vein. The inferior mesenteric vein joins the splenic vein. The arterial blood and portal blood mix in the hepatic sinusoids.

C. **Venous Drainage.** The venous drainage of the liver is to the **central veins** located at the center of a classic liver lobule (central veins → hepatic veins → IVC).

V Clinical Considerations

A. **Liver Biopsies** are frequently performed by needle puncture through the right intercostal space 8, 9, or 10 when the patient has exhaled. The needle will pass through the following structures: skin → superficial fascia → external oblique muscle → intercostal muscles → costal parietal pleura → costodiaphragmatic recess → diaphragmatic parietal pleura → diaphragm → peritoneum.

B. **Surgical Resection of the Liver** may be performed by removing one of the **liver segments** (five segments in total) or one of the **liver subsegments** (nine subsegments in total). **Hepatic veins** form the surgical landmarks that mark the periphery (or border) of a liver segment during segmental resection of the liver. Recall that **pulmonary veins** form the surgical landmarks that mark the periphery of a bronchopulmonary segment during segmental resection of the lung.

Gallbladder and Biliary Ducts

I General Features *(Figure 2-10)*

The gallbladder is a pear-shaped distensible sac that has the capacity to store ≈35 mL of bile (range: 15 to 60 mL). The gallbladder is divided into the **fundus** (anterior portion that projects below the inferior margin of the liver), **body** (which is in contact with the visceral surface of the liver), and the **neck** (posterior portion that is continuous with the **cystic duct**). A small pouch (**Hartmann pouch**) may extend from the neck as a sequela to pathologic changes and is a common site for gallstones to lodge. **Rokitansky–Aschoff sinuses** occur when the mucosa of the gallbladder penetrates deep into the muscularis externa. They are an early indicator of pathological changes (e.g., acute cholecystitis or gangrene). The **right and left hepatic ducts** join together after leaving the liver to form the **common hepatic duct**. The common hepatic duct is joined at an acute angle by the **cystic duct** to form the **common bile duct**. The cystic duct drains bile from the gallbladder. The mucosa of the cystic duct is arranged in a spiral fold with a core of smooth muscle known as the **spiral valve (valve of Heister)**. The spiral valve keeps the cystic duct constantly open so that bile can flow freely in either direction. The bile duct passes posterior to the superior portion of the duodenum and the head of the pancreas and ends at the **hepatopancreatic ampulla (ampulla of Vater)** where it joins the **pancreatic duct**. The **sphincter of Oddi** is an area of thickened smooth muscle that surrounds the bile duct as it traverses the ampulla. The sphincter of Oddi controls the bile flow.

II Vasculature of the Gallbladder

A. Arterial Supply

1. The arterial supply of the gallbladder is from the **cystic artery** (abdominal aorta→ celiac trunk → common hepatic artery→ proper hepatic artery → right hepatic artery → cystic artery).
2. The arterial supply (i.e., the cystic artery) to the gallbladder is highly variable and one of the most tricky/time-consuming steps in a lap/open cholecystectomy ensuring that the cystic artery has been ligated and not some other artery.

B. Venous Drainage

The venous drainage of the gallbladder is to the **cystic vein** (cystic vein → portal vein → hepatic sinusoids → central veins → hepatic veins → IVC).

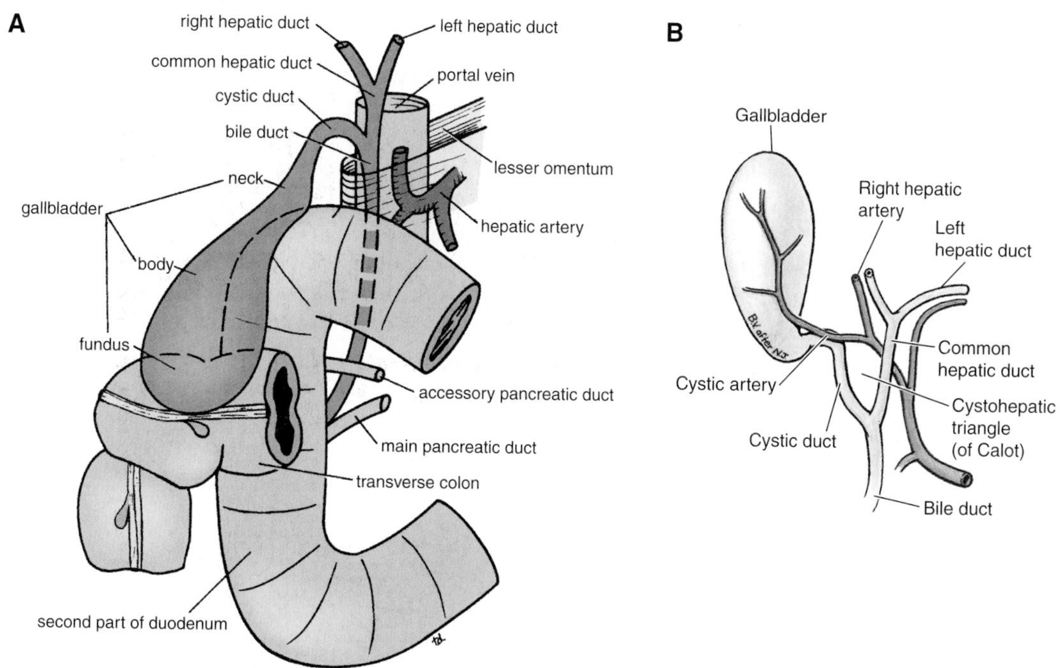

FIGURE 2-10. **Gallbladder and Biliary Ducts. (A) Relationships of the gallbladder and biliary ducts. (B) Arterial Supply of the Gallbladder.** Although variation in the arterial supply is quite common, the cystic artery most often arises from the right hepatic artery in the cystohepatic triangle of Calot.

Pancreas

I General Features *(Figure 2-11)*

The pancreas is a retroperitoneal organ that measures 15 to 20 cm in length and weighs about 85 to 120 gm. The normal pancreas is tan-pink to yellow in color and uniformly lobulated. A cut section of the pancreas reveals an extensive branching network of ducts extending into the lobules of the pancreas. The network of ducts involves the following: centroacinar cells of the intercalated duct → intralobular duct → interlobular duct → main pancreatic duct (duct of Wirsung) → joins the bile duct at the hepatopancreatic ampulla (ampulla of Vater) →duodenum. The sphincter of the pancreatic duct, the sphincter of the bile duct, and the sphincter of the hepatopancreatic ampulla (sphincter of Oddi) are smooth muscle sphincters that control the flow of bile and pancreatic juice. An **accessory pancreatic duct (duct of Santorini)** opens into the duodenum superior to the opening of the main pancreatic duct. In about 60% of cases, the accessory pancreatic duct communicates with the main pancreatic duct. In other cases, the main pancreatic duct is smaller than the accessory pancreatic duct and there is no communication between the two; in this situation, the accessory pancreatic duct carries the majority of the pancreatic juice. Gross anatomically, the pancreas consists of four parts as follows:

A. **Head of the Pancreas.** The head is the expanded part of the pancreas which lies in the concavity of the C-shaped curve of the duodenum and is firmly attached to the descending and horizontal parts of the duodenum. The **uncinate process** is a projection from the inferior portion of the pancreatic head. The head of the pancreas is related posteriorly to the IVC, right renal artery, right renal vein, and the left renal vein.

B. **Neck of the Pancreas.** The neck is related posteriorly to the confluence of the superior mesenteric vein and splenic to form the portal vein.

C. **Body of the Pancreas.** The body is related posteriorly to the aorta, superior mesenteric artery, left suprarenal gland, left kidney, renal artery, and renal vein.

D. **Tail of the Pancreas.** The tail is related to the splenic hilum and the left colic flexure.

II Vasculature of the Pancreas

A. **Arterial Supply.** The arterial supply of the pancreas is from the **anterior and posterior superior pancreaticoduodenal arteries** that supply the head and neck of the pancreas (abdominal aorta → celiac trunk → common hepatic artery → gastroduodenal artery → anterior and posterior superior pancreaticoduodenal arteries); **anterior and posterior inferior pancreaticoduodenal arteries** that supply the head and neck of the pancreas (abdominal aorta → superior mesenteric artery → anterior and posterior inferior pancreaticoduodenal arteries); **dorsal pancreatic artery** that supplies the body and tail of the pancreas (abdominal aorta → celiac trunk → splenic artery → dorsal pancreatic artery); **great pancreatic artery** that supplies the body and tail of the pancreas (abdominal aorta → celiac trunk → splenic artery → great pancreatic artery); and **caudal pancreatic arteries** that supply the body and tail of the pancreas (abdominal aorta → celiac trunk → splenic artery → caudal pancreatic arteries).

B. **Venous Drainage.** The venous drainage of the pancreas is to the **splenic vein** (splenic vein → portal vein → hepatic sinusoids → central veins → hepatic veins → IVC) and the **superior mesenteric vein** (superior mesenteric vein → portal vein → hepatic sinusoids → central veins → hepatic veins → IVC).

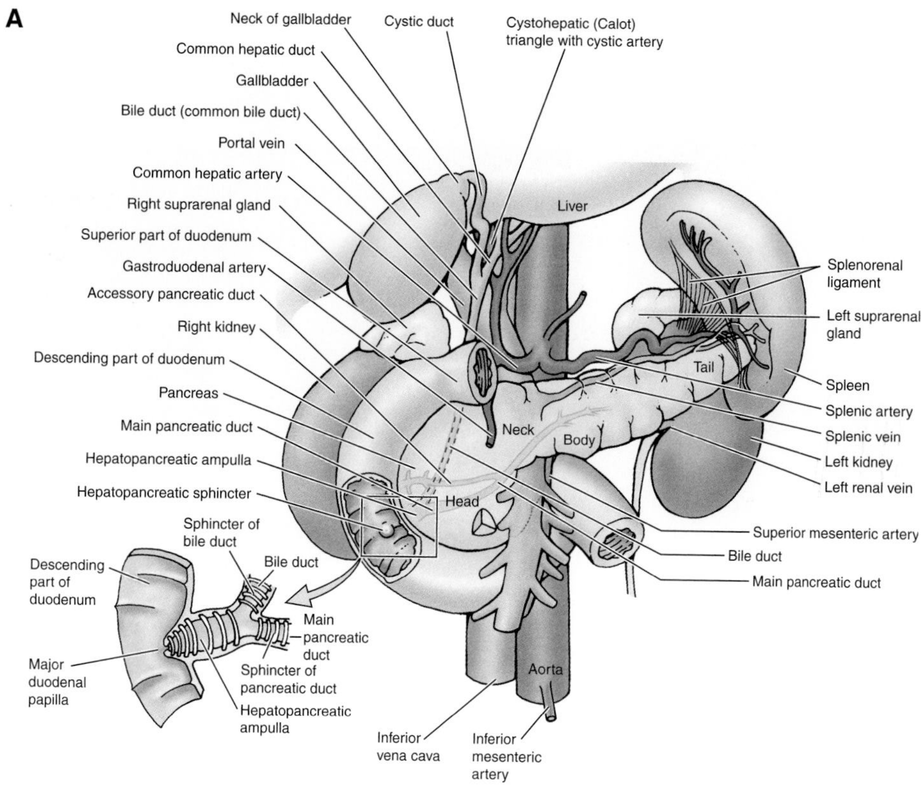
A
Neck of gallbladder
Cystic duct
Cystohepatic (Calot) triangle with cystic artery
Common hepatic duct
Gallbladder
Bile duct (common bile duct)
Portal vein
Common hepatic artery
Right suprarenal gland
Superior part of duodenum
Gastroduodenal artery
Accessory pancreatic duct
Right kidney
Descending part of duodenum
Pancreas
Main pancreatic duct
Hepatopancreatic ampulla
Hepatopancreatic sphincter
Liver
Splenorenal ligament
Left suprarenal gland
Tail
Spleen
Splenic artery
Splenic vein
Left kidney
Left renal vein
Neck
Body
Head
Superior mesenteric artery
Bile duct
Main pancreatic duct
Sphincter of bile duct
Bile duct
Descending part of duodenum
Main pancreatic duct
Major duodenal papilla
Sphincter of pancreatic duct
Hepatopancreatic ampulla
Aorta
Inferior vena cava
Inferior mesenteric artery

B
Aorta
Celiac artery
Dorsal pancreatic artery
Greater pancreatic artery
Common hepatic artery
Gastroduodenal artery
Right gastroomental artery
Splenic artery
Inferior pancreaticoduodenal artery (dividing into anterior and posterior branches)
Uncinate process of pancreas (posterior to superior mesenteric artery)
Anterior and posterior superior pancreaticoduodenal arteries
Superior mesenteric artery

FIGURE 2-11. **Pancreas. (A)** Relationships of the pancreas, duodenum, biliary ducts, and spleen. **(B)** Arterial supply of the pancreas.

Chapter 3

Radiology

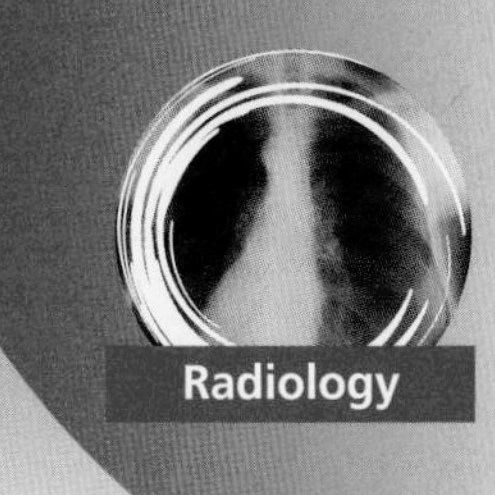

I Anterior–Posterior Supine Abdomen Radiograph

The film cassette is placed against the back and the X-ray beam is directed at the abdomen and travels in an anterior→ posterior direction (hence the name). This radiograph is taken with the patient supine either on a radiographic table or in bed (using a portable X-ray unit).

II Anterior–Posterior Upright Abdomen Radiograph

The film cassette is placed against the back and the X-ray beam is directed at the abdomen and travels in an anterior → posterior direction (hence the name). This radiograph is taken with the patient standing in the radiology department.

III Left Lateral Decubitus Abdomen Radiograph

The film cassette is placed against the back and the X-ray beam is directed at the abdomen and travels in an anterior → posterior direction.

IV The Acute Abdomen Series

The optimal series to evaluate an acute abdomen (sometimes called a three-way abdomen) includes a **posterior–anterior (PA) <u>chest</u> radiograph**, an **anterior–posterior (AP) supine abdomen radiograph**, and an **AP upright abdomen radiograph**. If the mobility of the patients is limited, then evaluation of an acute abdomen includes an **AP <u>chest</u> radiograph**, an **AP supine radiograph**, and a **left lateral decubitus abdomen radiograph**.

V Upper Gastrointestinal Endoscopy

Upper gastrointestinal (GI) endoscopy is a highly accurate method of evaluating the **esophagus, stomach**, and **duodenum**. The endoscopic examination of the esophagus, stomach, duodenal bulb (first part of the duodenum), and descending duodenum (second part of the duodenum) is carried out using a **videoendoscope**. The esophagus is studied from 20 to 40 cm where the junction between the pearly stratified squamous epithelium and the red gastric simple columnar epithelium is located (i.e., the Z line). The stomach is inspected with observations on the amount of mucus, fold thickness and pliability, pattern of peristaltic contraction waves, and appearance of blood vessels.

VI Small Bowel Examination

A. A **barium follow-through** is the routine small bowel examination.
B. A **small bowel barium enema** or the introduction of barium through a nasointestinal tube (**enteroclysis**) provides more detail of the small bowel than a follow-through. The increased detailing occurs because barium can be introduced into the lumen at a rate that distends the bowel optimally and methylcellulose can be introduced after the barium so that a double contrast examination of the jejunum is possible.
C. The introduction of **barium through an ileostomy** allows for the examination of the entire small bowel.

 Large Bowel (Colon) Examination

A. **A barium enema** is the routine large bowel examination.

B. **A single contrast barium enema** is used to detect fistulas, diverticulitis, or colon obstruction.

C. **A double contrast barium enema** is used to detect polyps, adenomas (cancer), and colitis.

D. **Evacuation Proctography.** A barium contrast medium of paste-consistency is introduced into the rectum followed by video fluoroscopy in lateral projection during evacuation. The indications for evacuation proctography include painful rectal evacuation and incontinence. Evacuation proctograph may reveal the following: speed and completeness of rectal evacuation, rectocele, intra-anal or rectal intussusception, rectal prolapse, enterocele, sigmoidocele, excessive pelvic floor descent, and anismus.

E. **Colonoscopy and Flexible Sigmoidoscopy.** A fiberoptic or video colonoscope gives a brilliant, high resolution, color view of the colonic mucosa. The benefits of inspecting the colonic mucosa by colonoscopy are that almost all colonic diseases begin on the mucosal surface and neoplasms project above the mucosal surface as visible polyps. Since the time course of most colonic pathology is slow, early diagnosis by colonoscopy leading to early treatment is worthwhile. Although the ascending colon and descending colon are normally retroperitoneal and therefore remain fixed in the paravertebral gutters, in ≈**15% of the subjects, the ascending colon and descending colon are intraperitoneal** (i.e., suspending by a mesentery) and are therefore mobile, which can increase the difficulty for the endoscopist. The colonoscope enters the sigmoid colon at ≈17 cm where frequent **transverse rectal folds (Houston valves,** which may be enlarged in patients with diverticular disease) increase the difficulty for the endoscopist. At the **rectosigmoid junction**, the sigmoid colon (which bends in an anterior direction and to the left) may be punctured if not negotiated properly. The lumen of the transverse colon appears triangular because of the presence of the **teniae coli** (three longitudinal bands of smooth muscle). The normal colorectal mucosa appears smooth and shiny with a fine, interlacing vascular pattern visible behind it.

VIII Hepatobiliary Scintigraphic Imaging

Hepatobiliary scintigraphic imaging (HIS) is performed using the radiotracer **99 m technetium-labeled iminodiacetic acid (HIDA)**, which is an analog of bilirubin. HIDA is endocytosed by hepatocytes and conjugated to glucuronide which is released into the bile. In a normal subject, HIDA will enter the gallbladder within 1 h after the intravenous administration. In a patient with acute cholecystitis (gallstone obstruction of the cystic duct), the gall bladder fails to fill with HIDA. False positives may result from prolonged fasting (3 days), ingestion of food with 2 h of the study, chronic cholecystitis, chronic alcohol abuse, or pancreatitis. The administration of morphine reduces the number of false positives. Morphine causes contraction of the sphincter of Oddi, leads to a rise in biliary system pressure, and augments bile movement through the cystic duct.

 Angiography

Angiography is a form of contrast imaging used to visualize the **lumen of blood vessels.** Angiography does not give one any information about the blood vessel itself per se except that it helps predict the course of the vessel and the caliber of the lumen. Angiography may be used to demonstrate the site of GI bleeding or to access the integrity or anomalies of blood vessels to various organs.

X Ultrasonography

Ultrasonography produces images of the body based on very high frequency sound waves that readily pass through fluids but are reflected back from acoustic interfaces (e.g., soft tissue, bone, gas, and stones).

XI Computerized Tomography

Computerized tomography (CT; plain or with contrast) produces computerized images of the body based on the amount of X-rays absorbed by different tissues at different angles in a series of body slices. CT is very effective at imaging soft tissues (e.g., tumors).

XII Magnetic Resonance Imaging

Magnetic resonance imaging (MRI) produces computerized images of the body based on the radio signals emitted by hydrogen atoms as they fall back into alignment in a series of body slices. Hydrogen atoms normally lie in random directions. However, MRI scanners align the nuclei of hydrogen atoms in a parallel direction. Subsequently, the hydrogen nuclei are temporarily knocked out of alignment by radio pulses and then emit radio signals as they fall back into alignment. Fatty tissue has a high density of hydrogen atoms and produces a bright MRI image. Bone tissue has a low density of hydrogen atoms and produces a dark MRI image.

XIII Radiology of the Esophagus Highlights

A. A radiographic study of a patient with **gastroesophageal reflux disease (GERD)** is to exclude any morphologic or functional sequelae of the condition, which includes thickened mucosal folds, granular appearance of the mucosa, ulceration, stricture, inflammatory polyps, and abnormal motility. GERD is caused by lower esophageal sphincter (LES) dysfunction that allows gastric acid reflux into the lower esophagus. **Scleroderma** may be a systemic cause of GERD.

B. The radiographic findings in **Barrett esophagus** include thickened mucosal folds, reticular appearance of the mucosa, ulceration, stricture, hiatal hernia, and reflux. Barrett esophagus can be defined as the replacement of esophageal stratified squamous epithelium with metaplastic "intestinalized" simple columnar (with Goblet cells) epithelium extending **at least 3 cm** into the esophagus. The clinical importance of this metaplastic invasion is that virtually all lower esophageal adenocarcinomas occur as a sequela.

C. The radiographic findings in **achalasia** include abrupt narrowing or stenosis of the distal esophagus (called "**beaking**"), absence of normal peristalsis, esophageal dilatation, and abnormally elevated LES tone. Achalasia is the failure of LES to relax during swallowing probably due to the absence of the myenteric plexus. **Chagas disease** (caused by *Trypanosoma cruzi*) may lead to achalasia.

D. The radiographic findings in **esophageal varices** include serpentine submucosal filling defects that are effaced when the esophagus is distended. Esophageal varices (EV) refer to the dilated subepithelial and submucosal venous plexuses of the esophagus that drain into the **left gastric (coronary) vein**. The left gastric vein empties into the portal vein from the distal esophagus and proximal stomach. **Uphill** EV are caused by **portal hypertension** due to cirrhosis of the liver and are located in the lower esophagus around the gastroesophageal junction. **Downhill** EV are caused by superior vena cava obstruction and are located in the middle esophagus.

E. The radiographic findings of **Zenker diverticulum** include a pouch or a sac located in the midline at the level of the pyriform sinuses, which extends inferiorly and posteriorly to the cervical esophagus. A Zenker diverticulum is a true esophageal diverticulum located at the upper esophageal sphincter. The cause of Zenker diverticulum is controversial and may include abnormal contraction and relaxation of the cricopharyngeus muscle, abnormal smooth muscle configuration, and an inflammatory cause due to its high association with a hiatal hernia and gastroesophageal reflux.

F. The radiographic findings of **Boerhaave syndrome** include extravasation of a water-soluble contrast agent from the distal esophagus usually just superior to the gastroesophageal junction on the left side, pneumomediastinum, pleural effusion on the left side, and pneumothorax on a chest radiograph. Boerhaave syndrome is a traumatic rupture of the lower esophagus usually following forceful retching through all layers of the esophageal wall. **Mallory–Weiss tears** involve only the mucosal and submucosal layers.

XIV Radiology of Gastrointestinal Hemorrhage Highlights

A. The most common causes of **gastric bleeding** include **gastric varices**, **gastric ulcer disease**, and **acute hemorrhagic gastritis**. The **left gastric artery** (a branch of the celiac trunk) is most commonly (85% of the cases) responsible for gastric bleeding.

B. The angiographic findings in **Mallory–Weiss syndrome** include acute extravasation of a contrast agent at the gastroesophageal junction with outlining of the distal esophagus or proximal stomach. Mallory–Weiss tears result in massive, painless bleeding from the submucosal venous plexus of the distal esophagus after a violent episode of retching.

C. The angiographic finding in **GI bleeding** is contrast extravasation of contrast agent into the bowel lumen. **Glucagon** is administered prior to contrast agent injection to reduce peristaltic activity of the bowel.

D. In upper and lower GI bleeding, **vasopressin** can be administered. Vasopressin causes smooth muscle contraction of the bowel wall so that tamponade occurs, which diminishes blood flow. In addition, vasopressin causes vasoconstriction, which also diminishes blood flow.

E. The scintigraphic findings in **lower GI bleeding** include extravasation of technetium-99 m labeled red blood cells or technetium sulfur colloid that results in focal accumulation of tracer activity with the lumen of the bowel. The **superior mesenteric artery** and the **inferior mesenteric artery** are most commonly responsible for lower GI bleeding.

XV Radiology of Peptic Ulcer Disease Highlights

A. The radiographic findings of a **benign gastric ulcer** include ulcer crater that projects beyond the normal boundaries of the gastric lumen; gastric folds that are regular shaped and extend to the margin of the ulcer; ulcer that is round, oval, or linear in shape; a thin, sharply demarcated line with parallel, straight margins at the base of the ulcer (called Hampton line); a lucent ring that separates the ulcer from the gastric mucosa (called an ulcer collar); and mucosal edema (called an ulcer mound).

B. The radiographic findings of a **malignant gastric ulcer** include ulcer crater that does not project beyond the normal boundaries of the gastric lumen; gastric folds that are irregular or club-shaped and do not extend to the margin of the ulcer; ulcer that is angular in shape; **Carmen meniscus** whereby the edges of the malignant ulcer trap barium is seen on a single contrast barium radiograph; and **Kirkland complex** whereby the heaped margins of the malignant ulcer touch and form a lucent rim around the ulcer.

XVI Radiology of the Large Bowel (Colon) Highlights

A. The plain film radiographic findings of **appendicitis** include a lower right quadrant calcification (called an appendicolith), abnormal gas pattern in the bowel, loss of right psoas major muscle shadow, and scoliosis of the vertebral columns (convex to the left).

B. The sonographic findings of **appendicitis** include dilatation of the appendix to >6 mm in cross section and noncompressible.

C. The contrast-enhanced CT findings of **appendicitis** include dilatation of the appendix to >6 mm and inflammatory changes in the adjacent adipose tissue. A contrast-enhanced CT is the best imaging technique to diagnose appendicitis.
D. The barium enema radiographic findings of **ulcerative colitis** include granular appearance of the mucosa, relatively deep ulcers (called **collar-button ulcers**), mucosal involvement beginning in the distal colon and proceeding to the proximal colon, "backwash" ileitis due to the chronic opening of the ileocecal valve, and "lead pipe" appearance of the colon occurring late in the disease process.
E. The barium enema radiographic findings of **Crohn disease** include small, bulls-eye, superficial mucosal ulcers (called **aphthous ulcers**), longitudinal and transverse ulcers that produce a "cobblestone" appearance of the mucosa, mucosal involvement that may extend from the pharynx to the anus, and deep ulcers often with "skip" areas (pathologic areas separated by normal areas), which occur late in the disease process.

XVII Radiology of Bowel Obstruction Highlights

A. The plain film radiographic findings of **small bowel obstruction** include multiple air–fluid levels, no colonic distention, a "stepladder" appearance of small bowel loops/air–fluid levels, and a "string of pearls" appearance whereby a small amount of residual air remains in the fluid-filled small bowel.
B. The "**rule of threes**" for the **normal small bowel** includes <3 mm thickness of the bowel wall, <3 mm thickness of the transverse bowel folds, <3 cm diameter of the bowel, and <3 air–fluid levels per radiograph.
C. The plain film radiographic findings of **large bowel obstruction** include dilatation of the cecum, dilatation of the small bowel due to reflux of gas through the ileocecal valve, and air–fluid levels distal to the hepatic flexure of the colon.
D. The "**coffee bean**" **sign** refers to volvulus of the large bowel where the two limbs of a colon loop are adjacent to each other. The adjacent colonic walls form a dense white line that is surrounded on both sides by a curved, gas-filled lumen.
E. **Ogilvie syndrome** occurs when the large bowel is markedly distended because of paralytic or adynamic ileus, a pseudoobstruction.

XVIII Radiology of Pancreatic Disease Highlights

A. The CT radiographic findings of **pancreatitis** include an enlarged and edematous pancreas, decreased density compared to a normal pancreas, and inflammatory changes in adjacent fat.
B. The "**colon cutoff**" **sign** in pancreatitis refers to gas in the transverse colon that is "cutoff" at the left upper quadrant due to inflammatory small bowel ileus in the left upper quadrant called a **sentinel loop**.
C. The plain film and barium radiographic findings of **pancreatitis** include a dilated C-loop of the duodenum due to inflammation of the pancreatic head, spiculation of the medial border of the duodenum, swollen ampulla of Vater, pleural effusions on the left side, and calcifications of the pancreas.
D. The "**double duct**" **sign** refers to the dilatation of both the pancreatic duct and the common bile duct due to the obstruction caused by the tumor of the pancreatic head.

XIX Radiology of Liver Disease Highlights

A. The "**starry sky**" sign refers to the relatively bright appearance of the portal triads against a decreased echogenicity of the remaining liver parenchyma seen on ultrasound due to **acute hepatitis**.
B. The ultrasound, CT, and MRI radiographic findings of **liver cirrhosis** include heterogeneous and coarse ultrasound appearance, small nodules representing liver regeneration, ascites, varices, splenomegaly, and portal vein abnormalities.
C. The CT and MRI radiographic findings of **hepatocellular cancer** include a focal lesion that may invade the portal vein or hepatic veins; multifocal or diffused lesion; and

increased enhancement in comparison to the remaining liver parenchyma after intravenous contrast agent is administered, especially during the hepatic arterial phase (within 20 s after the contrast agent is administered).

XX Radiology of GI Tumor Highlights

A. The upper GI series radiographic findings of **gastric cancer** include polypoid mass with or without ulceration or nodularity; a flat, superficial, spreading lesion; and an infiltrating, scirrhous appearance with linitis plastica ("**leather bottle**" stomach).

B. The barium radiographic findings of **small bowel adenocarcinoma** include an infiltrating circumferential mass, mucosal destruction and ulceration, and proximal dilatation that may be present.

C. The barium enema radiographic findings of **colon cancer** include polyps or a polypoid mass; circumferential narrowing ("**apple core**" appearance); flat, plaquelike lesions that produce a reticular surface appearance; and a long area of narrowing with tapered margins.

XXI Radiology of Gallbladder Disease Highlights

A. The ultrasound radiographic findings of **cholecystitis** include observation of gallstones, fluid around the gall bladder, and >3-mm thickness of the gall bladder wall.

B. **Murphy sign** refers to the interruption of the patient's deep inhalation upon pressure beneath the right costal margin.

C. **Mercedes-Benz sign** refers to the presence of gas-filled fissures within the gallstones seen on radiographs even though the gallstones may not be visible.

D. The HIS radiographic findings of **cholecystitis** include gall bladder failing to fill with radiotracer (HIDA) within 1 h after intravenous administration even though the common bile duct and duodenum have filled with radiotracer and morphine was administered.

XXII Selected Radiologic Photographs

A. **AP supine abdomen radiograph, AP upright abdomen radiograph, left lateral decubitus abdomen radiograph** (*Figure 3-1*)

B. **Esophagus and small bowel radiology** (*Figure 3-2*)

C. **Large bowel (colon) radiology** (*Figure 3-3*)

D. **HIS and angiography radiology** (*Figure 3-4*)

E. **CT and MRI images at the level of the portal vein** (*Figure 3-5*)

F. **CT and MRI images at the level of the celiac artery and upper poles of the kidneys** (*Figure 3-6*)

G. **CT and MRI images at the level of the hilum of the kidney and pancreas** (*Figure 3-7*)

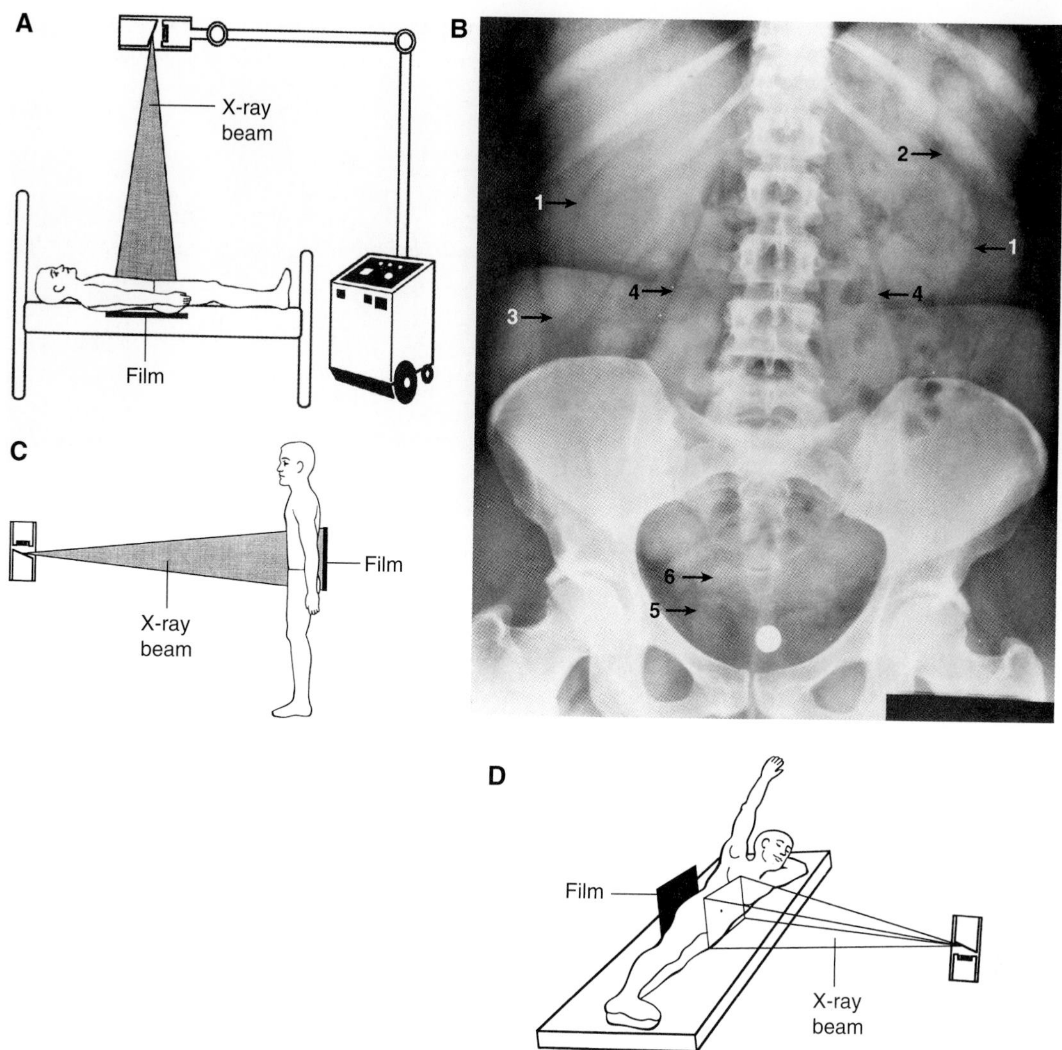

FIGURE 3-1. **Radiographs. (A,B) AP Supine Abdomen Radiograph. (A)** Diagram shows the patient positioning for an AP supine abdomen radiograph. **(B)** A normal AP supine abdomen radiograph shows an unremarkable bowel gas pattern and soft tissue shadows of the kidneys (1), spleen (2), liver margin (3), psoas major muscle (4), bladder (5), and uterus (6). **(C)** Diagram shows the patient positioning for an AP upright abdomen radiograph. **(D)** Diagram shows the patient positioning for a left lateral decubitus abdomen radiograph.

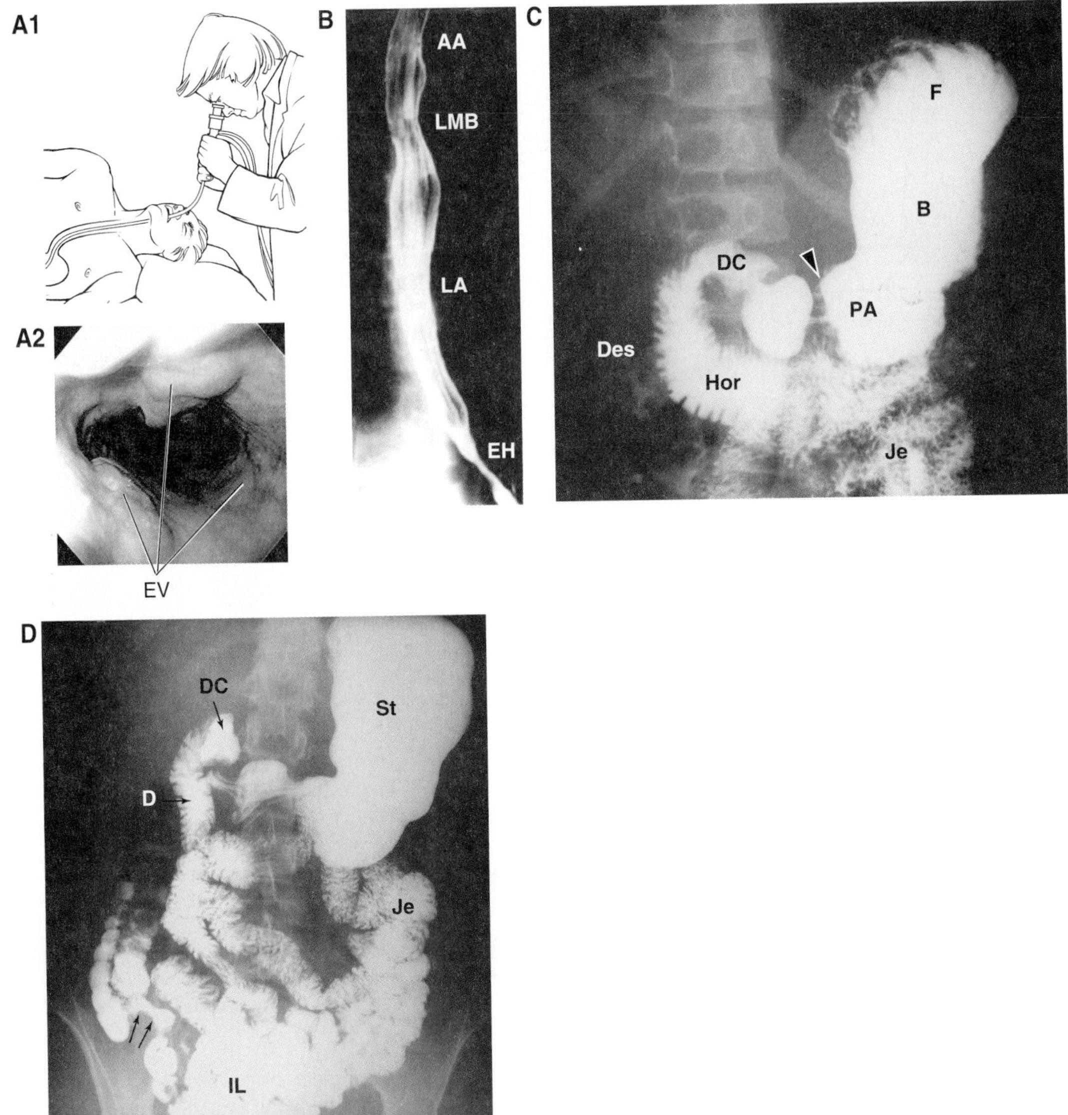

FIGURE 3-2. **Esophagus and Small Bowel Radiology. (A) Upper GI Endoscopy. (A1)** Diagram shows a physician performing an endoscopic examination of a patient. **(A2)** Endoscopic examination reveals esophageal varices (EV). **(B)** Barium contrast radiograph shows a normal esophagus with narrowing of the lumen at the following sites of constriction: aortic arch (AA), left main bronchus (LMB), left atrium (LA), and esophageal hiatus (EH). **(C)** Barium contrast radiograph shows a normal stomach and duodenum. Arrowhead indicates peristaltic wave. **(D)** Barium contrast radiograph shows a normal stomach, duodenum, jejunum, and ileum. Double arrows indicate terminal ileum entering the cecum. F — fundus; B — body; PA — pyloric antrum; DC — duodenal cap or superior part of the duodenum; Des — descending part of the duodenum; Hor — horizontal part of the duodenum; Je — jejunum; St — stomach; D — duodenal C-loop; IL — ileum.

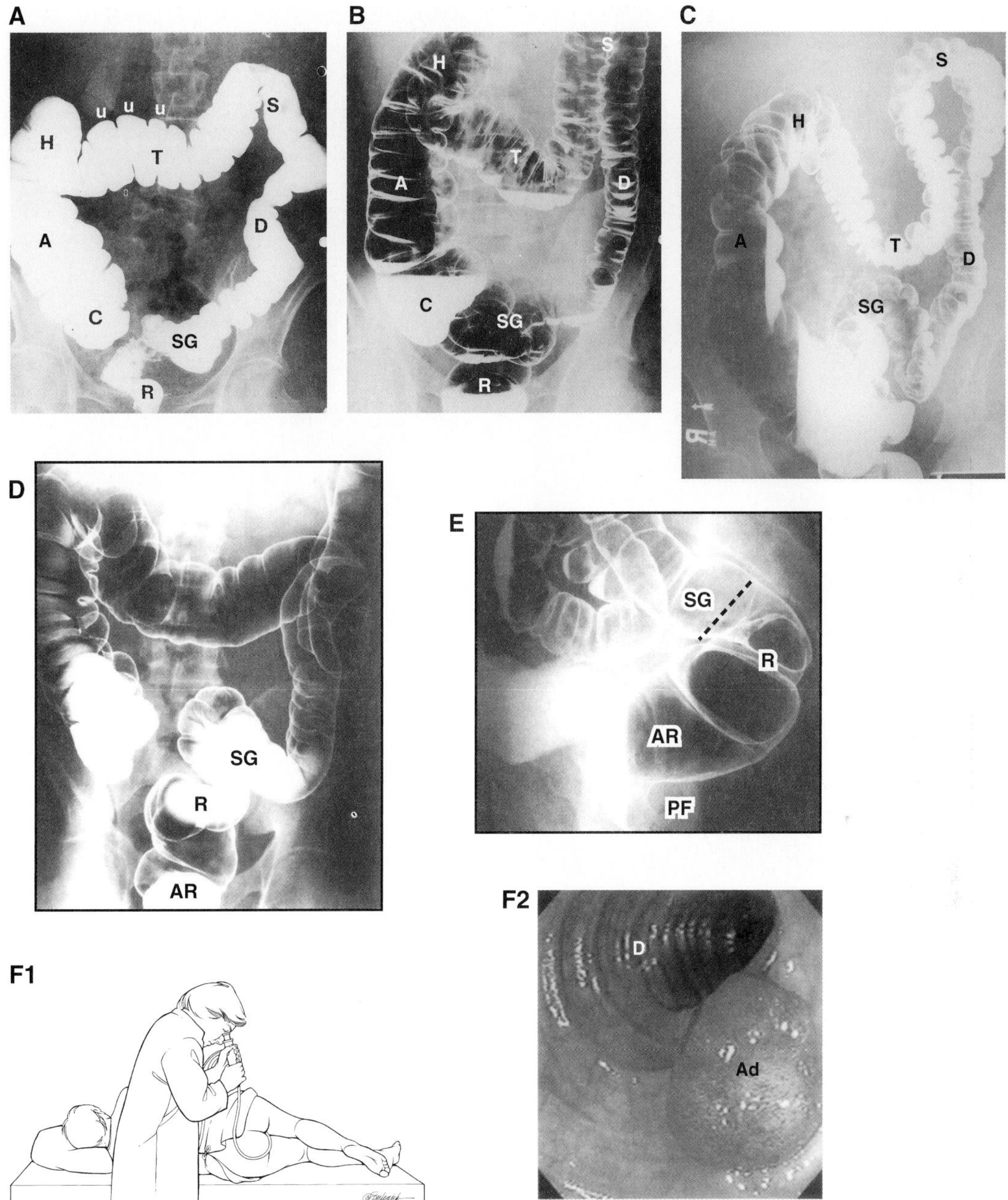

FIGURE 3-3. **Large Bowel (Colon) Radiology. (A)** Barium single contrast radiograph shows a normal colon. **(B)** Barium double contrast radiograph shows a normal colon. **(C)** Barium–air contrast radiograph with the patient in the left lateral decubitus position shows a normal colon. Note the barium–air interface. **(D,E) Large Bowel (Colon) Lying within the Pelvis Radiology**. **(D)** Barium contrast radiograph shows a normal sigmoid colon (SG), rectum (R), and ampulla of the rectum (AR). **(E)** Barium contrast radiograph (lateral view) shows a normal SG, rectosigmoid junction (dotted line), R, AR, and perineal flexure (PF). **(F) Colonoscopy. (F1)** Diagram shows a physician performing a colonoscopic examination of a patient. **(F2)** Colonoscopic examination of the descending colon (D) reveals a small adenoma (Ad). C — cecum; A — ascending colon; H — hepatic flexure; T — transverse colon; U — haustra; S — splenic flexure.

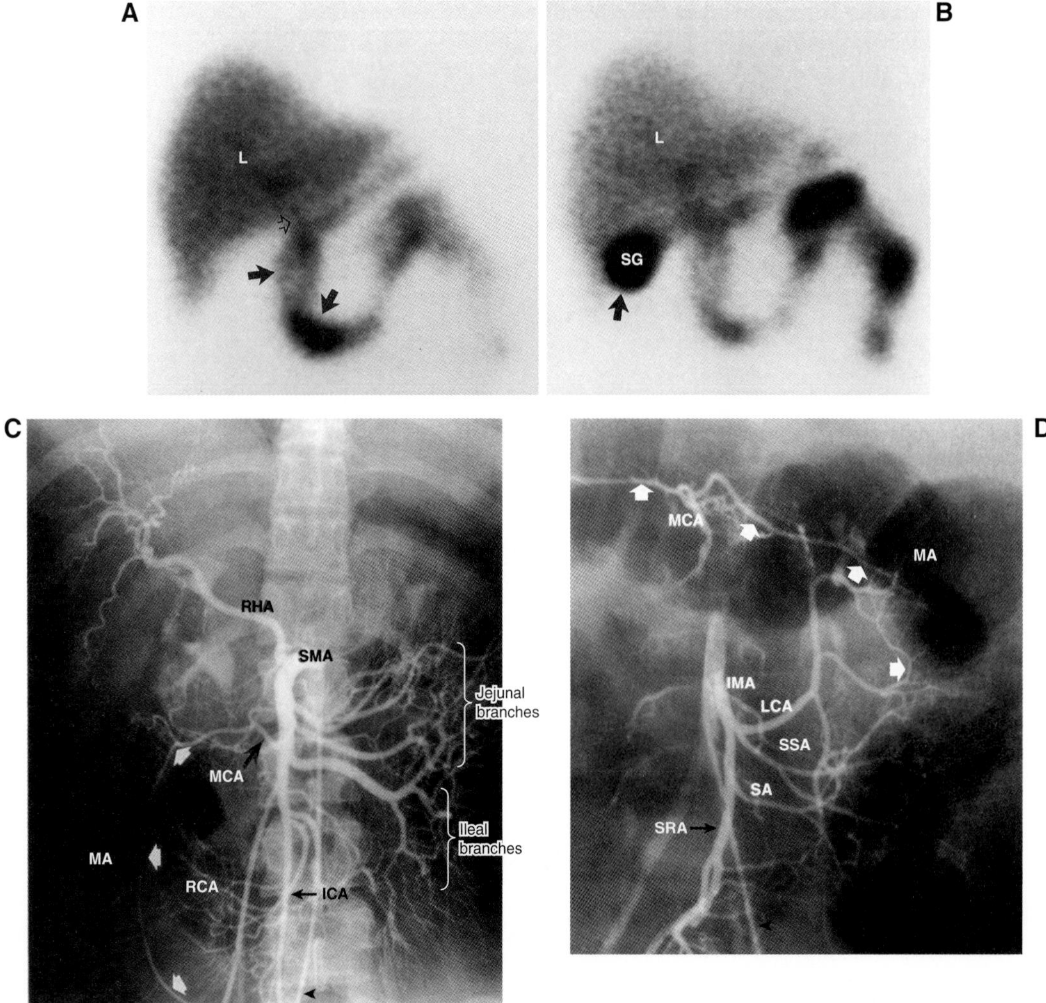

FIGURE 3-4. **HIS and Angiography Radiology. (A,B) HIS of a Normal Subject. (A)** At 30 min after injection of the radiotracer 99 m technetium-labeled mebrofenin, the radiotracer is excreted by the liver (L) through the bile duct (open arrow) into the duodenum (closed arrows). **(B)** At 60 min after injection of the radiotracer 99 m technetium-labeled mebrofenin, the radiotracer fills the gall bladder (gb; solid arrow). **(C,D) Arteriograms. (C) Arteriogram of the Superior Mesenteric Artery (SMA).** The SMA is catherized (arrowhead = catheter). In this subject, the right hepatic artery (RHA) arises anomalously from the SMA. Note the three main branches of the SMA: the middle colic artery (MCA), right colic artery (RCA), and the ileocolic artery (ICA). The MCA, RCA, and ICA form part of the marginal artery (MA; white arrows) that supplies the ascending colon. The participation of the ICA in the formation of the MA is not clearly shown. In addition, the SMA gives off various branches to the jejunum and ileum. **(D) Arteriogram of the Inferior Mesenteric Artery (IMA).** The IMA is catherized (arrowhead = catheter). Note the four main branches of the IMA: the left colic artery (LCA), superior sigmoid artery (SSA), sigmoidal arteries (SA), and the superior rectal artery (SRA). The LCA anastomoses with the MCA to form part of the marginal artery (MA; white arrows) that supplies the descending colon. Opacification of the MCA is due to the forceful injection of contrast medium into the IMA.

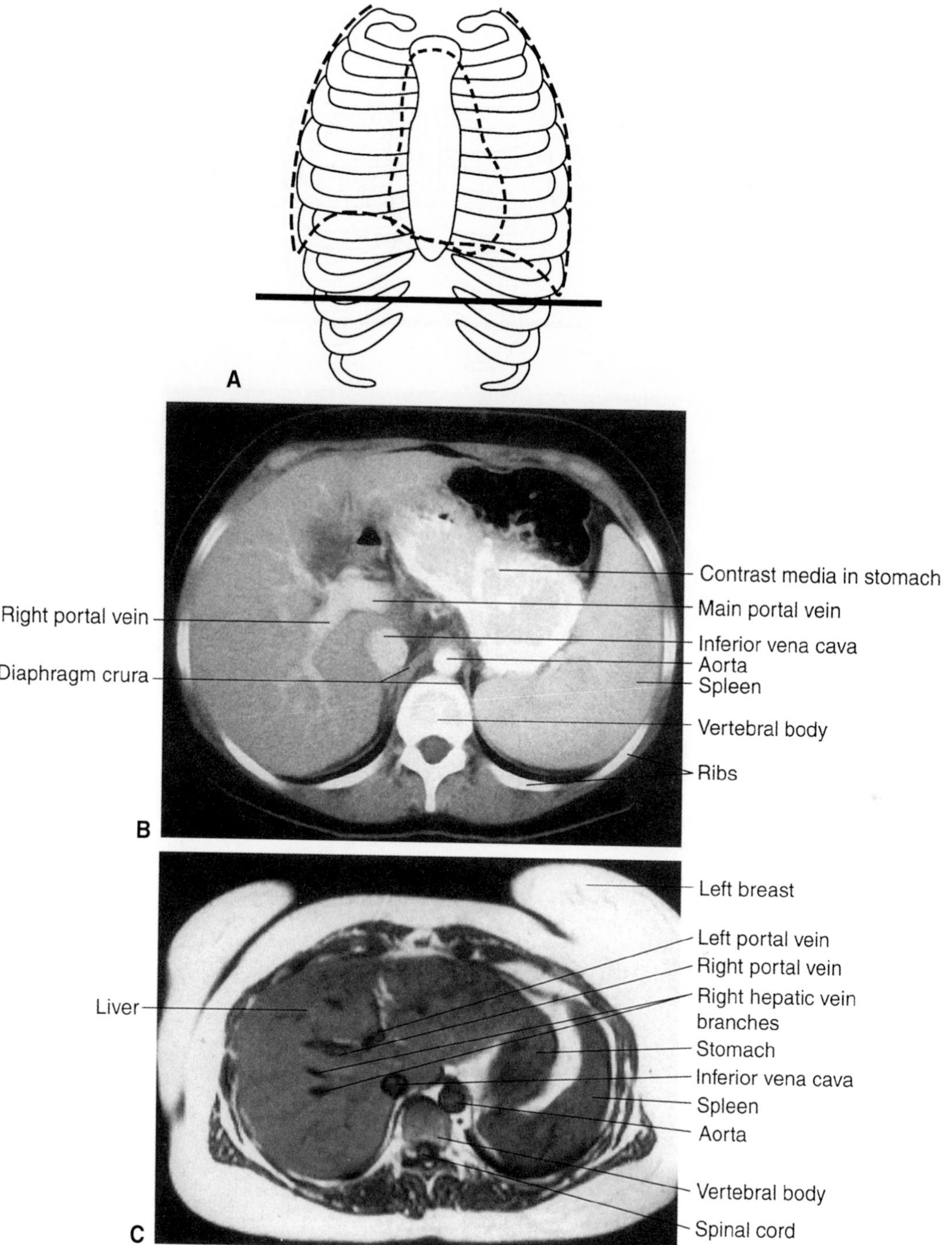

FIGURE 3-5. **CT and MRI Images at the Level of the Portal Vein. (A)** A schematic to show where the cross section was taken. **(B)** A normal abdominal axial CT image. **(C)** A normal abdominal axial MRI image.

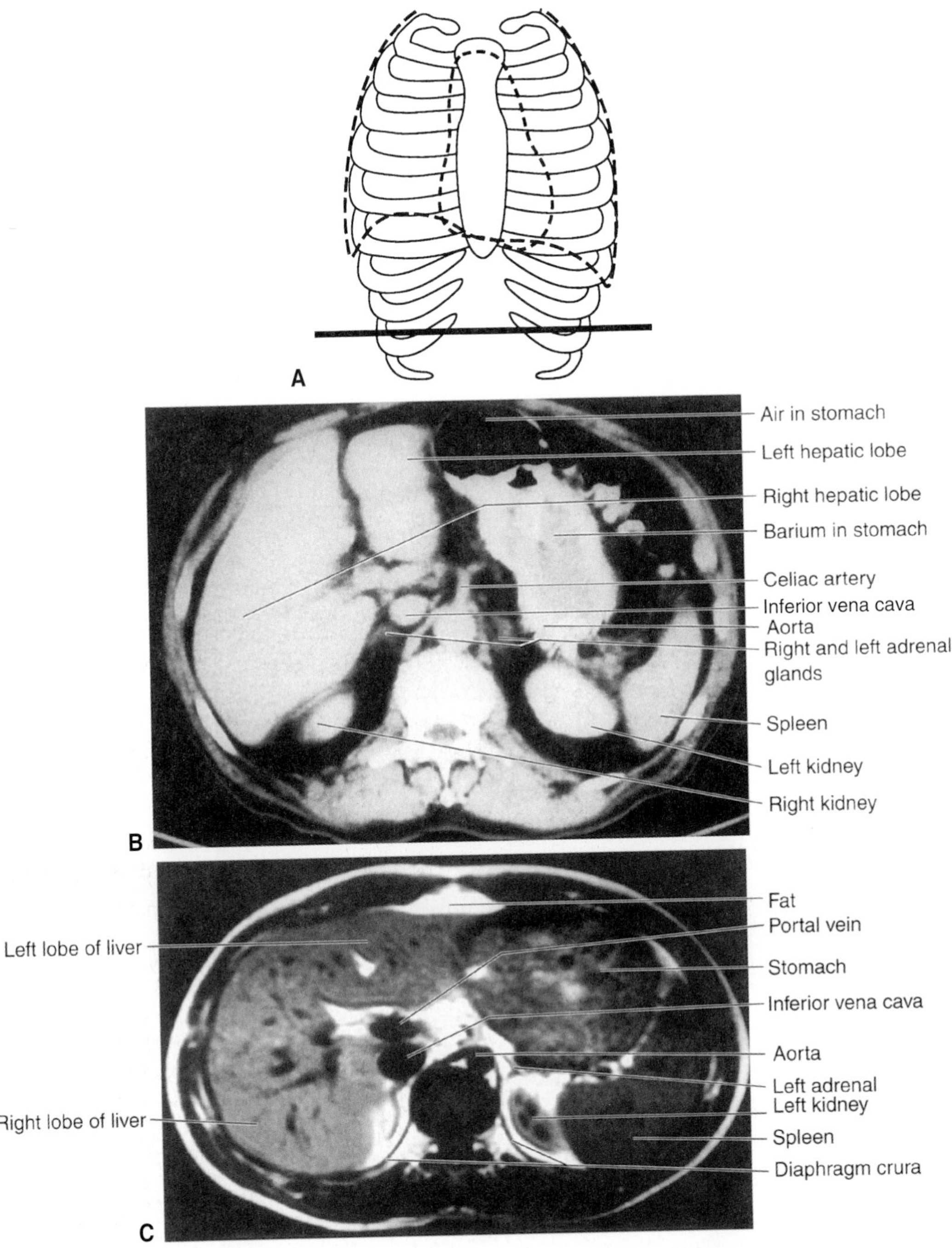

FIGURE 3-6. CT and MRI Images at the Level of the Celiac Artery and Upper Poles of the Kidneys. (A) A schematic to show where the cross section was taken. **(B)** A normal abdominal axial CT image. **(C)** A normal abdominal axial MRI image.

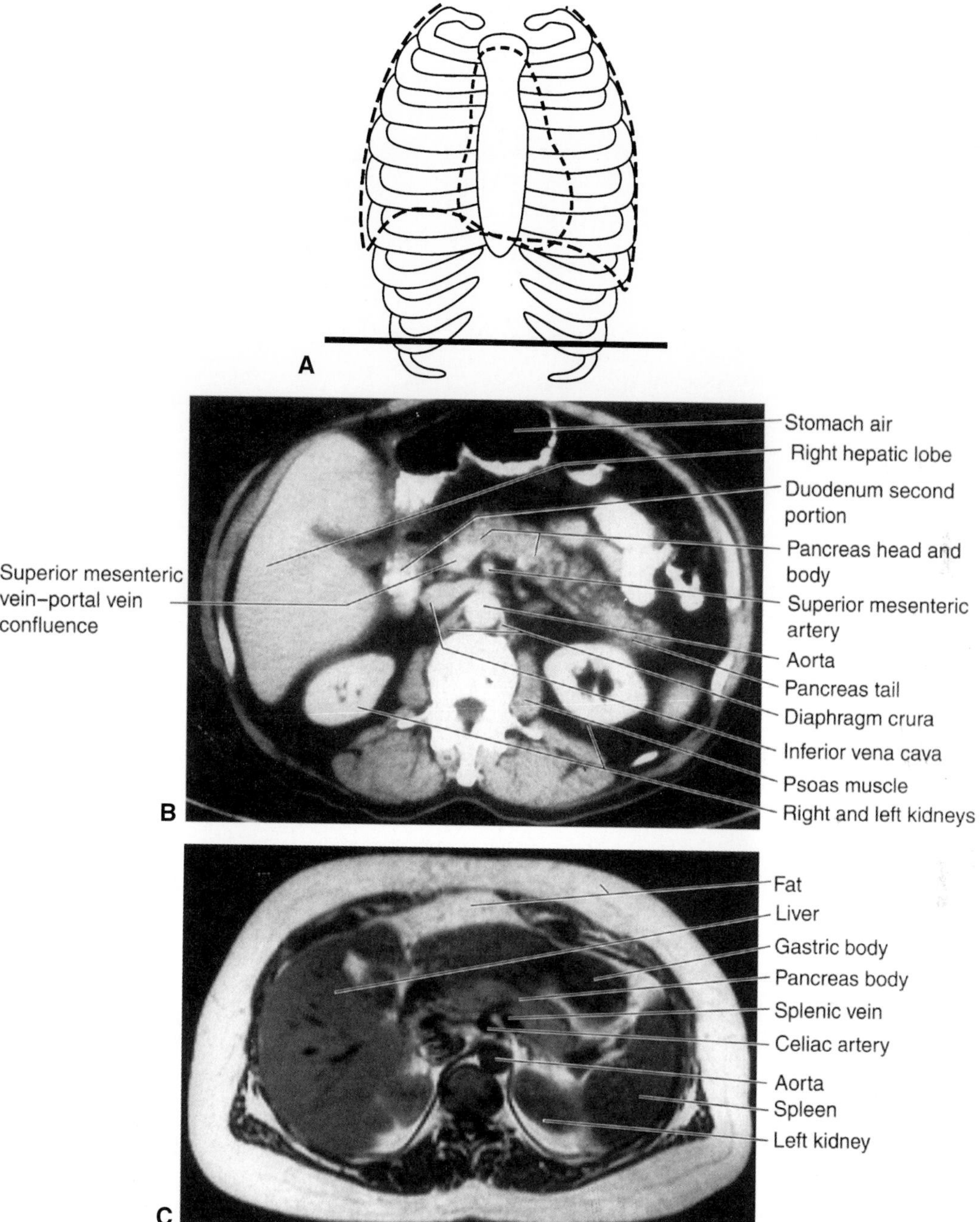

FIGURE 3-7. **CT and MRI Images at the Level of the Hilum of the Kidney and Pancreas. (A)** A schematic to show where the cross section was taken. **(B)** A normal abdominal axial CT image. **(C)** A normal abdominal axial MRI image.

Chapter 4

Histology

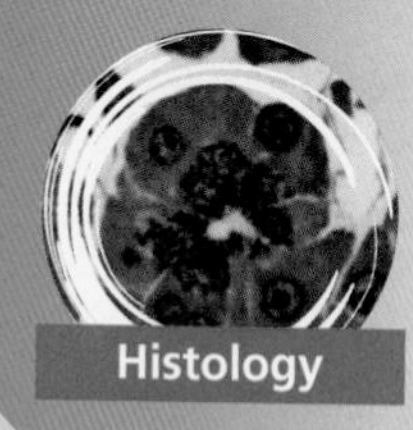

Esophagus (*Figure 4-1*)

I Mucosa

A. The mucosa consists of a **nonkeratinized stratified squamous epithelium** (except the distal 2 cm at the gastroesophageal (GE) junction that is lined by simple columnar epithelium), **lamina propria, and muscularis mucosae.**

B. Within the lamina propria, **mucosal glands (esophageal cardiac glands)** are found concentrated in the terminal portion of the esophagus near the GE junction. The esophageal cardiac glands secrete **neutral mucus** that protects the distal esophagus from damage due to gastric acid reflux.

II Submucosa

A. The submucosa along with the mucosa is thrown into a number of longitudinal folds. As a bolus of food passes down the esophagus, the longitudinal folds flatten, allowing dilation of the lumen to accommodate the food.

B. During endoscopy, inflation of the esophagus causes distention; so these longitudinal folds may not be appreciated.

C. The submucosa contains submucosal glands that are found throughout the esophagus but concentrated more in the proximal portion of the esophagus. The submucosal glands secrete acidic mucus that lubricates the lumen of the esophagus.

III Muscularis Externa

A. The **upper** 5% of the esophagus consists of skeletal muscle only.

B. The **middle** 45% of the esophagus consists of both skeletal muscle and smooth muscle interwoven together.

C. The **distal** 50% of the esophagus consists of smooth muscle only. In this area, the smooth muscle is organized into an **inner circular layer** and an **outer longitudinal layer.**

D. The esophagus has two sphincters as indicated below.
   1. The **upper esophageal sphincter** (UES) separates the pharynx from the esophagus. The UES is composed of **opening muscles**, specifically the **thyrohyoid muscle** and **geniohyoid muscle**. In addition, the UES is composed of **closing muscles**, specifically the **inferior pharyngeal constrictor muscle** and **cricopharyngeus muscle** (main player). The UES is **skeletal muscle**.
   2. The **lower esophageal sphincter** (LES) separates the esophagus from the stomach and **prevents GE reflux**, which is the reflux of acidic gastric contents into the esophagus (i.e., GE reflux disease [GERD]). The LES is composed of **smooth muscle** with the inner circular layer of smooth muscle being the major determinant of LES tone.

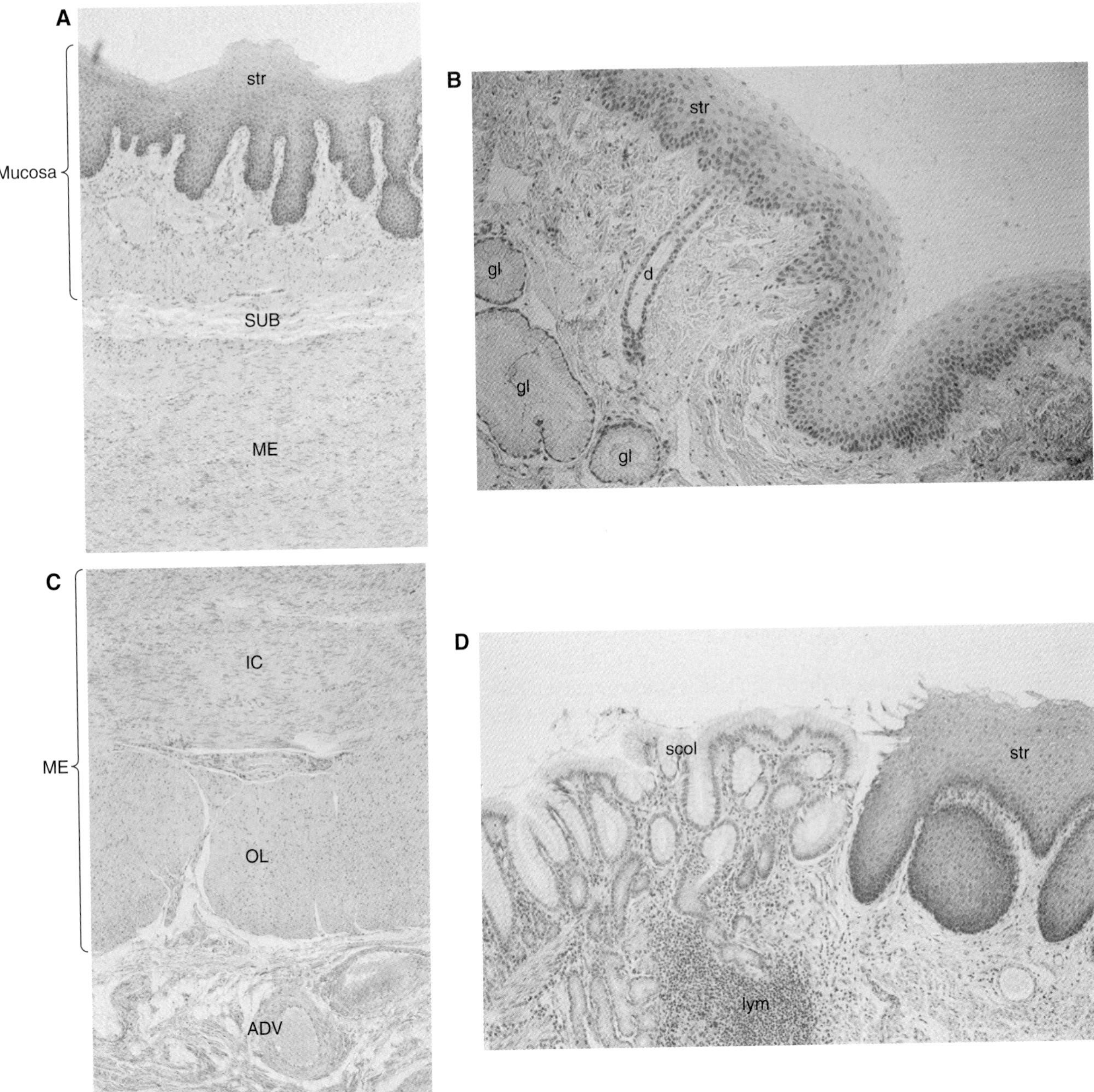

FIGURE 4-1. **Esophagus. (A)** A low power light micrograph shows the wall of the esophagus (sans adventitia). Note the mucosa with the nonkeratinized stratified squamous epithelium (str) lining the luminal surface of the esophagus, submucosa (SUB), and muscularis externa (ME). **(B)** Light micrograph shows submucosal glands (gl) and duct (d) which pierces the stratified squamous epithelium (str) and carries acidic mucus to the luminal surface of the esophagus. **(C)** Light micrograph shows muscularis externa (ME) with the inner circular (IC) layer and outer longitudinal (OL) layer of smooth muscle. Note also the adventitia (ADV). **(D) GE Junction.** The light micrograph shows junction where nonkeratinized stratified squamous epithelium (str) changes to simple columnar epithelium (scol). The simple columnar epithelium invaginates to form mucosal glands very similar to the cardiac glands found in the cardia region of the stomach. The mucosal lining of the cardiac region of the stomach extends about 2 cm into the esophagus such that the distal 2 cm of the esophagus is lined by a simple columnar epithelium. This junction can be seen macroscopically as a zigzag line (called the Z-line). Lymphatic infiltration (lym) is observed in the submucosa.

IV Adventitia

A. The adventitia consists of connective tissue that blends into the surrounding fascia of the head and neck region.

B. Short segments of the thoracic and abdominal esophagus may be associated with a serosa derived from the pleura or peritoneum.

V Gastroesophageal Junction

The histological GE junction does NOT correspond to the gross anatomical GE junction. The mucosal lining of the cardiac portion of the stomach **extends about 2 cm into the esophagus** such that the distal 2 cm of the esophagus is lined by a simple columnar epithelium. The junction where stratified squamous epithelium changes to simple columnar epithelium (or the mucosal GE junction) can be seen macroscopically as a **zigzag line** (called the **Z-line**). This distinction is clinically very important, especially when dealing with Barrett esophagus.

VI Clinical Considerations

A. **Barrett Esophagus.** Barrett esophagus can be defined as the replacement of esophageal stratified squamous epithelium with metaplastic "intestinalized" simple columnar epithelium with Goblet cells extending at least 3 cm into the esophagus. This metaplastic invasion is most commonly caused by GERD. The clinical importance of this metaplastic invasion is that virtually all lower esophageal adenocarcinomas occur as a sequela.

B. **Esophageal Strictures (Narrowing).** Caustic strictures are caused by ingestion of caustic agents (e.g., drain openers, oven cleaners, etc). Other strictures are caused by recurrent mucosal destruction due to gastric acid reflux. These strictures most often occur at the GE junction.

Stomach *(Figure 4-2)*

I Mucosa

The mucosa consists of a **simple columnar epithelium**, a **lamina propria**, and a **muscularis mucosae**. The epithelium of the gastric mucosa lines the lumen of the stomach and consists of **surface mucous cells** that secrete **mucus and HCO_3^-**. A surface mucous cell contains rough endoplasmic reticulum (rER), a well-developed Golgi, and numerous mucus-containing granules that are oriented toward the lumen of the stomach. The epithelium of the gastric mucosa also invaginates to form **mucosal glands**. The cellular composition of the mucosal glands changes (and therefore their function) depending on the gross area of the stomach considered.

A. **Cardia Region.** The cardia region is a 1 to 3 cm wide circular band located at the junction of the esophagus and stomach. In the cardia region, cardiac glands contain mucus-secreting cells. The cardiac glands probably aid in protecting the esophagus from the acidic chyme.

B. **Fundus and Body Regions.** In the fundus and body regions, gastric glands contain the following cells:

1. **Mucous neck cells.** Mucous neck cells are flower bouquet-shaped cells with basophilia located in the basal cytoplasm representing rER/polyribosomes, a well-developed Golgi, and mucous droplets (which appear as clear vacuoles because mucus dissolves in routine histological preparation) filling up the remainder of the cytoplasm. Mucous neck cells have a basally located nucleus. Mucous neck cells secrete mucus.
2. **Stem cells.** Stem cells are columnar-shaped cells with an oval, basally located nucleus. Stem cells demonstrate a high rate of mitosis. They migrate upward to replace surface mucous cells every 4 to 7 days and downward to replace other cell types.

3. **Parietal cells.** Parietal cells are triangular/round-shaped cells with an intense eosinophilic cytoplasm representing a large number of mitochondria, the canalicular membrane system (i.e., the intracellular canaliculi), and tubulovesicles. Parietal cells have a round, centrally located nucleus. Parietal cells secrete
   a. **HCl (gastric acid).** HCl is produced through the action of carbonic anhydrase, Cl^- ion channels located on the canalicular membrane system, and H^+–K^+ ATPases (H^+ pumps) located on the tubulovesicles. Because Cl^- is released by facilitated diffusion via Cl^- ion channels and H^+ is released by active transport via H^+–K^+ ATPases, the secretion product of parietal cells is HCl.
   b. **HCO_3^-.** HCO_3^- is secreted into the bloodstream causing a rise in the pH called the "alkaline tide."
   c. **Intrinsic factor.** Intrinsic factor is necessary for vitamin B_{12} absorption. Pernicious anemia may result from vitamin B_{12} deficiency caused by atrophic gastritis with decreased intrinsic factor production.
4. **Chief cells.** Chief cells are pyramidal-shaped cells with basophilia located in the basal cytoplasm representing the rER/polyribosomes, a well-developed Golgi, and eosinophilia located in the supranuclear cytoplasm representing secretory (zymogen) granules. Chief cells have a round, centrally located nucleus. Chief cells secrete
   a. **Pepsinogen.** Pepsinogen (inactive) is converted to pepsin (active) on contact with the acid pH of the gastric juice
   b. **Lipase.** Lipase cleaves fatty acids from triglycerides.
5. **Enteroendocrine cells.** Enteroendocrine cells are pyramidal-shaped cells with microvilli extending into the lumen of the gastric gland, basophilia located in the apical cytoplasm representing rER/polyribosomes, and secretory granules that are oriented toward blood vessels (i.e., away from the lumen of the gastric gland) that are typically lost during routine histological preparation so that the cytoplasm may appear clear. Enteroendocrine cells have a round, centrally located nucleus. Enteroendocrine cells include the following:
   a. **G cells.** G cells secrete gastrin (in response to a meal) that stimulates HCl secretion from the parietal cells. They are found predominately in the antrum of the stomach so that, in the case of ulcers, the antrum may be resected to reduce the amount of HCl secretion.
   b. **Enterochromaffinlike (ECL) cells.** ECL cells secrete serotonin which increases gut motility and histamine which stimulates HCl secretion.
   c. **D cells.** D cells secrete somatostatin which inhibits secretion of nearby enteroendocrine cells.

C. **Pyloric Antrum Region.** In the pyloric antrum region, pyloric glands contain mucus-secreting cells and G cells. The pyloric glands probably aid in protecting the duodenum from the acidic chyme.

II Submucosa

The submucosa along with the mucosa is thrown into a number of longitudinal folds called **rugae**.

III Muscularis Externa

The muscularis externa consists of **randomly arranged smooth muscle**. Some authors describe circular, longitudinal, and oblique layers of smooth muscle. The muscularis externa is thin in the orad region but much thicker in the caudad region.

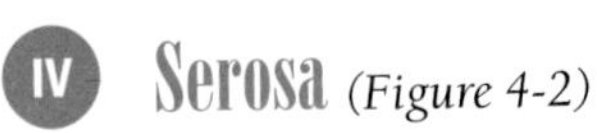

IV Serosa *(Figure 4-2)*

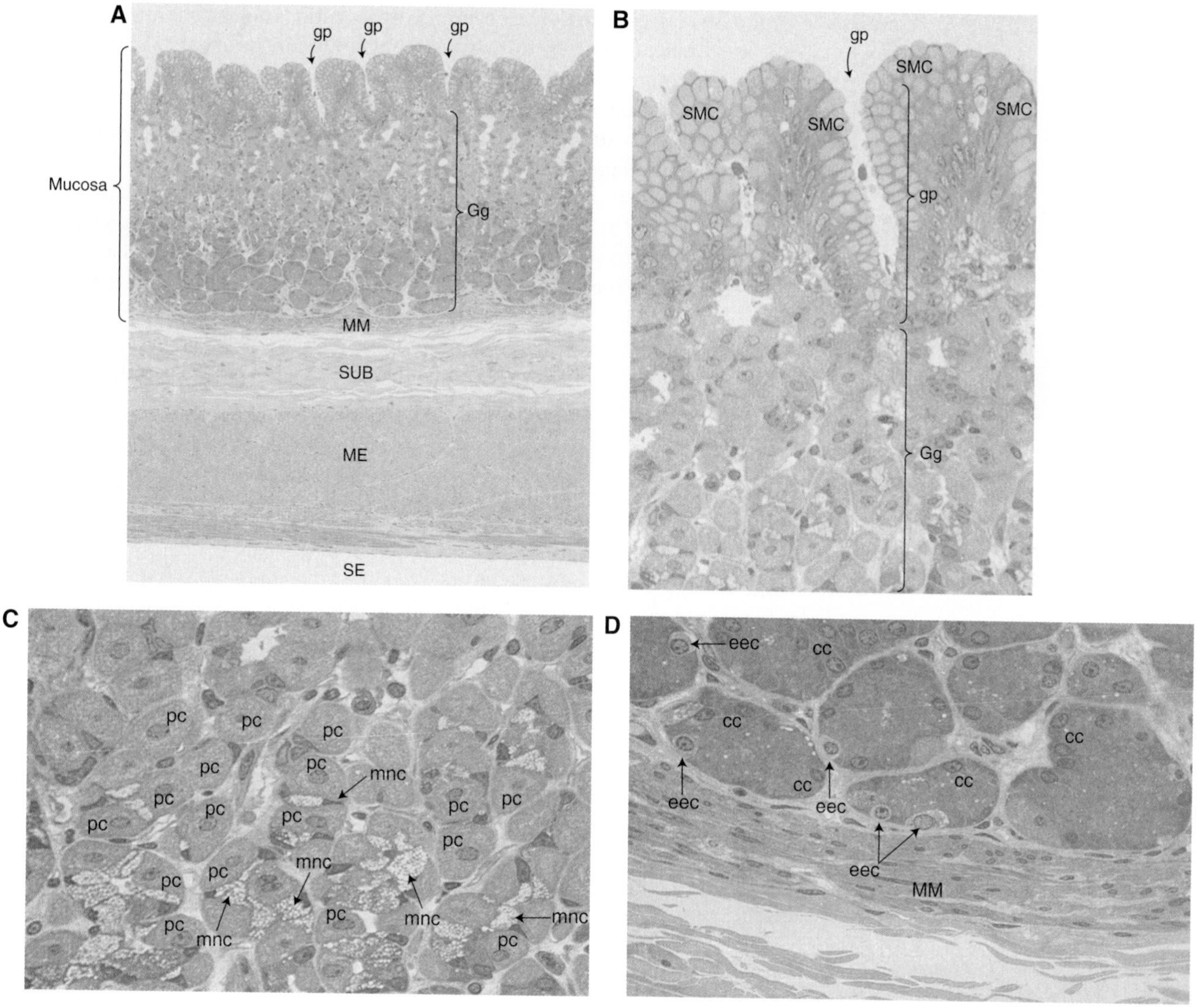

FIGURE 4-2. **Light Microscopy of the Stomach. (A)** A low power light micrograph shows the entire stomach wall from the fundus or body region. Note the mucosa containing the gastric glands (Gg) and the openings of the gastric pits (gp) onto the luminal surface of the stomach. **(B)** Light micrograph shows an opening of a gp onto the luminal surface of the stomach along with numerous surface mucous cells (smc) that line the luminal surface of the stomach. **(C)** Light micrograph shows a portion of a gastric gland that contains numerous parietal cells (pc) and mucous neck cells (mnc). **(D)** Light micrograph shows the lower portion of a gastric gland that contains numerous chief cells (cc) and enteroendocrine cells (eec). MM — muscularis mucosa; SUB — submucosa; ME — muscularis externa; SE — serosa.

Small Intestine *(Figure 4-3)*

Mucosa

The mucosa consists of **simple columnar epithelium**, a **lamina propria**, and a **muscularis mucosa**. The epithelium of the small intestinal mucosa covers the villi and consists of **enterocytes (surface absorptive cells)**, **Goblet cells**, and **M cells**. Enterocytes are joined by juxtaluminal **junctional complexes (i.e., zonula occludens** or **tight junction and zonula adherens)** and possess **microvilli** that are coated by filamentous glycoproteins called the **glycocalyx.** The glycocalyx contains important enzymes that include **maltase**, **α-dextrinase**, **sucrase**, **lactase**, **trehalase**, **aminopeptidases**, and **enterokinase.** Enterocytes absorb carbohydrates, protein, lipids, vitamins, Ca^{2+}, and Fe^{2+} from the intestinal lumen and transport them to the blood or lymph. **Goblet cells** secrete glycoproteins called

mucins (i.e., mucus). **M cells** are antigen-transporting cells. The epithelium of the small intestinal mucosa also invaginates to form **intestinal glands (or the crypts of Lieberkühn).** The cellular composition of the intestinal glands includes the following:

A. **Stem Cells.** Stem cells demonstrate a high rate of mitosis and migrate upward to replace enterocytes and goblet cells every 3 to 6 days.

B. **Paneth Cells** are found at the base of the intestinal glands and secrete the following:
   1. Lysozyme is a proteolytic enzyme that degrades the peptidoglycan coat of bacteria, thereby increasing membrane permeability of bacteria so that they swell and rupture.
   2. Tumor necrosis factor-α (TNF-α) is a proinflammatory substance.
   3. Defensin (cryptidin) increases the membrane permeability of bacteria and other parasites by formation of ion channels.

C. **Enteroendocrine Cells**
   1. I cells secrete cholecystokinin (CCK) in response to small peptides, amino acids, and fatty acids within the gut lumen. CCK stimulates enzyme secretion from pancreatic acinar cells, stimulates release of bile from the gall bladder (by contraction of gall bladder smooth muscle and relaxation of the sphincter of Oddi), decreases HCl secretion and gastric emptying, and increases pepsinogen secretion from the stomach.
   2. S cells secrete secretin (SEC) (called nature's antacid) in response to H^+ and fatty acids within the gut lumen. SEC stimulates release of HCO_3^- from the pancreas and the liver biliary tract.
   3. K cells secrete gastric-inhibitory peptide (GIP) in response to orally administered glucose, amino acids, and fatty acids in the gut lumen. GIP stimulates insulin secretion from pancreatic islets. This explains why an oral glucose load produces higher serum insulin levels than an IV glucose load.
   4. L cells secrete glucagonlike peptide-1 (GLP-1) in response to orally administered glucose, amino acids, and fatty acids in the gut lumen. GLP-1 stimulates insulin secretion in the presence of hyperglycemia and inhibits postprandial glucagon secretion from pancreatic islets. GLP-1 may be an effective therapeutic agent for Type 2 diabetes since the stimulatory effect of GLP-1 on insulin secretion is preserved in Type 2 diabetic patients.
   5. Mo cells secrete motilin.

II Submucosa

The submucosa consists of connective tissue containing blood vessels, nerves, and the submucosal plexus of Meissner.

III Muscularis Externa

The muscularis externa consists of an inner circular and outer longitudinal layer of smooth muscle and the myenteric plexus of Auerbach.

IV Serosa

The serosa consists of connective tissue covered by mesothelium of the peritoneum.

V Gut-Associated Lymphatic Tissue (Peyer Patches)

Gut-associated lymphatic tissue (GALT) are lymphatic follicles found in the intestinal mucosa and submucosa that are covered by an epithelial lining containing **M cells.** M cells are **antigen-transporting cells** that have **microfolds** on their luminal surface.

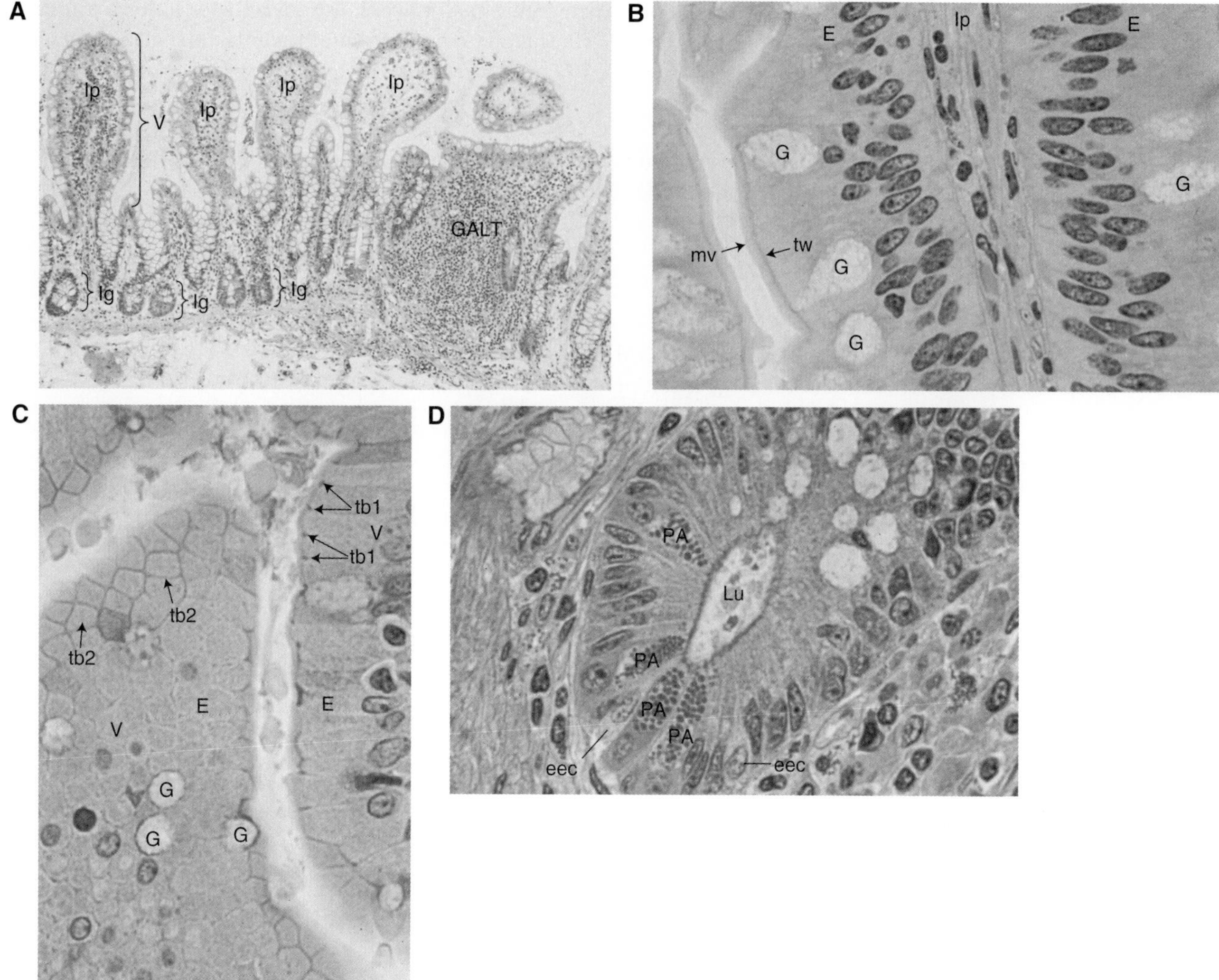

FIGURE 4-3. Light Microscopy of the Small Intestine. (A) A low power light micrograph shows villi (V) of the small intestine along with the intestinal glands (lg) or crypts of Lieberkühn. The core of all villi contains connective tissue called the lamina propria (lp). In addition, GALT can be observed. **(B)** Light micrograph shows a portion of a villus with lamina propria (lp) in its core that is lined by enterocytes (E) with a microvillus (mv) border and goblet cells (G). In addition, the thin, conspicuous, eosinophilic line represents the terminal web (tw) of the enterocytes. **(C)** Light micrograph shows a portion of two villi (V) lined by enterocytes (E) and goblet cells (G). The enterocytes are joined by junctional complexes (i.e., zonula occludens or tight junctions and zonula adherens) that extend around the entire perimeter of the enterocyte. Depending on the way these junctional complexes are cut, they may appear as eosinophilic bars called terminal bars (tb1) or as a eosinophilic spider-web pattern (tb2). **(D)** Light micrograph shows the lower portion of an intestinal gland with its lumen (Lu) that is lined by Paneth cells (PA) and enteroendocrine cells (eec). GALT — gut-associated lymphatic tissue.

Large Intestine *(Figure 4-4)*

I Mucosa

The mucosa consists of a **simple columnar epithelium**, a **lamina propria**, and a **muscularis mucosa**. The epithelium of the large intestinal mucosa consists of **enterocytes (surface absorptive cells)** and **Goblet cells.** Enterocytes absorb Na^+, Cl^-, and H_2O by facilitated diffusion using ion channels under the regulation of aldosterone. Aldosterone increases the number of Na^+ ion channels, thereby increasing the amount of Na^+ absorbed. Sedatives, anesthetics, and steroids are also absorbed, which is clinically important when medication cannot be delivered orally. Goblet cells secrete glycoproteins called **mucins** (i.e., mucus). The epithelium of the large intestinal mucosa also invaginates to form intestinal glands (crypts of Lieberkühn). The cellular composition of the intestinal glands includes the following:

A. Stem cells
B. Enterocytes
C. Goblet cells
D. Enteroendocrine cells

 Submucosa

The submucosa consists of connective tissue containing blood vessels, nerves, and submucosal plexus of Meissner. GALT is prominent within the submucosa (and lamina propria) throughout the large intestine.

 Muscularis Externa

The muscularis externa consists of an inner circular and three outer longitudinal bands of smooth muscle (called **teniae coli**) and the myenteric plexus of Auerbach. The contractions of the teniae coli form sacculations called **haustra**.

 Serosa

The serosa consists of connective tissue covered by mesothelium of the peritoneum. The serosa is distinguished by the presence of fatty tags called **appendices epiploicae**.

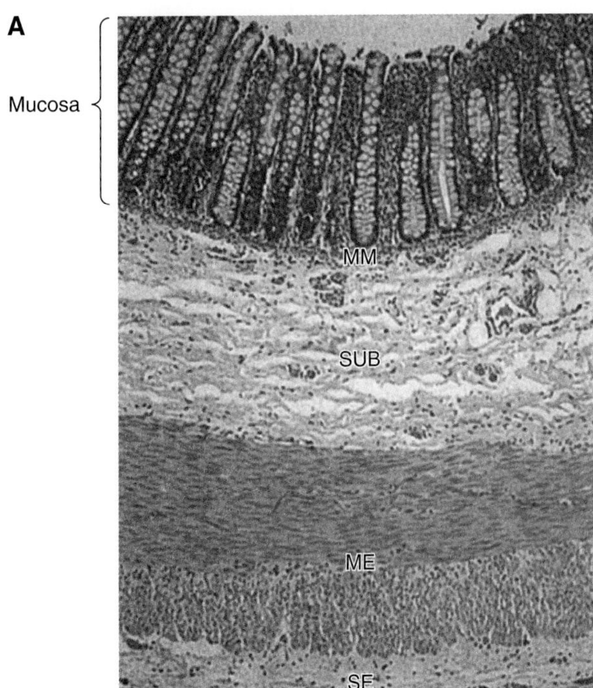

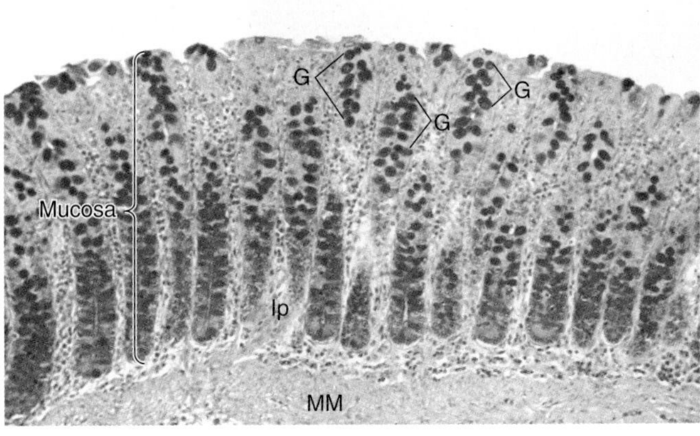

FIGURE 4-4. **Light Microscopy of the Large Intestine. (A)** A low power light micrograph shows the entire wall of the large intestine including the mucosa, submucosa (SUB), muscularis externa (ME), and serosa (SE). This tissue was routinely prepared so that the mucus is dissolved and the goblet cell cytoplasm appears clear. **(B)** Light micrograph shows mucosa of the large intestine including the intestinal glands (crypts of Lieberkühn) of the large intestine, lamina propria (lp), and muscularis mucosa (MM). Note the large number of goblet cells (G) lining the intestinal glands. This tissue was specially prepared so as to preserve the mucus within the goblet cells which generally dissolves in routine histological preparation. MM — muscularis mucosa.

Appendix *(Figure 4-5)*

Mucosa

The mucosa consists of a **simple columnar epithelium**, a **lamina propria**, and a **muscularis mucosa** (poorly developed and focally absent). The epithelium of the large intestinal mucosa consists of **enterocytes (surface absorptive cells)** and **Goblet cells.** Goblet cells secrete glycoproteins called **mucins** (i.e., mucus). GALT is prominent within the mucosa. The epithelium of the large intestinal mucosa also invaginates to form intestinal glands (crypts of Lieberkühn). The cellular composition of the intestinal glands includes the following:

A. Stem cells
B. Enterocytes
C. Goblet cells
D. Enteroendocrine cells

Submucosa

The submucosa consists of connective tissue containing blood vessels, nerves, and submucosal plexus of Meissner. GALT is also prominent within the submucosa.

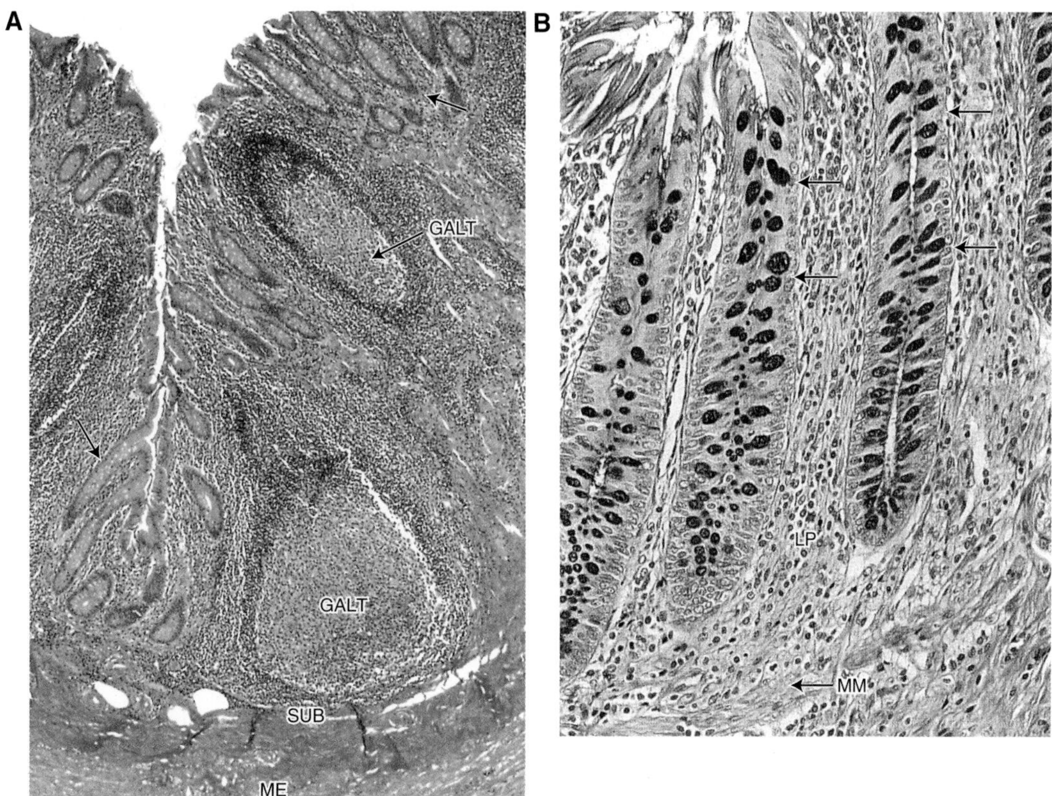

FIGURE 4-5. **Light Microscopy of the Appendix. (A)** This low power light micrograph shows the simple columnar epithelium which invaginates to form intestinal glands or crypts of Lieberkühn (arrows), lamina propria, and a poorly developed muscularis mucosa. GALT is present within the lamina propria and may extend into the submucosa (SUB). **(B)** This light micrograph shows the mucosa of the appendix consisting of simple columnar epithelium which invaginates to form intestinal glands or crypts of Lieberkühn, lamina propria (LP), and a poorly developed muscularis mucosa (MM). The crypts of Lieberkühn contain numerous goblet cells (arrows) which stain dark with this particular histological staining technique. ME — muscularis externa; GALT — gut-associated lymphatic tissue.

III Muscularis Externa

The muscularis externa consists of an inner circular layer and outer longitudinal layer of smooth muscle and the myenteric plexus of Auerbach.

IV Serosa

The serosa consists of connective tissue covered by mesothelium of the peritoneum.

Anal Canal *(Figure 4-6)*

The anal canal is divided into the upper and lower anal canals by the **pectinate line**.

I Upper Anal Canal

The upper anal canal extends from the anorectal junction (perineal flexure) to the pectinate line. The mucosa is thrown into longitudinal folds called the anal columns (or columns of Morgagni). The base of the anal columns defines the pectinate line. At the base of the anal columns are transverse folds of mucosa called the anal valves. Behind the anal valves are small, blind pouches called the anal sinuses into which mucous anal glands open.

A. **Colorectal Zone.** The upper anal canal is lined by a typical simple columnar epithelium (colonic epithelium) and intestinal glands called the colorectal zone.

B. **Transitional Zone.** The colonic epithelium undergoes a transition to a nonkeratinized stratified squamous epithelium at the pectinate line called the transitional zone where both colonic epithelium and nonkeratinized stratified squamous epithelium can be observed.

II Lower Anal Canal

The lower anal canal extends from the pectinate line to the anal verge. The lower anal canal is lined by a nonkeratinized stratified squamous epithelium called the squamous zone.

III Anal Verge

Anal verge is the point where the perianal skin begins and is lined by a keratinized stratified squamous epithelium.

Liver *(Figures 4-7 and 4-8)*

I General Features

The liver is the largest internal gland in the body. The functions of the liver are highly numerous and varied all of which primarily depend on the activity of hepatocytes. The **liver parenchyma** consists of radially arranged plates of **hepatocytes**. Hepatocytes contain the Golgi complex, rER, smooth endoplasmic reticulum (sER), mitochondria, lysosomes, peroxisomes, lipid, and glycogen. The **liver stroma** consists of **reticular fibers (Type III collagen)**. The stroma begins as a thin connective tissue capsule called **Glisson capsule** that extends into the liver around the portal triads, around the periphery of hepatic lobules, extends into the perisinusoidal space of Disse to surround hepatocytes, and then terminates around the central vein.

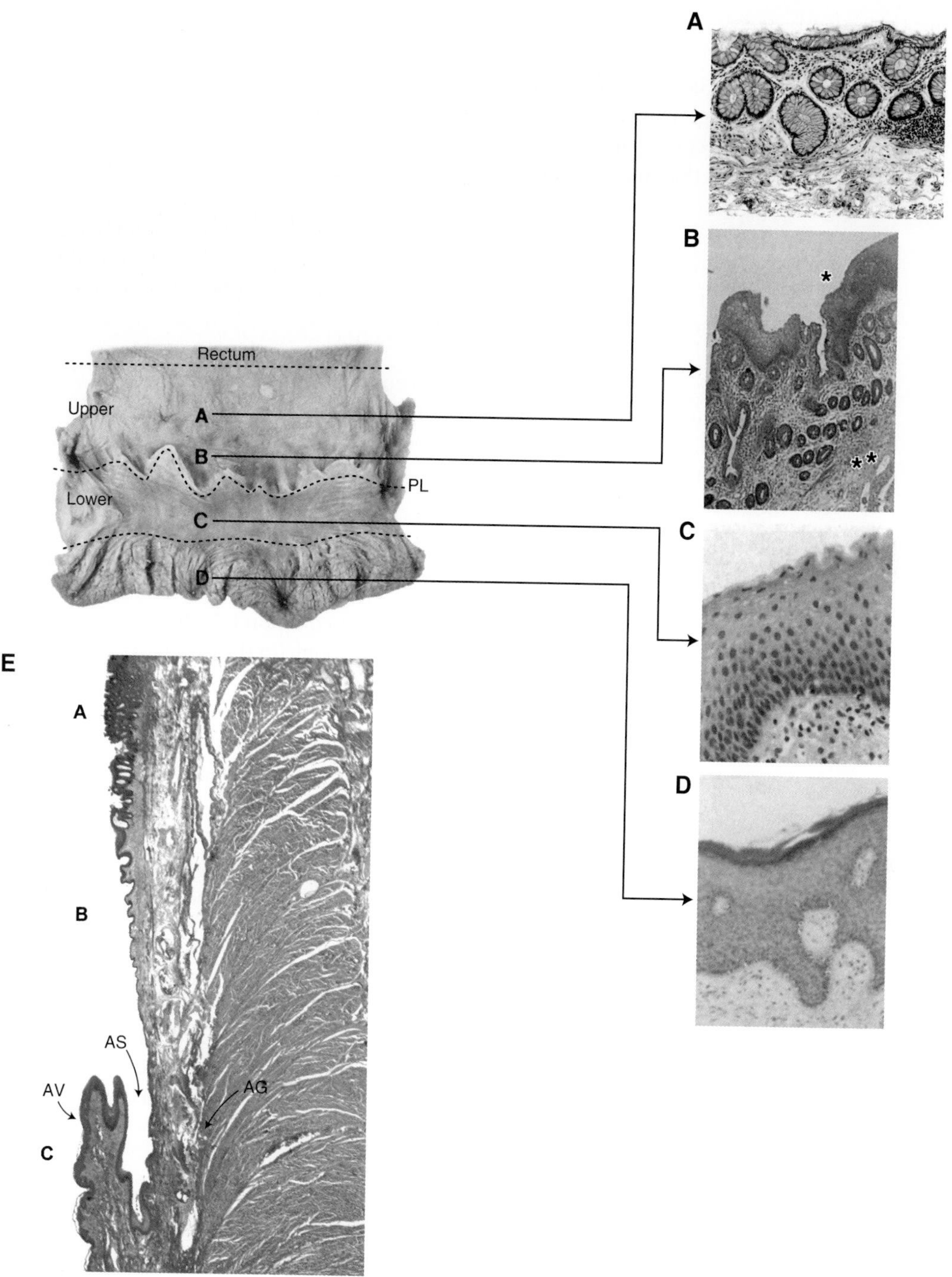

FIGURE 4-6. **The Anal Canal. (A–D) Photograph of a Human Surgical Specimen of the Rectum, Anal Canal (A–C), and Anal Verge (D).** A — colorectal zone; B — transitional zone; C — squamous zone; D — anal verge; PL — pectinate line. **(A)** Light micrograph shows the colorectal zone lined by simple columnar epithelium (colonic epithelium) and intestinal glands. **(B)** Light micrograph shows the transitional zone lined by both a simple columnar epithelium (**) and a nonkeratinized stratified squamous epithelium (*). **(C)** Light micrograph shows the squamous zone lined by a nonkeratinized stratified squamous epithelium. **(D)** Light micrograph shows the anal verge lined by keratinized stratified squamous epithelium. **(E)** Light micrograph of a longitudinal section of the anal canal shows the colorectal zone (A), transitional zone (B), and squamous zone (C). In addition, note the anal valves (AV) and the anal sinus (AS) into which mucous anal glands (AG) open.

Gross anatomically, one can identify, at the **porta hepatis**, components of the (a) common bile duct, (b) portal vein, (c) hepatic artery, and (d) lymphatics. The hepatic bile duct, portal vein, and hepatic artery are referred to as the **portal triad** (the lymphatics are forgotten about in this designation). Histologically, branches of the same components can be found within the substance of the liver as they help define a **classic hepatic lobule**.

II Classic Hepatic Lobule

This is the traditional description of the liver. The classic hepatic lobule consists of a **hexagon-shaped** block of tissue with a **central vein** at its center and **six portal triads** at each corner of the hexagon. The parenchyma is arranged radially as the plates of hepatocytes that are separated by sinusoids. A portal triad consists of the following:

A. **Hepatic Arteriole.** The hepatic arterioles (terminal branches of the right and left hepatic arteries) carry oxygen-rich blood and contribute 20% of the blood within the liver sinusoids. The blood flows from the periphery to the center of the lobule (i.e., centripetal flow).

B. **Portal Venule.** The portal venules (terminal branches of the portal vein) carry nutrient-rich blood and contribute 80% of the blood within the liver sinusoids. The blood flows from the periphery to the center of the lobule (i.e., centripetal flow).

C. **Bile Ductule**
   1. Bile follows this route: bile canaliculi → cholangioles → canals of Hering → bile ductules in the portal triad → right and left hepatic ducts → common hepatic duct → gall bladder and cystic duct → common bile duct.
   2. Bile flows from the center of the lobule to the periphery (i.e., centrifugal flow).

D. **Lymphatic Vessel**
   1. Lymph follows this route: space of Disse → lymphatic vessels in the portal triad → lymphatic vessels that parallel the portal vein → thoracic duct.
   2. Lymph flows from the center of the lobule to the periphery of a liver lobule (i.e., centrifugal flow).

III Liver Acinus

The concept of the liver acinus was introduced to correlate blood flow through the liver sinusoids and parenchyma with hepatocyte metabolic activity and pathology. The liver acinus consists of a **diamond-shaped** block of tissue whose **long axis** is defined by a line drawn between two central veins and whose **short axis** is defined by terminal branches of portal venules and hepatic arterioles. This arrangement creates three zones of hepatocytes (i.e., Zone 1, Zone 2, Zone 3) whose functions are listed in *Table 4-1*.

A. **Zone 1.** Hepatocytes in Zone 1 receive nutrient-rich blood (glucose, galactose, fructose, amino acids, short- and medium-chain fatty acids, glycerol), $\uparrow O_2$, and ↑toxins. Hepatocytes in Zone 1 are the first to undergo necrosis in bile duct occlusion (bile stasis).

B. **Zone 2.** An intermediate zone.

C. **Zone 3.** Hepatocytes in Zone 3 receive nutrient-poor blood, $\downarrow O_2$, and ↓toxins. Hepatocytes in Zone 3 are the first to undergo necrosis in an ischemic injury (called ischemic centrilobular necrosis) or right-sided cardiac failure.

IV Portal Lobule

The concept of the portal lobule emphasizes the bile secretion function of the liver in terms comparable to other exocrine glands. The portal lobule consists of a **triangle-shaped** block of tissue with a portal triad at its center and three central veins at each corner of the triangle.

TABLE 4-1 CHARACTERISTICS OF HEPATOCYTES IN THE ZONES OF THE LIVER

Zones	Characteristics of Hepatocytes
1	**Are exposed to nutrient-rich blood, ↑O_2, and ↑toxins**
	In the fed-state:
	Glycogen deposits appear first in Zone 1
	Bile most concentrated in Zone 1
	TCA Cycle activity highest in Zone 1
	Undergo necrosis due to: **bile duct occlusion**, primary biliary cirrhosis, chronic hepatitis, and pre-eclampsia/eclampsia (Note: Hepatic disease is very common in pre-eclamptic women and monitoring of platelet count and serum liver enzymes is standard practice.
	Undergo necrosis in poisoning due to: phosphorus, manganese, ferrous sulphate, allyl alcohol, and endotoxin of *Proteus vulgaris*
	Zone 1 hepatocytes have more rER and therefore are involved in protein synthesis
2	Are exposed to blood intermediate in nutrients, oxygen, and toxins
	Undergo necrosis due to yellow fever
3	**Are exposed to nutrient-poor blood, ↓O_2, and ↓toxins**
	In the fed-state:
	Hexose shunt activity highest in Zone 3
	Peroxisome activity highest in Zone 3
	Undergo necrosis due to: **ischemic injury** and **right-sided cardiac failure**
	Undergo necrosis in poisoning due to: carbon tetrachloride, chloroform, L-amanitine, pyrrolizidine alkaloids (bush tea), tannic acid, and copper
	Zone 3 hepatocytes have more sER and therefore are involved in drug/alcohol/toxin catabolism

V The Sinusoidal Domain of the Hepatocyte

When two hepatocytes abut one another, the cell membranes (or surfaces) form a bile canaliculus sealed by a zonula occludens ("tight junction") and that domain of the hepatocytes becomes specialized for bile production. The other surfaces of the hepatocyte interface with a hepatic sinusoid (blood) and that domain (sinusoidal domain) interacts with the blood.

A. **The Perisinusoidal Space (or Space of Disse).** The space of Disse lies between the hepatocyte and the sinusoidal endothelium. Numerous microvilli from the hepatocyte surface extend into the space of Disse, which is a site of exchange between the blood and the hepatocytes. Type III collagen (reticular fibers) of the stroma is found in the space of Disse. Hepatic stellate cells (fat-storing cells; Ito cells) are found in the space of Disse and play a role in liver inflammation. These cells contain fat, store and metabolize vitamin A, and secrete Type I collagen (during inflammation; cirrhosis). In liver cirrhosis, increased deposition of Type I collagen (along with laminin and proteoglycans) in the perisinusoidal space narrows the diameter of the sinusoid causing portal hypertension.

B. **Hepatic Sinusoids.** The hepatic sinusoids are **discontinuous capillaries** that consist of a single layer of endothelial cells joined by a fascia occludens creating wide gaps between cells and contain fenestrae. They are surrounded by a discontinuous basal lamina.

C. **Within the Sinusoid.** **Kupffer cells** are **macrophages** derived from circulating monocytes that are found in the hepatic sinusoids. These cells secrete proinflammatory cytokines: **TNF-α** (causes a slowdown in bile flow called cholestasis), **interleukin-6** (causes synthesis of acute phase proteins by hepatocytes), and **TGF-β** (causes synthesis of Type I collagen by hepatic stellate cells). Kupffer cells may also phagocytize damaged or senile RBCs missed by splenic macrophages.

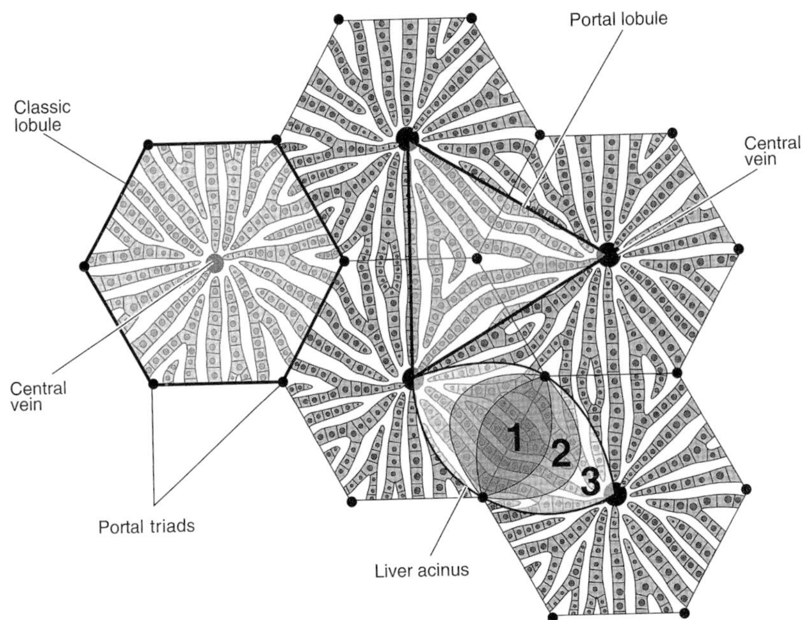

FIGURE 4-7. **Liver Architecture.** Diagram of a classic liver lobule, liver acinus, and portal lobule. The classic liver lobule (hexagon shaped) contains a central vein at its center with six portal triads at the periphery. The liver acinus (diamond shaped) defines three zones (Zones 1, 2, and 3) on the basis of the location of hepatocytes to incoming blood. Hepatocytes in Zone 1 are nearest to the incoming blood, hepatocytes in Zone 2 are intermediate, and hepatocytes in Zone 3 are the farthest from the incoming blood. The portal lobule (triangle shaped) consists of a triangle-shaped block of tissue with a portal triad at its center and three central veins at each corner of the triangle.

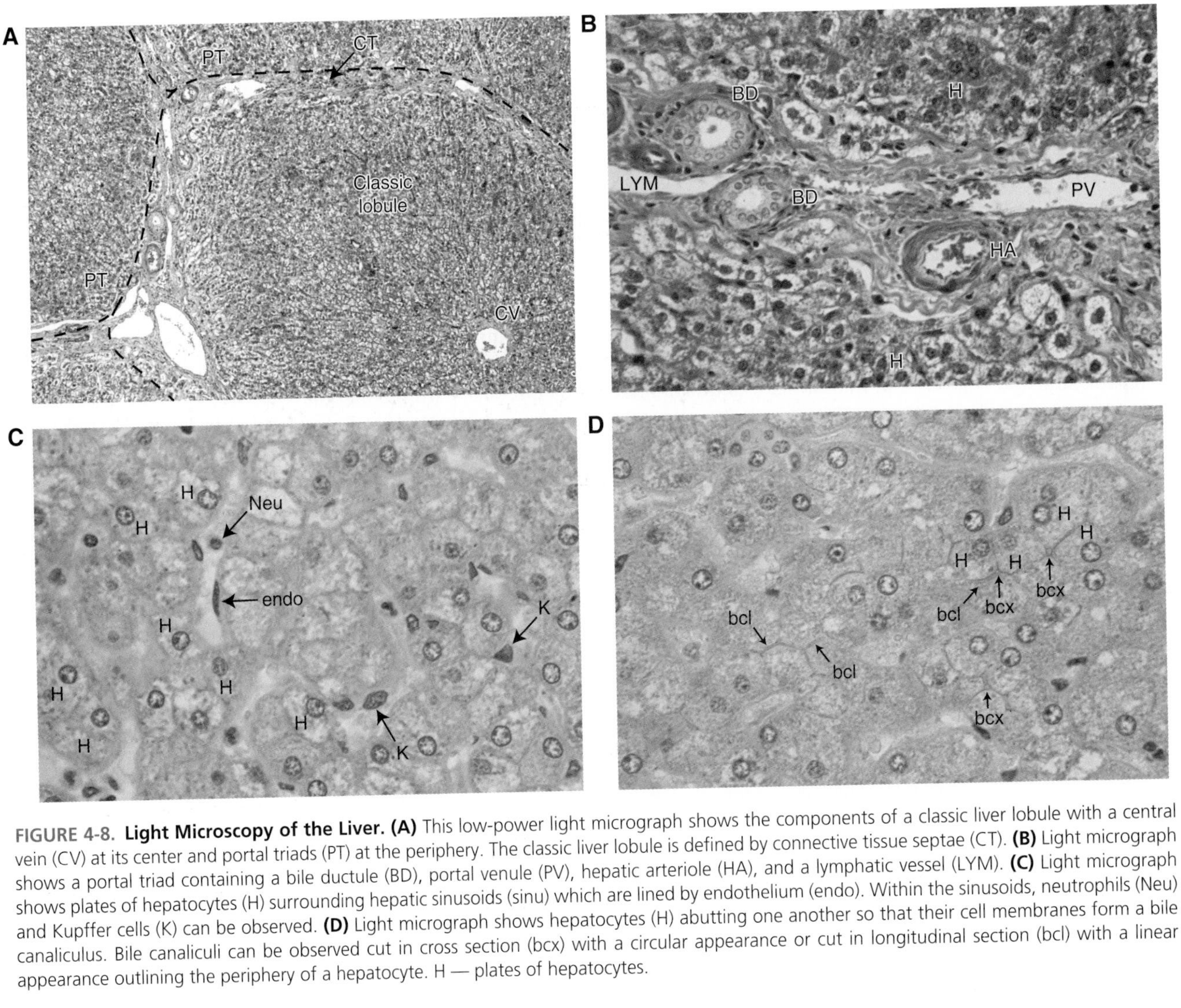

FIGURE 4-8. **Light Microscopy of the Liver. (A)** This low-power light micrograph shows the components of a classic liver lobule with a central vein (CV) at its center and portal triads (PT) at the periphery. The classic liver lobule is defined by connective tissue septae (CT). **(B)** Light micrograph shows a portal triad containing a bile ductule (BD), portal venule (PV), hepatic arteriole (HA), and a lymphatic vessel (LYM). **(C)** Light micrograph shows plates of hepatocytes (H) surrounding hepatic sinusoids (sinu) which are lined by endothelium (endo). Within the sinusoids, neutrophils (Neu) and Kupffer cells (K) can be observed. **(D)** Light micrograph shows hepatocytes (H) abutting one another so that their cell membranes form a bile canaliculus. Bile canaliculi can be observed cut in cross section (bcx) with a circular appearance or cut in longitudinal section (bcl) with a linear appearance outlining the periphery of a hepatocyte. H — plates of hepatocytes.

Gall Bladder and Biliary Ducts *(Figure 4-9)*

I Gall Bladder

A. **Mucosa.** The mucosa consists of a **simple tall columnar epithelium** and a **lamina propria** (the muscularis mucosa is absent). The epithelium of the gall bladder is joined by juxtaluminal **junctional complexes (i.e., zonula occludens** or **tight junction and zonula adherens)**, possesses numerous short **microvilli**, and has complex **lateral interdigitations**. The simple columnar epithelium **concentrates bile ≈10-fold** through the absorption of H_2O and electrolytes and **secretes mucus** that is added to the bile (called "white bile"). Numerous mucosal folds project into the lumen of the gall bladder and flatten out as the gall bladder is distended by bile. The mucosa may penetrate deep into the muscularis externa to form **Rokitansky-Aschoff sinuses**, which are early signs of pathological changes within the mucosa.

B. **Submucosa.** The submucosa is absent in the gall bladder.

C. **Muscularis Externa.** The muscularis externa consists of randomly arranged smooth muscle cells.

D. **Adventitia or Serosa.** The adventitia consists of a thick layer of connective tissue found in the area where the gall bladder attaches to the liver surface. The serosa consists of a thick layer of connective tissue covered by mesothelium of the peritoneum found in the area that is not attached to the liver surface.

II Biliary Ducts

A. **Bile Canaliculus.** A bile canaliculus is lined by hepatocytes. When two hepatocytes abut one another, the cell membranes (or surfaces) form a bile canaliculus sealed by a zonula occludens ("tight junction"). Microvilli of the hepatocytes extend into the lumen of the bile canaliculus.

B. **Cholangiole.** A cholangiole is lined by simple cuboidal epithelium.

C. **Canal of Hering.** A canal of Hering is lined by simple cuboidal epithelium.

D. **Bile Ductules in the Portal Triad.** The bile ductules in the portal triad are lined by simple cuboidal epithelium.

E. **Right and Left Hepatic Ducts.** The right and left hepatic ducts are lined by simple columnar epithelium. In addition, these larger ducts acquire a wall consisting of connective tissue and some smooth muscle cells.

F. **Common Hepatic Duct, Cystic Duct, and Common Bile Duct**
   1. **Mucosa.** The mucosa consists of a simple tall columnar epithelium and a lamina propria (the muscularis mucosa is absent). The mucosa of the cystic duct is arranged in a spiral fold with a core of smooth muscle known as the spiral valve (valve of Heister) that keeps the cystic duct open constantly so that bile can flow freely in either direction.
   2. **Submucosa.** The submucosa is absent.
   3. **Muscularis externa.** The muscularis externa consists of randomly arranged smooth muscle cells that thicken near the duodenum as the sphincter of Oddi forms.
   4. **Adventitia.** The adventitia consists of connective tissue.

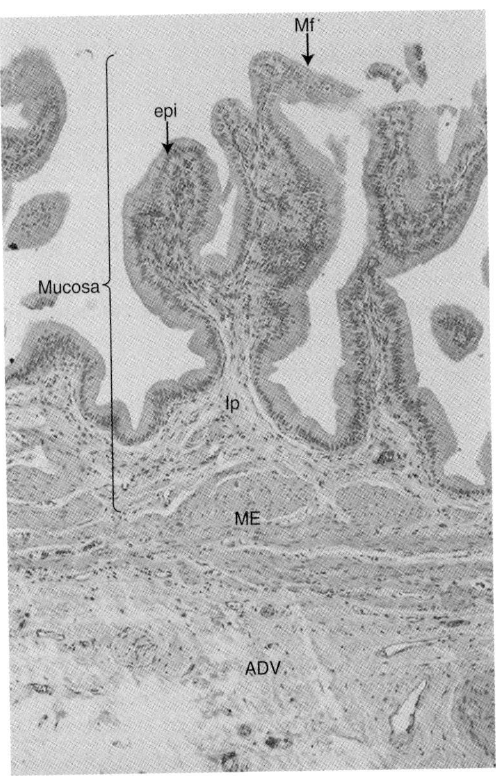

FIGURE 4-9. **Light Microscopy of the Gall Bladder and Biliary Ducts.** This low power light micrograph shows the mucosa of the gall bladder which consists of simple tall columnar epithelium (epi) and the connective tissue of the lamina propria (lp). In addition, the smooth muscle cells of the muscularis externa (ME) and the connective tissue of the adventitia (ADV) are shown. Note the numerous mucosal folds (Mf) that project in the lumen.

Pancreas *(Figure 4-10)*

The pancreas is both an exocrine gland and an endocrine gland.

I Exocrine Pancreas

A. The exocrine pancreas is a compound tubuloacinar gland, which contains pancreatic (secretory) acini and a network of ducts.

B. The functional unit of the exocrine pancreas is the pancreatic **acinus**.
   1. A pancreatic acinus consists of **acinar cells** that contain rER, Golgi, and zymogen granules.
   2. Acinar cells secrete digestive enzymes that include **trypsinogen, chymotrypsinogen, procarboxypeptidase, lipase, amylase, elastase, ribonuclease, deoxyribonuclease, cholesterol esterase**, and **phospholipase**.
   3. The secretion of digestive enzymes is stimulated by CCK released by I cells of the small intestine.

C. The exocrine pancreas also contains a **network of ducts**.
   1. The network of ducts consists of centroacinar cells of the intercalated duct → intralobular duct → interlobular duct → main pancreatic duct (duct of Wirsung) → joins the common bile duct at the hepatoduodenal ampulla (ampulla of Vater) → duodenum.
   2. The duct network delivers digestive enzymes to the duodenum and secretes HCO_3^-.
   3. Secretion of HCO_3^- by the intercalated and intralobular ducts is stimulated by SEC released by S cells of the small intestine.

II Endocrine Pancreas

A. The endocrine pancreas constitutes only 2% of the entire pancreas and consists of the **islets of Langerhans** that are scattered throughout the pancreas. The islets of Langerhans consist mainly of the following cell types:

1. **Alpha (α) Cells** (20% of the islet) secrete **glucagon** (29 amino acids; 3.5 kDa) in response to hypoglycemia which will elevate blood glucose, free fatty acid, and ketone levels. Glucagon binds to the **glucagon receptor** which is a **G-protein linked receptor** present on hepatocytes and adipocytes. About 30% to 40% of glucagon within the blood is derived from α cells; the remainder is derived from cells within the gastrointestinal tract called **enteroglucagon.**
2. **Beta (β) Cells** (75% of the islet) secrete **insulin** [51 amino acids consisting of **chain** A (21 amino acids) and **chain B** (30 amino acids) held together by **disulfide bonds**; 6 kDa] in response to hyperglycemia which will lower blood glucose, free fatty acid, and ketone levels. Insulin binds to the **insulin receptor** which is a **receptor tyrosine kinase** present on hepatocytes, skeletal muscle cells, and adipocytes.
3. **Delta (δ) Cells** (5% of the islet) secrete **somatostatin** (14 amino acids) which inhibits hormone secretion from nearby cells in a paracrine manner. Somatostatin binds to the **somatostatin receptor** which is a **G-protein-linked receptor.**

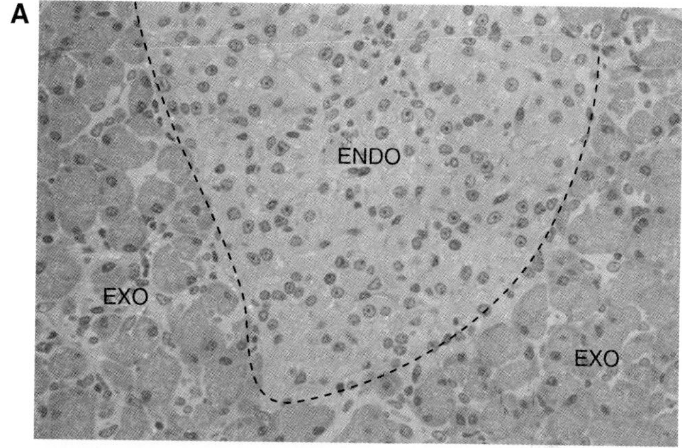

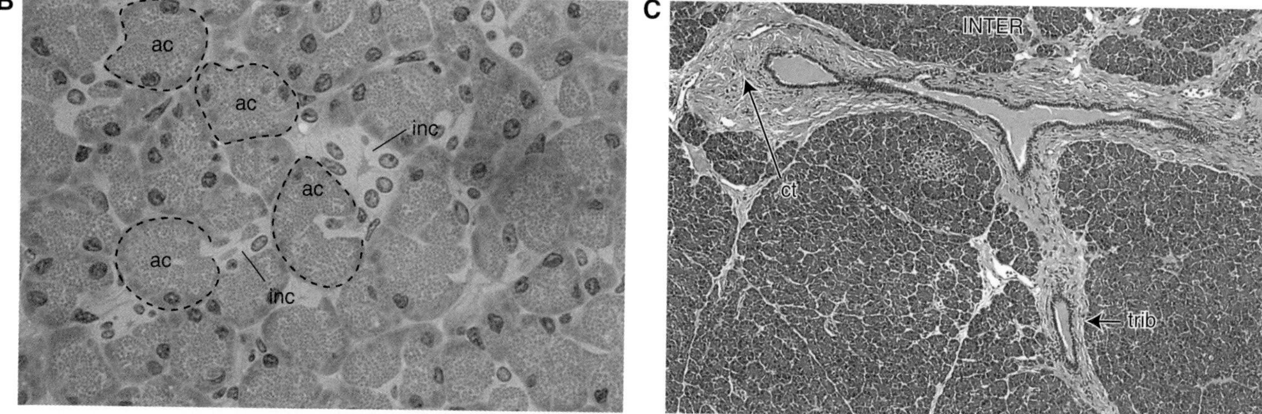

FIGURE 4-10. **Light Microscopy of the Pancreas. (A)** This light micrograph shows the exocrine pancreas (EXO) and the endocrine pancreas (ENDO) which appear as a pale-staining island of cells (dotted line circle). The endocrine pancreas (or islets of Langerhans) consists of α, β, and δ cells which are readily identifiable only using immunocytochemical staining techniques. **(B)** This light micrograph shows numerous pancreatic (secretory) acini (ac) consisting of acinar cells. The acinar cells secrete digestive enzymes into the lumen lined by centroacinar cells. This lumen is continuous with intercalated ducts (inc). Intercalated and intralobular ducts of the pancreas are not surrounded by connective tissue. **(C)** This light micrograph shows a fairly large interlobular duct (INTER) of the exocrine pancreas surrounded by connective tissue (ct). The larger interlobular ducts receive tributaries (trib) of smaller interlobular ducts as they course through the exocrine pancreas.

Chapter 5

Physiology

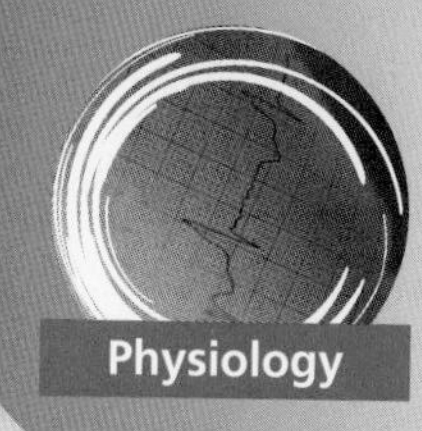

Esophagus

I Sphincters

A. **The Upper Esophageal Sphincter (UES)** separates the pharynx from the esophagus. The UES relaxes (opens) during swallowing (deglutition), belching, and vomiting. The UES maintains closure of the upper end of the esophagus, prevents air from entering the esophagus, and, with severe gastric acid reflux, prevents refluxed material from entering the pharynx.

B. **The Lower Esophageal Sphincter (LES)** separates the esophagus from the stomach and **prevents gastroesophageal reflux**, which is the reflux of acidic gastric contents into the esophagus (i.e., gastroesophageal reflux disease). The LES is composed of **smooth muscle** with the inner circular layer of smooth muscle being the major determinant of LES tone. At rest, the LES is tonically contracted at a pressure 12 to 30 mm Hg > gastric pressure, which is maintained even in the absence of neural input (e.g., a bilateral vagotomy does not eliminate LES tonic contraction).
1. **LES contraction** involves CN X and postganglionic enteric neurons that release **acetylcholine (Ach)**.
2. **LES relaxation** involves CN X and postganglionic enteric neurons that release either **nitric oxide (NO)** or **vasoactive intestinal polypeptide (VIP)**.

II Swallowing

Swallowing is coordinated by the swallowing center located in the medulla which receives sensory information via CN V, IX, and X. Humans swallow about 600 times per day. Swallowing occurs in two phases as indicated below.

A. **Oropharyngeal Phase.** A number of events occur during this phase.
1. The bolus of food is pushed upward and backward against the hard palate which forces the bolus of food into the pharynx.
2. The soft palate elongates to close off the nasopharynx.
3. The epiglottis tips over to close off the larynx.
4. The hyoid bone and larynx move upward.
5. Respiration is stopped.
6. The UES relaxes and opens for about 0.5 to 1 s to allow the bolus of food to pass into the esophagus. Subsequently, the UES contracts tightly.

B. **Esophageal Phase.** A number of events occur during this phase which lasts about 6 to 10 s.
1. A **primary peristaltic wave** sweeps down the entire esophagus and pushes the food bolus toward the stomach aided by gravity.
2. A **secondary peristaltic wave** clears the esophagus of any residual food.

3. The LES relaxes within 2 s after swallowing at a time when the primary peristaltic wave is observed in the middle portion of the esophagus.
4. When the food bolus reaches the LES, the LES is relaxed but closed. The food bolus with the aid of peristalsis forces the LES open.

III Vomiting (Emesis)

Vomiting is coordinated by the **vomiting center** located in the medulla (dorsolateral reticular formation), which receives sensory information from the **vestibular system** (e.g., motion sickness), **limbic system** (sights, smells, and emotions can induce vomiting), **chemoreceptor trigger zone** in the area postrema (activated by certain chemicals, drugs like emetics, radiation, certain metabolic states, and the vestibular system), **touch receptors in the pharynx**, and CN X **sensory neurons and sympathetic sensory neurons** from the GI tract that sense distention and mucosal irritation. Vomiting occurs in a number of steps as indicated below:

1. Nausea accompanied by sweating, pallor, and hypersalivation is experienced.
2. **Reverse peristalsis** is observed in the small intestine and moves intestinal contents toward the stomach.
3. A **forced inspiration** occurs so that the epiglottis tips over to close off the larynx. At the same time, a **giant retrograde contraction** begins in the small intestine and moves the intestinal contents into the stomach.
4. The **abdominal muscles contract** while the breath is held thereby increasing the intra-abdominal pressure.
5. The **UES and LES relax,** which allows the expulsion of gastric contents through the oral cavity as vomitus. If the UES remains closed, **retching** occurs.

IV Clinical Consideration

Forceful vomiting is commonly seen in alcoholics, bulimia, and pregnancy which may tear the posterior wall of the esophagus. Clinical findings include severe retrosternal pain after vomiting and extravasated contrast medium. **Mallory–Weiss tears** involve only the mucosal and submucosal layers. **Boerhaave syndrome** involves tears through all layers of the esophagus.

Stomach

I Gastric Motility *(Figure 5-1)*

A. Receptive Relaxation

1. With each swallow of food, the thin muscularis externa of the orad stomach relaxes to receive the food bolus (called **receptive relaxation**) so that the stomach can accommodate ≈1.5 L of food.
2. Receptive relaxation is a **vagovagal reflex** whereby visceral stretch sensory information from mechanoreceptors in the stomach travels with CN X to the CNS and motor impulses (i.e., preganglionic parasympathetic axons) travel with CN X to the muscularis externa. The neurotransmitter **VIP** released from postganglionic axons seems to play an important role in receptive relaxation.

B. Gastric Mixing

1. **Fed state**
   a. In the fed state after a large meal, the stomach enters a **lag phase** in which contractions are absent but gastric secretion is high.

b. After the lag phase, the thick muscularis externa of the caudad stomach contracts to grind the food bolus into smaller particles and to mix the food bolus with the gastric secretions to form **chyme**.
c. The frequency of slow waves (3 slow waves/min in the stomach) sets the maximum frequency of smooth muscle contractions.
d. Strong peristaltic contractions begin in the caudad stomach and sweep distally toward the pyloric antrum where the contractions are the strongest, thereby moving the chyme toward the pyloric sphincter. The contractions occur at a rate of **3 to 5 contractions/min** and last between **2 and 20 s**.
e. Chyme with small particles of food is emptied into the duodenum through the pyloric sphincter. Chyme with large particles of food is propelled back into the stomach (called **retropulsion**).
f. The peristaltic contractions involved in gastric mixing are increased by the parasympathetic nervous system (CN X). The peristaltic contractions involved in gastric mixing are decreased by the sympathetic nervous system.

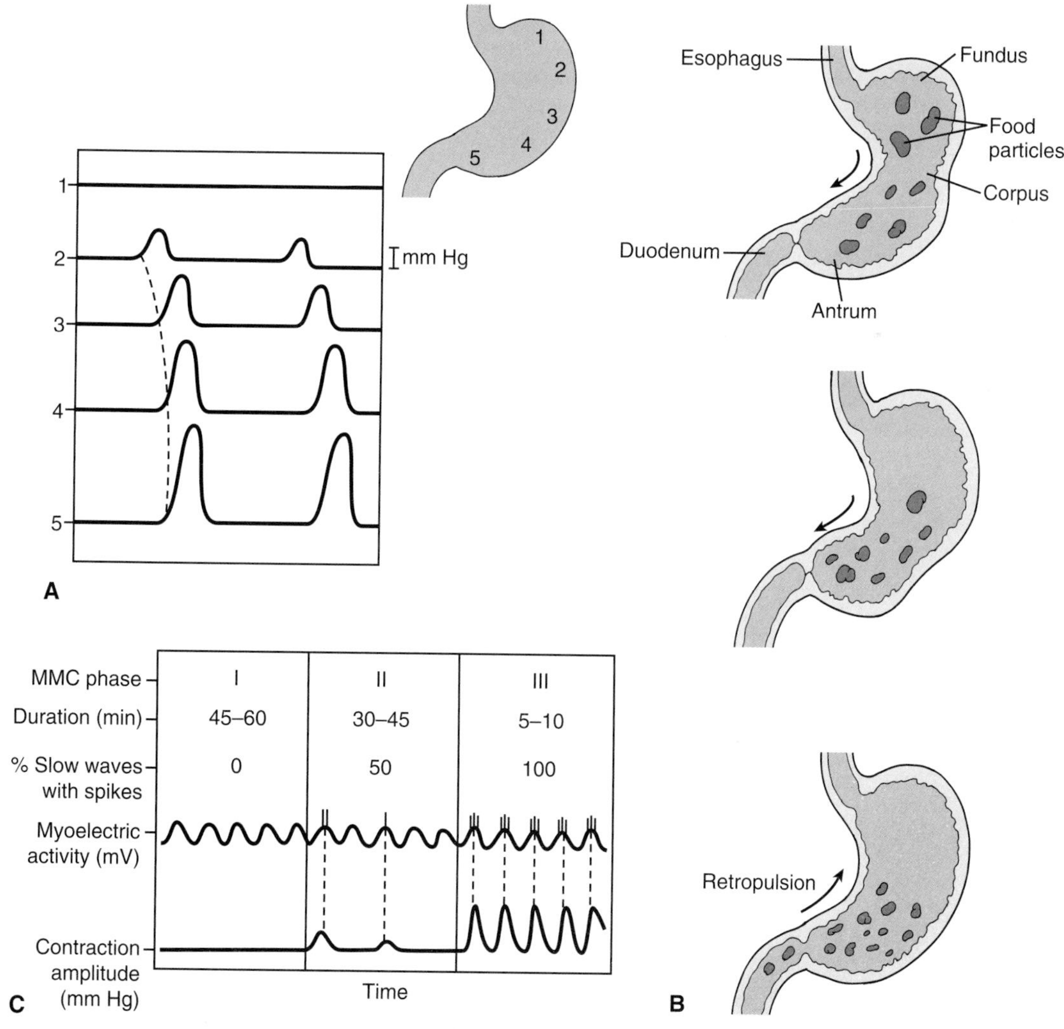

FIGURE 5-1. **Stomach Motility. (A) Intraluminal Pressures Measured from Five Regions of the Stomach (1–5).** The increase in intraluminal pressure is caused by peristaltic contractions of the muscularis externa. In Region 1, no increase in intraluminal pressure is observed. In Region 2, periodic spikes in intraluminal pressure are first observed. The periodic spikes increase in intensity as they sweep distally toward the pyloric antrum (Region 5). **(B) Diagram of Retropulsion.** Chyme with large particles of food is propelled back into the stomach. **(C) Stomach Motility in the Fasting or Interdigestive State.** The MMCs have three phases. In Phase I (quiescent phase), no action potentials at the crest of the slow waves are observed and therefore, no smooth muscle contraction occurs. In Phase II, action potentials at the crest of ≈50% of the slow waves are observed, and therefore, some smooth muscle contraction occurs. In Phase III, action potentials at the crest of 100% of the slow waves are observed, and therefore, strong smooth muscle contraction occurs that lasts ≈5 to 10 min. In Phase III, gastric contents are moved a long distance.

2. **Fasting or interdigestive state**
   a. In the fasting or interdigestive state, periodic peristaltic contractions, called **migrating motor complexes (MMCs)**, are observed, which occur at **90 to 120 min intervals** and are mediated by **motilin** (secreted by enterochromaffinlike [ECL] cells in the small intestine).
   b. The MMCs move chyme through the small intestines to the ileocecal valve during an overnight fast.
   c. The MMCs also move gastric HCl through the small intestines to control bacterial growth. The pyloric sphincter is open during the MMC.

C. Gastric Emptying.

After a meal, the stomach contains ≈**1.5 L** and it takes ≈**3 h** to empty this amount into the duodenum.

1. When the stomach contents are **isotonic**, the rate of emptying is **fast**.
2. When the stomach contents are **hypertonic or hypotonic**, the rate of emptying is **slow**.
3. When the stomach contents contain ↑**fat**, the rate of empting is **slow**. This is mediated by **cholecystokinin (CCK)** that is secreted by **I cells** when fatty acids arrive in the duodenum. This provides adequate time for fat digestion and absorption by the small intestine. CCK also stimulates enzyme secretion from the pancreas and stimulates bile release from the gallbladder.
4. When the duodenal contents contain ↑**H^+ ions (low pH)**, the rate of emptying is **slow**. Chemo-sensitive receptors in the duodenum sense H^+ ions and relay this information back to the muscularis externa of the stomach via the myenteric plexus of Auerbach. This provides adequate time for H^+ ions neutralization by pancreatic HCO_3^-.

II Gastric Secretion

The cells of the gastric mucosa secrete a fluid called **gastric juice** which consists mainly of **mucus**, HCO_3^-, **intrinsic factor (IF)**, **pepsinogen**, and **HCl**. The average adult produces ≈**2 to 3 L/day** of gastric juice. The resting gastric juice is an **acidic (pH 2 to 2.5) isotonic solution**. After a meal, the buffering capacity of the food raises the pH of the gastric juice to ≈**pH 4 to 5**.

III Gastric Mucus

A. Function of Gastric Mucus

1. Gastric mucus acts as a **lubricant** for the mucosa and the food to minimize frictional forces and prevent tissue injury.
2. Gastric mucus acts as a **protectant** against the acidic and proteolytic properties of the gastric juice by

B. Regulation of Gastric Mucus Secretion

1. Gastric mucus secretion is increased by both the **parasympathetic nervous system** (CN X) which increases **soluble mucus** secretion from mucous neck cells and **chemical/mechanical irritation** which increases **gel-forming mucus** from surface mucous cells.
2. The production of gel-forming mucus as a result of chemical/mechanical irritation is mediated via the generation of **prostaglandins (PGE_1, PGE_2, $PGF_{2\alpha}$)**.
3. Prostaglandin biosynthesis involves phospholipase A_2 and cyclooxygenase (COX). The ability of **nonsteroidal anti-inflammatory drugs (NSAIDs**; e.g., aspirin, ibuprofen, naproxen, indomethacin) to inhibit COX may explain the ulcerogenic side effect of NSAIDs.

IV HCO_3^-

A. Function of HCO_3^-. Gastric HCO_3^- becomes trapped in the gel mucus and forms part of the mucus–HCO_3^- barrier, thereby maintaining a **pH gradient** of pH 2 of gastric acid in the lumen → pH 7 of mucosal epithelium.

B. Regulation of HCO_3^- Secretion. HCO_3^- secretion is increased by the **parasympathetic nervous system (CN X)**, **chemical irritation** (i.e., presence of HCl in the lumen), and **prostaglandins**.

V Intrinsic Factor

IF is secreted by parietal cells in the stomach.

A. Function of Intrinsic Factor. IF binds to and promotes the absorption of **vitamin B_{12}** in the terminal ileum by receptor-mediated endocytosis. **Pernicious anemia** may result from vitamin B_{12} deficiency caused by atrophic gastritis with decreased IF production.

B. Regulation of Intrinsic Factor Secretion. IF secretion is increased by **parasympathetic nervous system (CN X)**, **gastrin**, and **histamine** (i.e., the same factors that increase gastric HCl secretion).

VI Pepsinogen

A. Function of Pepsinogen

1. Pepsinogen isozymes are converted to **pepsin isozymes (active)** on contact with the acid pH of the gastric juice. The pH optimum for pepsin isozymes falls between pH 1.5 and 5.0.
2. Pepsin isozymes are endopeptidases that cleave peptide bonds between hydrophobic amino acids and are particularly active in the proteolysis of collagen, a major constituent of meat.
3. The small peptides generated by this proteolytic process serve as signals for the secretion of GI hormones (e.g., gastrin, CCK).

B. Regulation of Pepsinogen Secretion. Pepsinogen secretion is increased by **parasympathetic nervous system (CN X)** mediated by ACh and gastrin-releasing peptide (GRP), **chemical irritation** (i.e., presence of HCl in the lumen), **secretin** (SEC), and **CCK**.

VII HCl *(Figure 5-2)*

Gastric HCl is secreted by the parietal cells in the stomach. **Cl^- ion channels** are present on the canalicular membrane system and **H^+–K^+ ATPases** are present on the tubulovesicles. The fusion of the canalicular membrane system and the tubulovesicles brings the Cl^- ion channels and H^+–K^+ ATPases together, bordering the luminal space. The parietal cells contain **carbonic anhydrase** which generates H^+ ($CO_2 + H_2O \rightarrow H^+ + HCO_3^-$). The key event in HCl secretion is the **cAMP-dependent opening of Cl^- ion channels**, which allows both Cl^- and K^+ to move into the luminal space. K^+ plays an important role because a **K^+ gradient** in the opposite direction of H^+ movement is necessary in order for the H^+–K^+ ATPase to pump H^+.

A. Function of HCl. Gastric HCl aids in the digestion of food, converts pepsinogen (inactive) → pepsin (active), and provides a defense mechanism by killing ingested microorganisms.

B. **Stimulation of HCl Secretion.** Gastric HCl secretion is increased by the **parasympathetic nervous system (CN X; Ach)**, **gastrin**, and **histamine (a major stimulus)**.

C. **Inhibition of HCl Secretion.** Gastric HCl secretion is decreased by **CCK**, **secretin**, **glucose insulinotropic peptide (GIP)**, **somatostatin**, **prostaglandins (PGE_1)**, **hypertonic solutions**, **emptying of the stomach**, and **distention of the duodenum**.

VIII Phases of HCl Secretion

A. **Cephalic Phase**

1. The cephalic phase is initiated by **sight**, **smell**, **taste**, and **conditioned reflexes**.
2. The cephalic phase accounts for **30%** of the total HCl secreted in response to a meal and lasts ≈**30 min** into the meal.
3. The cephalic phase is controlled by the **parasympathetic nervous system** (CN X).
4. **GRP** released from postganglionic enteric neurons binds to receptors on the G cells and stimulates gastrin secretion which then activates the parietal cell.

B. **Gastric Phase**

1. The gastric phase is initiated by **stomach distention** and the presence of **amino acids/small peptides** in the stomach lumen.
2. The gastric phase accounts for **60%** of the total HCl secreted in response to a meal and lasts ≈**2.5 h** after the start of the meal.
3. The gastric phase is controlled by the **parasympathetic nervous system** (CN X) and a **direct effect on G cells.**
4. **GRP** released from postganglionic enteric neurons binds to receptors on the G cells and stimulates gastrin secretion, which then activates the parietal cell.
5. Amino acids/small peptides directly effect G cells and stimulate gastrin secretion, which then activates the parietal cell.

C. **Intestinal Phase**

1. The intestinal phase is initiated by the **presence of chyme in the duodenum**.
2. The intestinal phase accounts for **10%** of the total HCl secreted in response to a meal.
3. Amino acids/small peptides within the duodenum directly effect G cells and stimulate gastrin secretion which then activates the parietal cell.
4. However, the intestinal phase can also inhibit HCl secretion via somatostatin, SEC, GIP, and CCK.

IX Other Gastric Secretions

A. **HCO_3^-.** HCO_3^- is secreted into the bloodstream by the parietal cells in the stomach. This causes a rise in blood pH called the **alkaline tide**. For every H^+ that is pumped into the stomach lumen during the formation of gastric HCl, an OH^- remains in the parietal cell cytoplasm. To prevent intracellular alkalization and cell death, the enzyme carbonic anhydrase ($CO_2 + H_2O \rightarrow H^+ + HCO_3^-$) catalyzes the formation of HCO_3^- from CO_2 and the OH^-. The HCO_3^- is transported across the basolateral cell membrane in exchange for Cl^-. Thus, an HCO_3^- enters the bloodstream for every H^+ produced. In addition, some of this HCO_3^- may find its way into the mucus-HCO_3^- barrier via the paracellular route.

B. **Gastrin.** Gastrin is secreted into the bloodstream (endocrine mechanism) by G cells in the pyloric antrum of the stomach/proximal duodenum. Two major forms of gastrin are secreted, called **G17** (containing 17 amino acids; little gastrin) and **G34** (containing 34 amino acids; big gastrin). The common feature of all gastrins is a **C-terminal tetrapeptide (Try–Met–Asp–Phe)** which has full biological activity. Gastrin binds to the CCK2 receptor which is a G protein-linked receptor using the IP_3 + DAG pathway.

1. **Function of gastrin.** Gastrin stimulates HCl secretion from parietal cells, stimulates histamine release from ECL cells, and promotes growth of the gastric mucosa.
2. **Regulation of gastrin secretion.** Gastrin secretion is increased by the **parasympathetic nervous system (CN X; GRP), stomach distention**, and the presence of **amino acids/small peptides** in the stomach lumen.

C. **Histamine.** Histamine is secreted into the extracellular space (paracrine mechanism) by ECL cells in the stomach. Histamine is derived from the amino acid histidine and contains an imidazole containing a characteristic five member ring with two nitrogen atoms. Histamine binds to the H_2 receptor which is a G protein-linked receptor using the ↑cAMP pathway.

1. **Function of histamine.** Histamine stimulates HCl secretion from parietal cells.
2. **Regulation of histamine secretion.** Histamine secretion is increased by **gastrin** released from G cells in the stomach/proximal duodenum. Histamine secretion is decreased by **somatostatin** released from D cells in the stomach.

D. **Somatostatin.** Somatostatin is secreted into the extracellular space (paracrine mechanism) by D cells in the stomach. Two major forms of somatostatin are secreted, called SS-14 and SS-28.

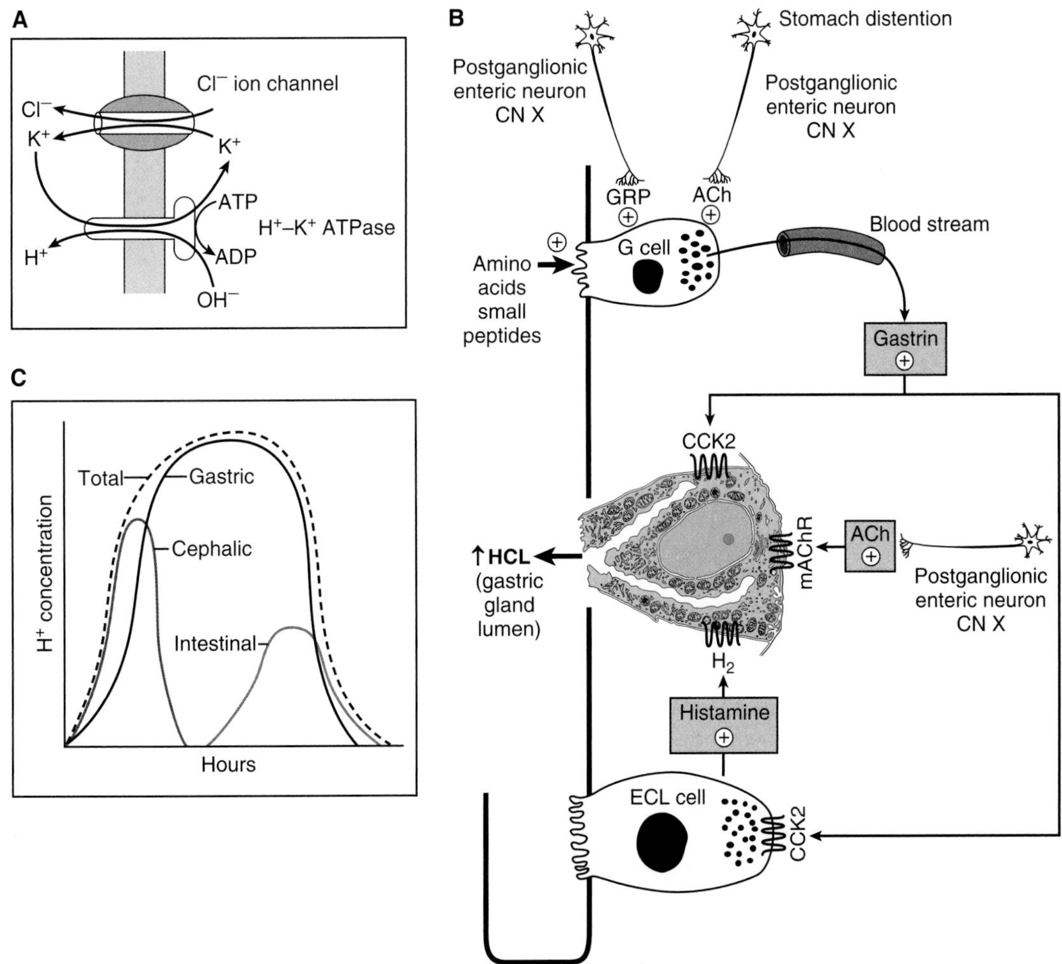

FIGURE 5-2. **Parietal Cell and HCl Secretion. (A)** Diagram shows the ion flow through the Cl^- ion channel and the H^+–K^+ ATPase. **(B)** Diagram shows the factors that increase HCl secretion from the parietal cell. **(C)** Graph shows the three phases of HCl secretion. Ach — acetylcholine; GRP — gastrin-releasing peptide; ECL — enterochromaffin-like cell; CCK2 — cholecystokinin 2 receptor; H_2 — histamine 2 receptor; mAChR — muscarinic acetylcholine receptor.

X Clinical Considerations

A. **Dumping Syndrome** refers to the abnormally rapid emptying of **hyperosmotic** stomach contents (especially high carbohydrate foods) into the jejunum within 30 min ("early dumping") or 1 to 3 h ("late dumping") after a meal. The dumping syndrome usually occurs after a partial gastrotectomy or vagotomy for treatment of obesity or an ulcer. Clinical findings include epigastric discomfort, borborygmi (rumbling sounds due to gas movement), palpitations, dizziness, diarrhea, and hypoglycemia.

B. **Gastroparesis.** Gastroparesis is delayed gastric emptying in the absence of mechanical obstruction and is the most common gastric motor dysfunction. The failure to generate enough force to empty the stomach may be caused by abnormal slow wave progression, vagotomy, or peripheral neuropathy due to diabetes. The most common cause of delayed gastric emptying in adults is pyloric antrum obstruction caused by scarring from a peptic ulcer.

Small Intestine

I Small Intestine Motility *(Figure 5-3)*

Small intestine motility mixes the chyme, brings it into contact with the absorptive mucosal surface, and propels it forward. Chyme takes about 2 to 3 h to pass through the small intestine. As in the stomach, the frequency of slow waves (12 slow waves/min in the duodenum → 8 slow waves/min in the ileum) sets the maximum frequency of smooth muscle contractions.

A. **Fed State.** In the fed state after a large meal, two types of contractions are observed in the small intestine: **segmentation (mixing) contractions** and **peristaltic (propulsion) contractions**.

1. In a segmentation contraction, a small section of small intestine contracts (i.e., the inner circular layer of smooth muscle), which sends chyme in both the orad and caudad directions. Subsequently, the same section then relaxes and the chyme returns with no net caudad movement of chyme.
2. In a peristaltic contraction, a small section of small intestine contracts (i.e., the outer longitudinal layer of smooth muscle) behind a bolus of chyme while simultaneously a small section of small intestine relaxes ahead of the bolus of chyme. This results in a rapid caudad movement of chyme at a rate of 2 to 25 cm/s.
3. In the fed state, smooth muscle contraction is modulated by the **parasympathetic nervous system** (CN X), whereby postganglionic parasympathetic neurons release **Ach** and other postganglionic enteric neurons release **substance P**. In the fed state, smooth muscle relaxation is modulated by the **parasympathetic nervous system** (CN X), whereby postganglionic enteric neurons release **NO** and **VIP**.

B. **Fasting or Interdigestive State.** In the fasting or interdigestive state, periodic peristaltic contractions are observed, called **MMCs**, which are a continuation of the MMCs initiated in the stomach.

1. MMCs occur at **90 to 120 min intervals** and are mediated by **motilin** (secreted by ECL cells in the small intestine).
2. The MMCs sweep the small intestine clean of undigestible food residua, bacteria, and desquamated epithelial cells.
3. As soon as feeding occurs, the MMCs stop and the fed-pattern of motility returns.

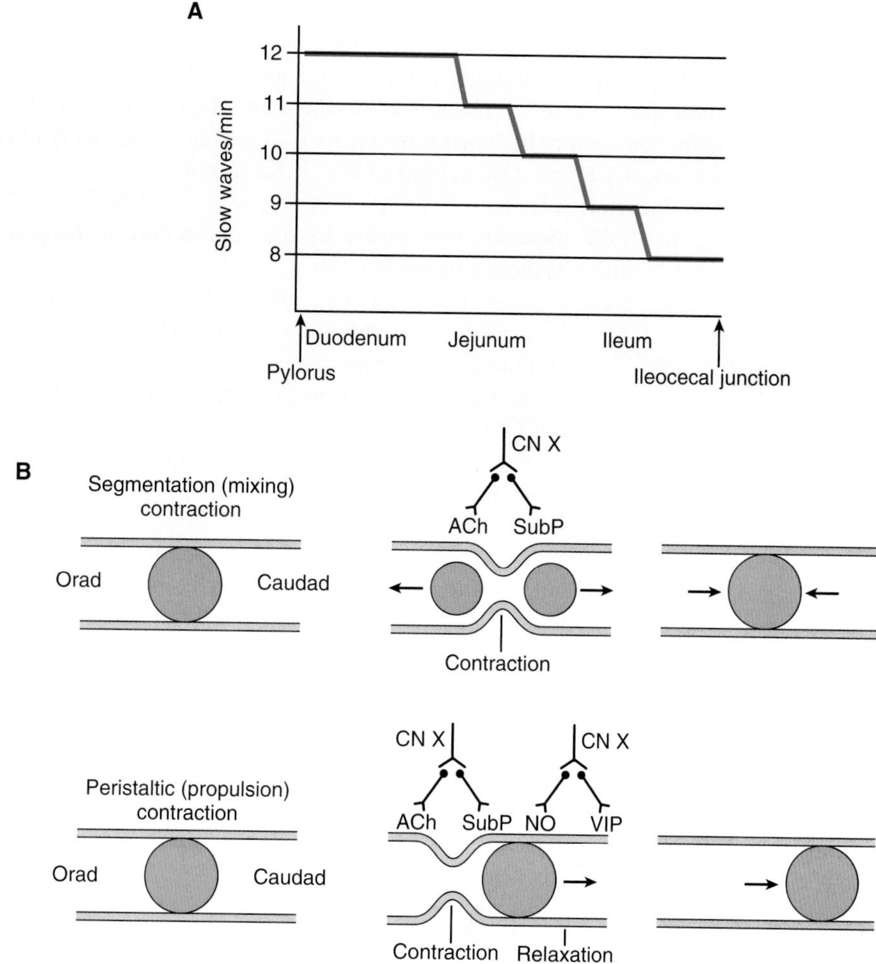

FIGURE 5-3. **Small Intestine Motility. (A)** Graph shows the slow wave frequency decreasing in a step-wise pattern from the duodenum to the ileum. **(B)** Diagram shows a segmentation contraction and a peristaltic contraction. Note the neurotransmitters involved in the contraction and relaxation of the smooth muscle. Ach — acetylcholine; SubP — substance P; NO — nitric oxide; VIP — vasoactive intestinal polypeptide.

C. **Ileocecal Sphincter.** The ileocecal sphincter separates the terminal ileum from the cecum.

1. This sphincter is normally closed. When it opens, small amounts of chyme enter the colon at a rate that is compatible with the ability of the colon to absorb H_2O and electrolytes.
2. This sphincter is incompetent so that the build up of gas or feces in the colon is prevented.
3. The ileocecal sphincter opens in response to the following: distension of the terminal ileum, peristaltic contractions in the terminal ileum, and the **gastroileal reflex** which causes the emptying of the ileum after a meal.

II Small Intestine Secretion *(Table 5-1)*

A. **Aqueous Solution.** The enterocytes of the small intestine secrete an aqueous solution during the course of digestion. Under normal circumstances, the enterocytes absorb more than they secrete. Under pathological circumstances (e.g., cholera infection), aqueous secretion greatly exceeds absorption and diarrhea results.

B. **Mucus.** Mucus is secreted by Goblet cells in the small intestine.

C. **Cholecystokinin.** CCK is secreted into the bloodstream (endocrine mechanism) by the enteroendocrine I-cells in the intestinal glands (crypts of Lieberkuhn). CCK is a

33-amino acid peptide and a member of the gastrin–CCK family. The C-terminal five amino acids of CCK (CCK5) are identical to those of gastrin and include the tetrapeptide that is minimally necessary for gastrin activity, which means that CCK has some gastrin activity. The minimum fragment of CCK necessary for biological activity is the C-terminal heptapeptide (CCK7). CCK binds selectively to the CCK1 receptor whereas CCK and gastrin bind to the CCK2 receptor.

1. **Function of CCK**
   a. CCK increases bile release by the contraction of the gallbladder and relaxation of the sphincter of Oddi.
   b. CCK increases pancreatic enzyme and HCO_3^- secretion.
   c. CCK decreases HCl secretion by parietal cells.
   d. CCK inhibits gastric emptying.
   e. CCK exerts a growth effect on the pancreas and gallbladder.
2. **Regulation of CCK secretion.** CCK secretion is increased by the presence of amino acids (tryptophan and phenylalanine)/small peptides and fatty acids/monoglycerides in the small intestinal lumen.

D. **Secretin (Called "Nature's Antacid").** SEC is secreted into the bloodstream (endocrine mechanism) by the enteroendocrine S cells in the intestinal glands (crypts of Lieberkuhn). SEC is a 27-amino acid peptide and a member of the SEC–glucagon family. All 27 amino acids are necessary for biological activity.

1. **Function of SEC**
   a. SEC increases HCO_3^- release from the pancreas and liver biliary tract.
   b. SEC inhibits the effect of gastrin on the parietal cell.
   c. The neutralization of acidic chyme by HCO_3^- is essential for fat digestion because pancreatic lipases have a pH 6 to 8 optimum.
2. **Regulation of SEC secretion.** SEC secretion is increased by the presence of H^+ (<pH 4.5) and fatty acids in the intestinal lumen.

E. **Gastric Inhibitory Peptide or Glucose Insulinotropic Peptide.** GIP is secreted into the bloodstream (endocrine mechanism) by the enteroendocrine K cells in the intestinal glands (crypts of Lieberkuhn). GIP is a 42-amino acid peptide and a member of the SEC–glucagon family.

1. **Functions of GIP**
   a. GIP inhibits the effect of gastrin on the parietal cell.
   b. GIP increases insulin secretion under conditions of hyperglycemia by pancreatic β cells.
   c. The action of GIP to increase insulin secretion explains why an oral glucose load is utilized by cells more rapidly than an intravenous glucose load. An oral glucose load stimulates insulin secretion from pancreatic β cells via both GIP and blood glucose levels. An intravenous glucose load stimulates insulin secretion from pancreatic β cells via only blood glucose levels.
2. **Regulation of GIP secretion.** GIP secretion is increased by the presence of glucose, amino acids/small peptide, and fatty acids in the small intestinal lumen.

F. **Glucagonlike Peptide-1.** Glucagonlike peptide-1 (GLP-1) is secreted into the bloodstream (endocrine mechanism) by the enteroendocrine L cells in the intestinal glands (crypts of Lieberkuhn). GLP-1 is a 30-amino acid peptide with a 50% sequence homology to glucagon. The glucagon gene is composed of six exons that yield preproglucagon. In the pancreatic α cells, preproglucagon is processed to glucagon and glucagon-related polypeptide. In the intestinal L cells, preproglucagon, is processed to GLP-1, GLP-2, and glycentin.

1. **Functions of GLP-1**
   a. GLP-1 increases insulin secretion in the presence of hyperglycemia.
   b. GLP-1 decreases postprandial glucagon secretion.
   c. GLP-1 inhibits gastric emptying.

d. GLP-1 reduces food intake.
e. GLP-1 stimulates pancreatic β-cell growth.
f. GLP-1 has a 1 to 2 min half-life due to the rapid degradation of the N-terminus by **dipeptidyl peptidase IV (DPP-IV)**. A naturally occurring peptide in the saliva of the Gila monster called **exendin-4** shares sequence homology with GLP-1. However, exendin-4 has a prolonged half-life because it is resistant to DPP-IV degradation. The drug **exenatide** is synthetic exendin-4 and is the first GLP-1 based diabetes therapy approved in the United States by the FDA.

2. **Regulation of GLP-1 secretion.** GLP-1 secretion is increased in the presence of glucose, amino acids/small peptide, and fatty acids in the small intestinal lumen.

TABLE 5-1 SUMMARY TABLE OF GASTROINTESTINAL HORMONES

Hormone	Cell	Functions	Regulation
Gastrin	G cell in stomach	Stimulates HCl secretion from parietal cells Stimulates histamine release from ECL cells Promotes growth of gastric mucosa	Increased by CN X (GRP), stomach distention, presence of amino acids in the stomach lumen
Histamine	ECL cell in stomach (paracrine mechanism)	Stimulates HCl secretion from parietal cells	Increased by gastrin released from G cells Decreased by somatostatin released from D cells
Somatostatin	D cell in stomach (paracrine mechanism)	Inhibits histamine secretion from ECL cells A major inhibitory peptide	Increased by the presence of HCl in the stomach lumen Increased by gastrin
CCK	I cell in small intestine	Increases bile release by contraction of the gallbladder and relaxation of the sphincter of Oddi Increases pancreatic enzyme and HCO_3^- secretion Decreases HCl secretion by parietal cells Inhibits gastric emptying Exerts a growth effect on pancreas and gallbladder	Increased by presence of amino acids/small peptides and fatty acids/monoglycerides in the small intestinal lumen
SEC	S cell in small intestine	Increases HCO_3^- release from the pancreas and liver biliary tract Inhibits the effect of gastrin on the parietal cell	Increased by the presence of H^+ (<pH 4.5) and fatty acids in the intestinal lumen
GIP	K cell in small intestine	Inhibits the effect of gastrin on the parietal cell Increases insulin secretion under conditions of hyperglycemia	Increased by the presence of glucose, amino acids/small peptide, and fatty acids in the small intestinal lumen
GLP-1	L cell in small intestine	Increases insulin secretion under conditions of hyperglycemia Decreases postprandial glucagon secretion Inhibits gastric emptying Reduces food intake Stimulates pancreatic β-cell growth	Increased by the presence of glucose, amino acids/small peptide, and fatty acids in the small intestinal lumen

III Digestion and Absorption of Carbohydrates *(Figure 5-4)*

A. Digestion

1. The digestion of carbohydrates begins in the oral cavity and then continues in the small intestine.
2. Starch contains both α-1,4 and α-1,6 glycosidic bonds. The α-1,4 glycosidic bonds are hydrolyzed by salivary amylase in the oral cavity (plays a minor role because

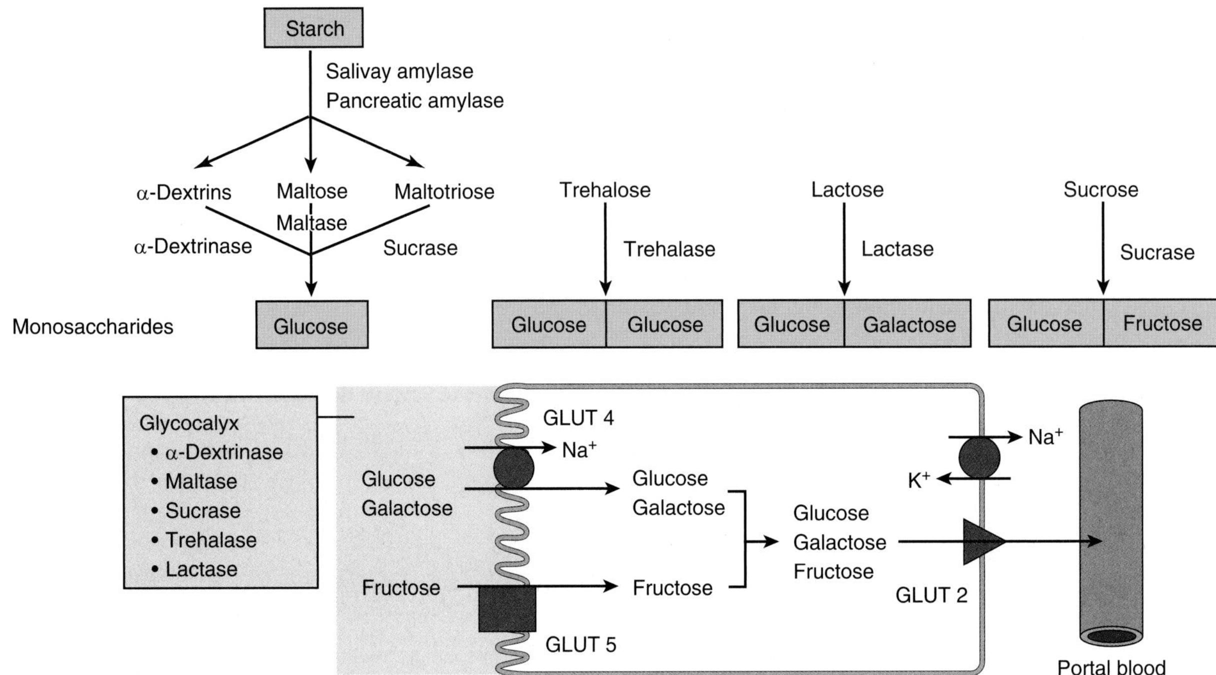

FIGURE 5-4. **Digestion and Absorption of Carbohydrates.** GLUT — glucose.

salivary amylase is inactivated by ↓pH in the stomach) and pancreatic amylase in the small intestine. This yields three disaccharides: **α-dextrins**, **maltose**, and **maltotriose**.

3. These three disaccharides are further digested to **glucose** by **α-dextrinase**, **maltase**, and **sucrase**.
4. There are three main disaccharides in the US diet: **trehalose**, **lactose**, and **sucrose**.
5. Trehalose is digested to two molecules of glucose by **trehalase**. Lactose is digested to glucose and galactose by **lactase**. Sucrose is digested to glucose and fructose by **sucrase**.
6. The enzymes α-dextrinase, maltase, sucrase, trehalase, and lactase are all located in the glycocalyx of the enterocytes.
7. In short, carbohydrates are digested to the monosaccharides called **glucose**, **galactose**, and **fructose**.

B. Absorption

1. Only monosaccharides can be absorbed by enterocytes.
2. Glucose and galactose enter enterocytes by secondary active transport using a **Na^+ dependent-glucose transporter**. The energy for this process is derived from a Na^+ gradient across the apical membrane which is created by the **Na^+–K^+ ATPase** located on the basolateral membrane.
3. Fructose enters enterocytes by facilitated diffusion using **Glucose Transporter 5 (GLUT5)**. Glucose, galactose, and fructose exit enterocytes by facilitated diffusion using **GLUT2** to enter portal blood.

IV Digestion and Absorption of Proteins *(Figure 5-5)*

A. Digestion

1. The protein requirement for a normal healthy adult is ≈40 g of protein/day. Humans do not have a storage mechanism for proteins (like, for example, glycogen), and, therefore, we synthesize about 300 g of protein/day.

2. The digestion of protein begins in the stomach by the action of pepsin which has a pH optimum of pH 1.5 → 5.0. However, the action of pepsin is terminated in the small intestine as the pH rises above pH 5.0.
3. The digestion of protein continues in the small intestine by the action of pancreatic proteases and proteases in the glycocalyx of enterocytes.
4. **Trypsinogen (inactive)** is secreted by the exocrine pancreas and is converted to its active form **trypsin (active)** by **enterokinase** located in the glycocalyx of enterocytes.
5. Trypsin then converts all other inactive pancreatic precursors to their active form (**trypsinogen → trypsin, chymotrypsinogen → chymotrypsin, proelastase → elastase, procarboxypeptidase A → carboxypeptidase A, and procarboxypeptidase B → carboxypeptidase B**).
6. These five active pancreatic proteases then hydrolyze dietary protein to **amino acids, dipeptides, tripeptides**, and **oligopeptides**.
7. Oligopeptides are further digested to amino acids, dipeptides, and tripeptides by **aminopeptidases** located in the glycocalyx of enterocytes.
8. Most of the dipeptides and tripeptides are further hydrolyzed to amino acid by **cytoplasmic peptidases** within enterocytes.
9. In short, proteins are digested to **amino acids, dipeptides**, and **tripeptides**.

B. Absorption

1. Only amino acids, dipeptides, and tripeptides can be absorbed by enterocytes. Dipeptides and tripeptides are absorbed faster than amino acids by enterocytes.
2. L-amino acids enter enterocytes by secondary active transport using **Na^+-amino acid cotransporters**.
3. There are four separate Na^+-amino acid cotransporters which handle either neutral, acidic, basic, or imino amino acids.
4. The energy for this process is derived from a Na^+ gradient across the apical membrane which is created by **Na^+–K^+ ATPase** located on the basolateral membrane.
5. Dipeptides and tripeptides enter enterocytes by secondary active transport using **H^+-dipeptide/tripeptide cotransporters**.
6. The energy for this process is derived from an H^+ gradient across the apical membrane which is created by **Na^+–H^+ exchanger** located on the apical membrane.

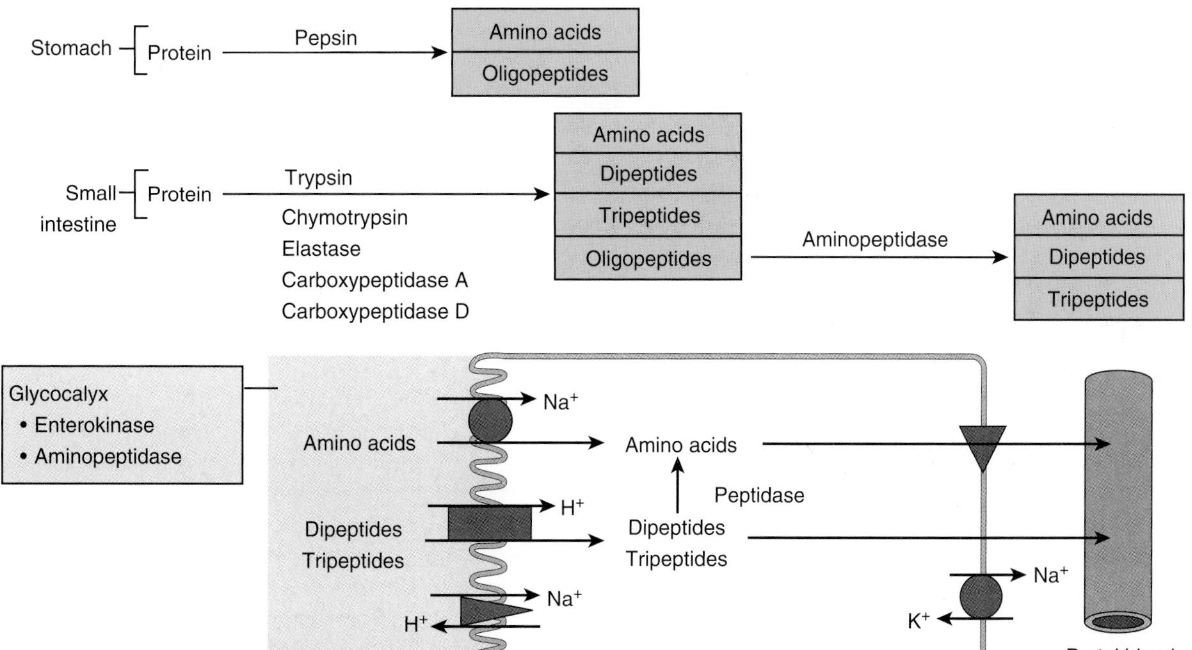

FIGURE 5-5. **Digestion and Absorption of Proteins.**

7. Amino acids exit enterocytes by facilitated diffusion to enter portal blood.
8. Dipeptides and tripeptides exit enterocytes to enter portal blood.

V Digestion and Absorption of Lipids *(Figure 5-6)*

A. Digestion

1. **Triacylglycerols** are the main lipid in the human diet.
2. The digestion of lipids begins in the stomach by the action of **lingual lipase** and **gastric lipase** and then continues in the small intestine by the action of **pancreatic lipase** and **colipase** (which is necessary to stabilize pancreatic lipase at the surface of the lipid droplet), **cholesterol ester hydrolase**, and **phospholipase** A_2.
3. Ten percent of ingested triacylglycerols are hydrolyzed in the stomach to **fatty acids** and **glycerol** by lingual lipase and gastric lipase.
4. The remaining 90% of ingested triacylglycerols are hydrolyzed in the small intestine to **monoacylglycerols** and **fatty acids** by pancreatic lipase/colipase.
5. Ingested **cholesterol esters** are hydrolyzed in the small intestine to **cholesterol** and **fatty acids** by cholesterol ester hydrolase.
6. **Phospholipids** are hydrolyzed in the small intestine to **lysolecithin** and **fatty acids** by phospholipase A_2.

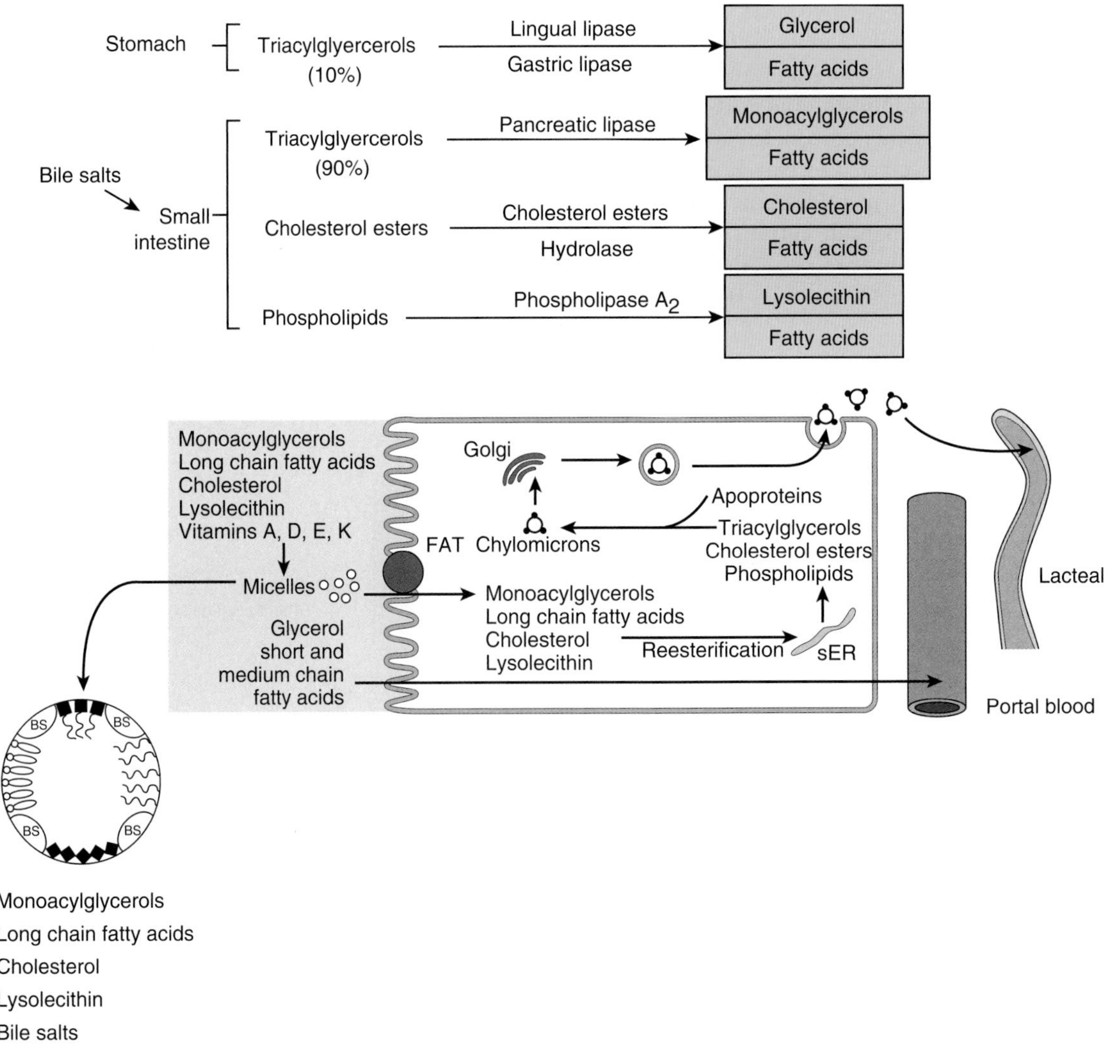

FIGURE 5-6. **Digestion and Absorption of Lipids.** FAT — fatty acid transporter; sER — smooth endoplasmic reticulum.

7. Lipid digestion in the small intestine is aided by **bile salts** that are secreted into the small intestine from the gallbladder. Bile salts surround and emulsify lipids (i.e., produce small droplets of lipid dispersed in an aqueous solution) which assists pancreatic enzyme action.
8. In short, lipids are digested to **monoacylglycerols, short, medium**, and **long-chain fatty acids, cholesterol, lysolecithin**, and **glycerol**.

B. Absorption

1. The hydrophobic products of lipid digestion (i.e., monoacylglycerol, >12 carbon long chain fatty acids, cholesterol, and lysolecithin) are packaged into the center of the **micelles** which travel to the microvillus border of the enterocytes.
2. The hydrophobic products enter enterocytes by diffusion assisted by **fatty acid transporters**.
3. Within the enterocytes, **reesterification** occurs in the **smooth endoplasmic reticulum** to form triacylglycerols, cholesterol esters, and phospholipids.
4. Within the enterocytes, the reesterified lipids are packaged with **apoproteins** (e.g., ApoB) into **chylomicrons**.
5. The chylomicrons are processed by the **Golgi** into **secretory vesicles** which bind to the basolateral membrane.
6. The hydrophobic products exit enterocytes by **exocytosis** of chylomicrons into **lacteals** of the lymph system.
7. The hydrophilic product of lipid digestion (i.e., glycerol) along with short and medium chain fatty acids enter the enterocyte directly by diffusion and exit the enterocyte by diffusion to enter portal blood.

VI Absorption of Vitamins

A. Fat-Soluble Vitamins (A, D, E, and K). The fat-soluble vitamins A, D, E, and K are processed in the same manner as other lipids in the diet.

B. Water-Soluble Vitamins (B_1, B_2, B_6, B_{12}, Biotin, C, Folic Acid, Nicotinic Acid, and Pantothenic Acid).

1. All water-soluble vitamins (except B_{12}) enter enterocytes by secondary active transport using **Na^+-amino acid cotransporters**. All water-soluble vitamins exit enterocytes probably by diffusion to enter portal blood.
2. **Vitamin B_{12} (cobalamin)**
   a. In the stomach, vitamin B_{12} binds to **R protein** (secreted by the salivary glands).
   b. In the duodenum, pancreatic proteases degrade R protein so that B_{12} then binds to **IF** secreted by parietal cells forming B_{12} + IF that is resistant to pancreatic proteases.
   c. Vitamin B_{12} enters enterocytes when a **B_{12} + IF dimer** binds to the **cubilin receptor** located on enterocytes in the **ileum**.
   d. Vitamin B_{12} exits enterocytes by diffusion to enter portal blood where it circulates bound to **transcobalamin II.**

VII Absorption and Secretion of Fluid and Electrolytes

The enterocytes of the GI tract (small intestine and colon) **absorb fluids (≈9 L of fluid/day) and electrolytes**. The source of the 9 L of fluid is ≈2 L from the diet and ≈7 L from salivary, gastric, pancreatic, biliary, and intestinal secretions. Approximately, 100 to 200 mL of fluid is not absorbed and is excreted in the feces. In addition, epithelial cells lining the intestinal glands (crypts of Lieberkühn) **secrete fluids and electrolytes.** In normal circumstances, absorption is greater than secretion so that any disturbance in absorption can lead to excessive fluid loss via the GI tract causing diarrhea.

A. **Absorption of Fluid and Electrolytes.** Absorption occurs by enterocytes lining the villi of the small intestine. The absorption of NaCl occurs by an **electroneutral mechanism** (versus the electrogenic mechanism discussed in the next section on the large intestine) in the small intestine and proximal colon wherein the net reaction is the absorption of Na^+ and Cl^- in exchange for H^+ and HCO_3^- efflux.

1. **Absorption of Na^+ in the jejunum.** Na^+ is absorbed in the jejunum by various transporters which include **Na^+–K^+ ATPase, GLUT4, Na^+-amino acid Cotransporters, Na^+–H^+ Exchanger**, and the **HCO_3^- Transporter**.
2. **Absorption of Na^+ in the Ileum.** Na^+ is absorbed in the ileum by various transporters which include **Na^+–K^+ ATPase, GLUT4, Na^+-amino acid Cotransporters, Na^+–H^+ Exchanger, Cl^-–HCO_3^- Exchanger**, and the **Cl^- Transporter**.
3. **Absorption of Cl^-.** Cl^- is absorbed in the small intestine via the paracellular route and by various transporters which include **Na^+–K^+ ATPase, Na^+–Cl^- Cotransporter, Cl^-–HCO_3^- Exchanger**, and the **Cl^- Transporter**.
4. **Absorption of H_2O.** H_2O is absorbed in the small intestine by **diffusion** using **aquaporin H_2O channels** and by **diffusion via the paracellular route** across a zonula occludens between enterocytes. The absorption of electrolytes and H_2O occur in proportion to each other (i.e., in an **isosmotic fashion**). The diffusion of H_2O occurs because of the osmolarity difference between the intestinal fluid and interstitial fluid. The osmolarity difference is created by the reabsorption of solutes (e.g., Na^+). At the start, the intestinal fluid is isosmotic with the interstitial fluid. Then, solutes are reabsorbed from the intestinal fluid which lowers the osmolarity of the intestinal fluid (i.e., hyposmotic or raises H_2O concentration) compared to the interstitial fluid and also raises the osmolarity of the interstitial fluid (i.e., hyperosmotic or lowers H_2O concentration) compared to the intestinal fluid. The osmolarity difference causes net diffusion of H_2O.
5. **Absorption of HCO_3^- in the jejunum.** HCO_3^- is absorbed in the jejunum by various transporters which include **Na^+–K^+ ATPase, Na^+–H^+ Exchanger**, and the **HCO_3^- Transporter**.
6. **Absorption of K^+.** K^+ is absorbed (≈85% of ingested K^+) in the small intestine by **diffusion via the paracellular route** across the zonula occludens between enterocytes.

B. **Secretion of Fluid and Electrolytes.** Secretion occurs by epithelial cells lining the intestinal glands (crypts of Lieberkuhn).

1. **Secretion of Cl^-.** Cl^- is the primary ion secreted by the small intestine. Cl^- is secreted into the intestinal fluid of the small intestine by transporter proteins and two ion channel proteins which include **Na^+–K^+ ATPase, Na^+–K^+–$2Cl^-$ Cotransporter, Cl^- ion-channel protein (cystic fibrosis transmembrane conductance regulator; CFTR)**, and the **Cl^- ion-channel.**
2. **Secretion of Na^+.** Na^+ is secreted via the paracellular route by passively following Cl^- into the intestinal fluid.
3. **Secretion of H_2O.** H_2O is secreted via the paracellular route by passively following Na^+ and Cl^- into the intestinal fluid.
4. **Secretion of HCO_3^- in the Duodenum and Ileum.** HCO_3^- is secreted into the intestinal fluid of the duodenum and ileum by various transporter proteins and ion channel proteins which include **Na^+–K^+ ATPase, Na^+–H^+ Exchanger, Cl^-–HCO_3^- Exchanger, and the Cl^- ion-channel protein (CFTR).**

Large Intestine

 I Large Intestine Motility *(Figure 5-7)*

Material that is not absorbed in the small intestine enters the large intestine where it is called **feces**. The colon receives ≈**500 to 1,500 mL of chyme/day** from the ileum. A major-

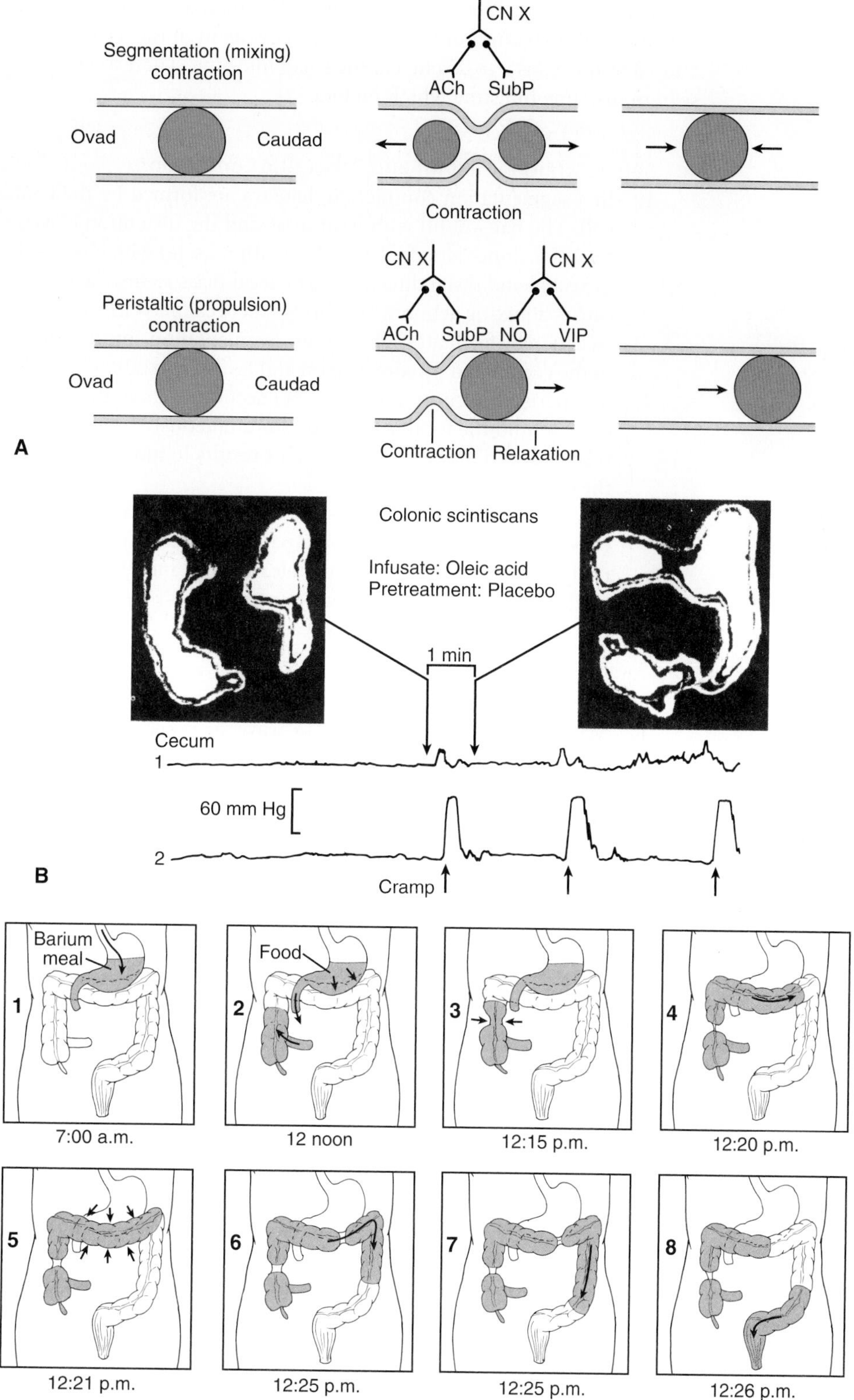

FIGURE 5-7. **Large Intestine Motility. (A) Diagram Shows a Segmentation Contraction and a Peristaltic Contraction.** Note the neurotransmitters involved in the contraction and relaxation of the smooth muscle. **(B) Diagram Shows Mass Movement Contractions.** The colonic scintiscans show a movement of the fecal mass from the ascending colon (on the left) to the splenic flexure (on the right). The pressure tracing (below) demonstrates the mass movement contractions associated with this fecal mass movement and abdominal cramps. **(C) Time Course of Mass Movement Contractions in the Large Intestine.** At 7:00 a.m., a barium breakfast is ingested (1). At noon, the barium breakfast is in the lower ileum and cecum, and the ingestion of lunch accelerates the emptying of the ileum (2). At 12:15 p.m., the tip of the barium breakfast is choked off (3). At 12:20 p.m., the barium breakfast fills the transverse colon (4). At 12:21 p.m., segmentation contractions begin (haustra form) and mix the contents (5). At 12:25 p.m. (still during the consumption of lunch), mass movement contractions occur around the leading end of the large intestinal contents and rapidly propels the contents to the sigmoid colon (6–8). Ach — acetylcholine; SubP — substance P; NO — nitric oxide; VIP — vasoactive intestinal polypeptide.

ity of the fluid and electrolytes that enter the colon are absorbed such that the fecal mass contains ≈**50 to 100 mL of H_2O/day**. The movement of the fecal mass through the colon is 5 to 10 cm/h versus 2 to 25 cm/s in the small intestine. There are three types of contractions seen in the large intestine which include.

A. Segmentation (Mixing) and Peristaltic Contractions

1. In a segmentation contraction, **haustra** are formed by the contraction of the **tenia coli**. The haustra fill with fecal mass and the distention causes the haustra to contract (i.e., inner circular layer of smooth muscle) which sends the fecal mass in both proximal and distal directions. The fecal mass returns with no net movement. This causes a mixing action which brings the fecal mass in contact with the mucosal surface thereby facilitating absorption. Segmentation contractions occur predominately in the cecum and proximal colon and last ≈12 to 60 s.
2. In a peristaltic contraction, a small section of large intestine contracts (i.e., tenia coli) behind the fecal mass while simultaneously, a small section of large intestine relaxes ahead of the fecal mass. This results in movement of the fecal mass toward the anal canal.
3. Smooth muscle contraction is modulated by the **parasympathetic nervous system (CN X)** whereby postganglionic parasympathetic neurons release **ACh** and other postganglionic enteric neurons release **substance P**. Smooth muscle relaxation is modulated by the **parasympathetic nervous system (CN X)** whereby postganglionic enteric neurons release **NO** and **VIP**.

B. Mass Movement Contractions

1. Mass movement contractions (a wave of peristaltic contractions) begin at mid-transverse colon and move the fecal mass a long distance toward the anal canal. Mass movement contractions occur 1 to 3 times/day, are responsible for colonic evacuation, and are associated with cramps.
2. During mass movement contractions, segmentation contractions and haustra temporarily disappear.
3. Mass movement contractions occur shortly after a meal (particularly after breakfast) and stimulate the urge to defecate if some fecal mass is present in the rectum. This is a result of the **gastrocolic reflex** whereby distention of the stomach by food increases the frequency of mass movement contractions in the large intestine.
4. The gastrocolic reflex involves visceral stretch sensory information from **mechanoreceptors** in the stomach which travel with CN X to the CNS and motor impulses mediated by the hormones **gastrin** and **CCK**.

II Defecation Reflex

A. The rectum is usually empty because it is more active in segmental contractions than the sigmoid colon so that the fecal mass tends to move into the sigmoid colon.

B. The internal anal sphincter (smooth muscle) is usually tonically contracted.

C. When mass movement contractions occur, the fecal mass distends the rectum to >25% of capacity and initiates a reflexive relaxation of the internal anal sphincter and a reflexive contraction of the external anal sphincter (striated muscle).

D. This is called the **retrosphincteric reflex**. Sensory impulses from **pressure-sensitive receptors** travel to sacral spinal cord levels. Motor impulses travel with the **pelvic splanchnic nerves (parasympathetic; S2 to S4)** and relax the internal anal sphincter. This causes the urge to defecate.

E. If the Person Decides to Defecate

1. Relaxation of the external anal sphincter (via the **pudendal nerve**) and puborectalis muscle (via the **nerve to the levator ani**) occurs.

2. Evacuation is preceded by a deep breath which moves the diaphragm down.
3. The glottis closes, and contraction of the respiratory muscles with full lungs elevates both intrathoracic and intra-abdominal pressures.
4. The abdominal muscles also contract, which further raises the intra-abdominal pressure.
5. The increased pressure helps to force the fecal mass through the relaxed external anal sphincter.
6. The muscles of the pelvic diaphragm also relax, allowing the pelvic floor to drop and straighten out the rectum.

F. If the Person Decides Not to Defecate

1. Contraction of the external anal sphincter (via the **pudendal nerve**) and puborectalis muscle (via the **nerve to the levator ani**) occurs.
2. Pressure-sensitive receptors accommodate relieving the sensation to defecate, the fecal mass moves back into the rectum, and the tone of the internal anal sphincter is regained by the **hypogastric plexus** and **lumbar splanchnic nerves (sympathetic)**.

III Absorption and Secretion of Fluid and Electrolytes

The enterocytes of the GI tract (small intestine and large intestine) absorb ≈9 L of fluid/day. The enterocytes of the small intestine absorb ≈7 L of fluid/day so that normally ≈2 L of fluid/day is delivered to the large intestine. If >2.5 L of fluid/day is delivered to the large intestine, diarrhea will occur.

A. Absorption of Fluid and Electrolytes. In the small intestine and proximal colon, the absorption of NaCl occurs by an **electroneutral mechanism** whereby the net reaction is the absorption of Na^+ and Cl^- in exchange for H^+ and HCO_3^- efflux. In the distal colon, the absorption of NaCl occurs by an **electrogenic mechanism.**

1. **Absorption of Na^+ in the proximal colon.** Na^+ is absorbed in the proximal colon (by an electroneutral mechanism identical to that of the ileum) by various transporters which include **Na^+–K^+ ATPase, GLUT4, Na^+-amino acid Cotransporters, Na^+–H^+ Exchanger, Cl^-–HCO_3^- Exchanger**, and the **Cl^- Transporter**.
2. **Absorption of Na^+ in the distal colon.** Na^+ is absorbed in the distal colon (by an electrogenic mechanism) by various transporter proteins and ion-channels proteins which include **Na^+–K^+ ATPase, Electrogenic Na^+ ion-channel protein, and the K^+ ion-channel protein.**
3. **Absorption of Cl^- in the proximal colon.** Cl^- is absorbed in the proximal colon (by an electroneutral mechanism identical to that of the small intestine) via the paracellular route and by various transporters which include **Na^+–K^+ ATPase, Na^+–Cl^- Cotransporter, Cl^-–HCO_3^- Exchanger, and the Cl^- Transporter.**
4. **Absorption of Cl^- in the distal colon.** Cl^- is absorbed in the distal colon via the paracellular route driven by the electrogenic Na^+ absorption.
5. **Absorption of H_2O in the colon.** H_2O is absorbed in the colon by the **standing osmotic gradient mechanism**. This is in contrast to the absorption of H_2O in the small intestine which occurs in an isosmotic fashion whereby the absorption of electrolytes and H_2O occur in proportion to each other. The standing osmotic gradient mechanism involves **Na^+–K^+ ATPase** located in the basolateral membrane of enterocytes near the apical end of the lateral intercellular space. Na^+ is pumped from the cytoplasm into the intercellular space and Cl^- and HCO_3^- follow to preserve electroneutrality. The hyperosmotic solution of NaCl near the apical end of the intercellular space causes the osmotic flow of H_2O into the intercellular space from the intestinal fluid and neighboring enterocytes.

6. **Absorption of K^+ in the colon.** K^+ is absorbed in the colon by a transporter protein and ion channel protein which include **H^+–K^+ ATPase** and **K^+ ion-channel protein.**

B. Secretion of Electrolytes

1. **Secretion of Cl^- in the colon.** Cl^- is secreted in the colon in a manner identical to that in the small intestine. Cl^- is secreted into the intestinal fluid of the colon by transporter proteins and two ion channel proteins which include **Na^+–K^+ ATPase, Na^+–K^+–$2Cl^-$ Cotransporter, Cl^- ion-channel protein (CFTR),** and the **Cl^- ion-channel protein.**
2. **Secretion of HCO_3^- in the colon.** HCO_3^- secretion in the colon is somewhat enigmatic. Some HCO_3^- secretion in the colon is stimulated by the short chain fatty acids and seems to involve HCO_3^- diffusion into the intestinal fluid in response to a pH gradient. In addition, some HCO_3^- is secreted in the colon in a manner identical to that in the small intestine. HCO_3^- is secreted into the intestinal fluid of the colon by various transporter proteins and ion channel proteins which include **Na^+–K^+ ATPase, Na^+–H^+ Exchanger, Cl^-–HCO_3^- Exchanger,** and the **Cl^- ion-channel protein (CFTR)**
3. **Secretion of K^+ in the Colon.** K^+ is secreted in the colon by transporter proteins and ion channel proteins which include **Na^+–K^+ ATPase, Na^+–K^+–$2Cl^-$ Cotransporter,** and the **K^+ ion channel protein.**

IV Intestinal Gas (Flatus)

A. Flatus is passed 10 to 14 times/day. The composition and frequency of flatus is a result of dietary intake of fermentable substrates (e.g., carbohydrates, nonabsorbable carbohydrates like stachyose and raffinose in beans and legumes, poorly absorbable carbohydrates like fructose and sorbitol in fruit, and starches) and the activity of the colonic bacterial flora.

B. The principal gases of flatus are **O_2, N_2, CO_2, H_2,** and **CH_4 (methane).**
   1. The O_2 and N_2 in flatus are derived mainly from swallowed air during eating and drinking and also by diffusion from the bloodstream.
   2. The CO_2 in flatus is derived from bacterial fermentation of dietary substrates and perhaps from the neutralization of HCl by HCO_3^- in the GI tract.
   3. The H_2 in flatus is derived from bacterial fermentation of dietary carbohydrates particularly.
   4. The CH_4 (methane) in flatus is derived from bacterial fermentation (by *Methanobrevibacter smithii*) of dietary carbohydrates and proteins.

C. The majority of the gas within flatus is odorless (i.e., O_2, N_2, CO_2, H_2, and CH_4 [methane]).

D. The gases within flatus that cause odor and are socially unacceptable are H_2S (hydrogen sulfide), NH_3 (ammonia), and volatile fatty acids and amino acids.

E. Flatulence can be treated by controlling aerophagia (i.e., the amount of swallowed air) by eliminating gum or candy chewing, stopping smoking, improving oral hygiene, and receiving treatment for anxiety.

F. Flatulence can also be treated by restricting the diet (i.e., reducing consumption of beans, legumes, fruits, and starches). Flatulence can also be treated by taking activated charcoal before meals or simethicone.

V Summary of Overall Fluid Balance in the Small and Large Intestine *(Figure 5-8)*

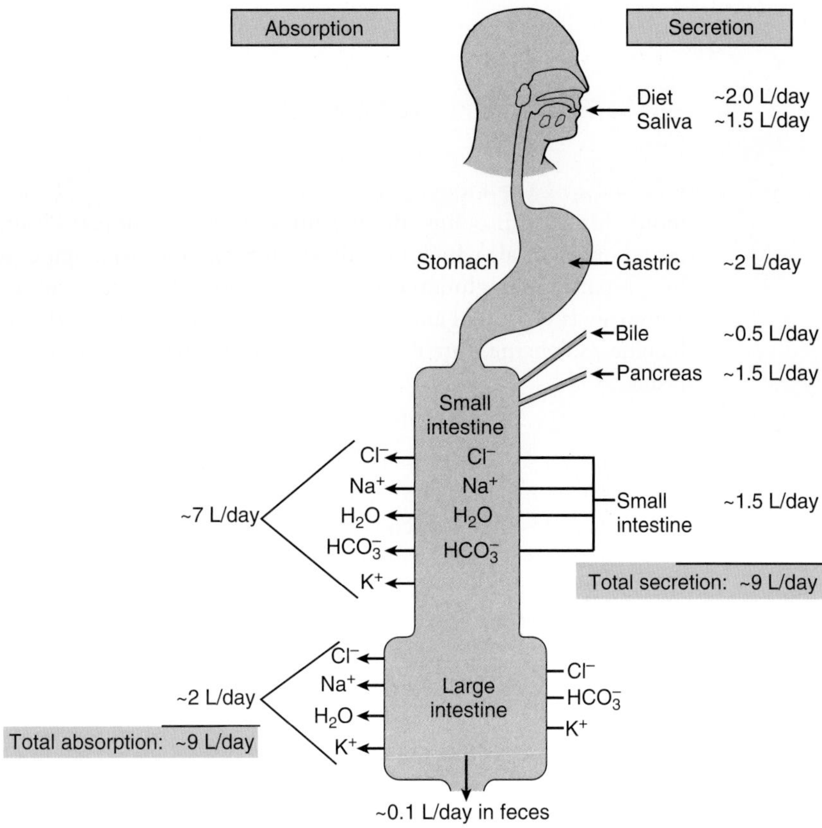

FIGURE 5-8. **Summary Diagram of the Overall Fluid Balance in the Small and Large Intestine.** A total of ≈9 L/day enters the GI tract with 2 L/day from the diet and 7 L/day from various secretions. Of this ≈9 L/day total, the small intestine absorbs ≈7 L/day which delivers ≈2 L/day to the large intestine. The large intestine absorbs ≈2 L/day leaving ≈100 mL/day to be excreted with the feces. If >2.5 L/day is delivered to the large intestine, diarrhea will occur.

Liver

The many varied functions of the liver include:

I Lymph Production

II Uptake and Release of IgA

III Storage of Iron

IV Storage of Vitamin A

V Carbohydrate Metabolism

A. **Synthesis of Glycogen**
B. **Degradation of Glycogen**
C. **Synthesis of Glucose (or Gluconeogenesis)**
D. **Degradation of Monosaccharides.** Hepatocytes metabolize glucose, fructose, and galactose.

VI Protein and Amino Acid Metabolism

A. **Synthesis of Proteins** (see Table 5-2)

B. **Synthesis of the Eleven Nonessential Amino Acids.** Of the 20 amino acids commonly found in proteins, the hepatocytes can synthesize 11 amino acids (hence, the term nonessential) which include glycine, alanine, asparagine, serine, glutamine, proline, aspartic acid, glutamic acid, cysteine, tyrosine, and arginine. The remaining nine amino acids (essential amino acids) must be consumed in the diet and include valine, leucine, isoleucine, threonine, phenylalanine, tryptophan, methionine, histidine, and lysine.

C. **Degradation of Ammonia (NH_3)**

1. NH_3 which is produced from protein and nucleic acid catabolism is highly neurotoxic and is therefore converted to nontoxic **urea** in hepatocytes by the **urea cycle**. The urea is released from the liver into the blood and excreted in the urine by the kidneys. Approximately 30 g of urea/day is excreted by a healthy adult eating a normal diet.

TABLE 5-2 SYNTHESIS OF PROTEINS BY THE LIVER

Protein	Function
Albumin	The liver synthesizes 3 g/day of albumin which plays an important role in plasma volume and colloid osmotic pressure of the plasma. The importance of albumin is emphasized that liver disease and long-term starvation result in generalized edema and ascites. Albumin acts as a carrier protein for many active substances and drugs.
Components of the complement system	Used in the inflammatory response
Fibrinogen, prothrombin, and factors V, VII, IX, X, XII	Cascade proteins used in blood clotting
VLDL, LDL, HDL	Lipoproteins used in the transport of lipids in the blood
Transferrin	Used in iron transport
Ceruloplasmin	Used in Cu^{2+} transport
Haptoglobin, hemopexin, and many other plasma proteins	Functions vary
α-Fetoprotein	Produced by the embryonic liver and regenerating liver which can be used as an indicator of liver carcinoma; sometimes called "fetal albumin"
α_1-Antitrypsin	A serum protease inhibitor. **α_1-antitrypsin deficiency** is an autosomal recessive disorder caused by a missense mutation where methionine 358 is replaced with arginine (i.e., the Pittsburgh variant), which destroys the affinity for elastase and results in pulmonary emphysema. Normally, methionine 358 in the reactive center of α_1-antitrypsin acts as a "bait" for elastase wherein elastase is trapped and inactivated. This protects the physiologically important elastic fibers present in the lung from destruction.
IGF-1 and IGF-2	Insulin-like growth factors which are involved in growth-hormone independent tissue growth in general and increase protein synthesis in chondrocytes at the epiphyseal growth plate and cause linear bone growth (i.e., the pubertal growth spurt).
Angiotensinogen	Is converted to angiotensin II by renin (release from the macula densa cells in the kidney), which plays a role in the regulation of blood pressure.
Retinol-binding protein	Binds retinol (vitamin A)
Apoproteins	Plays a role in lipid transport in the plasma

VII Lipid Metabolism

A. Synthesis of 25-Hydroxylation of Vitamin D

B. Synthesis of Fatty Acids

C. Degradation (or β-Oxidation) of Fatty Acids. Fatty acids are a major source of energy in the human and are oxidized by a process called **β-oxidation.** In the liver, acetyl CoA is converted to **ketone bodies** which can be oxidized by muscle, kidney, or the brain during starvation.

D. Synthesis of Ketone Bodies (Acetoacetate and 3-Hydroxybutyrate). The synthesis of ketone bodies (acetoacetate and 3-hydroxybutyrate) occurs mainly in the liver whenever fatty acid levels are high in the blood (e.g., fasting, starvation, or high-fat diet).

E. Synthesis of Cholesterol

F. Synthesis of Lipoproteins (*Figure 5-9*). Lipids (e.g., free cholesterol, cholesterol esters, and triacyglycerols) are insoluble in plasma and therefore are transported in the plasma as **lipoproteins**. Lipoproteins consist of a polar coat (composed of **phospholipids, free cholesterol**, and **apoproteins**) surrounding a central core (composed of **triacylglycerols** and **cholesterol esters**).

1. **Very low density lipoprotein** (*Figure 5-9C*)
   a. Hepatocytes synthesize and release very low density lipoprotein (VLDL), which is relatively rich in triacylglycerols (55%), into the plasma.
   b. VLDL travels to skeletal muscle and adipose tissue where the triacylglycerols are hydrolyzed by **lipoprotein lipase** (located on the endothelial cells of capillaries) to **fatty acids** and **glycerol**.
   c. The fatty acids are oxidized in skeletal muscle or stored as triacylglycerols in adipose tissue.
   d. As the triacylglycerols in VLDL are hydrolyzed, the core of VLDL is reduced, thereby generating intermediate density lipoprotein (IDL).
2. **Intermediate density lipoprotein** (*Figure 5-9C*)
   a. IDL returns to the liver, binds to LDL receptors or IDL receptors located on hepatocytes, and undergo lysosomal digestion.
   b. IDL may also undergo further hydrolysis of triacylglycerol by lipoprotein lipase or hepatic lipase and thereby be converted to LDL.
3. **Low density lipoprotein** (*Figure 5-9C*)
   a. LDL which is rich in cholesterol and cholesterol esters distributes cholesterol to cells throughout the body (i.e., both hepatic and nonhepatic cells) that have specific **LDL receptors**.
   b. LDL can also enter macrophages that have **scavenger receptors** which results in the intracellular accumulation of cholesterol and the formation of **foam cells**.
   c. LDL is internalized by a normal process called **receptor-mediated endocytosis**, which involves the following steps:
      i. Circulating serum LDL ("bad cholesterol") binds to the LDL receptor located on the cell membrane ($apoB_{100}$ is the ligand) and the complex undergoes endocytosis as clathrin-coated vesicles.
      ii. The clathrin-coated vesicles fuse with **endosomes**, where LDL disassociates from the LDL receptor due to pH↓, and the LDL receptor is recycled to the cell membrane.
      iii. **Endolysosomes** containing active lysosomal enzymes fuse and digest the LDL to cholesterol.
      iv. Cholesterol can then be used for the following processes: synthesis of cell membranes; synthesis of bile salts in hepatocytes; synthesis of steroid hormones in certain endocrine cells; inhibition of **3-hydroxy-3-methyglutaryl**

CoA reductase, which suppresses de novo cholesterol synthesis, and therefore maintains normal levels of serum cholesterol; activation of acyl cholesterol acyl transferase which converts cholesterol to cholesterol esters for storage.

d. Since LDL distributes cholesterol to cells throughout the body, LDL is called "**bad cholesterol**" and is the target in lipid lowering therapy.

e. **Familial Hypercholesterolemia** is a genetic disease involving a mutation in the **LDL receptor** in which patients have greatly elevated levels of serum cholesterol and suffer myocardial infarctions early in life. The mutation in the LDL receptor blocks receptor-mediated endocytosis.

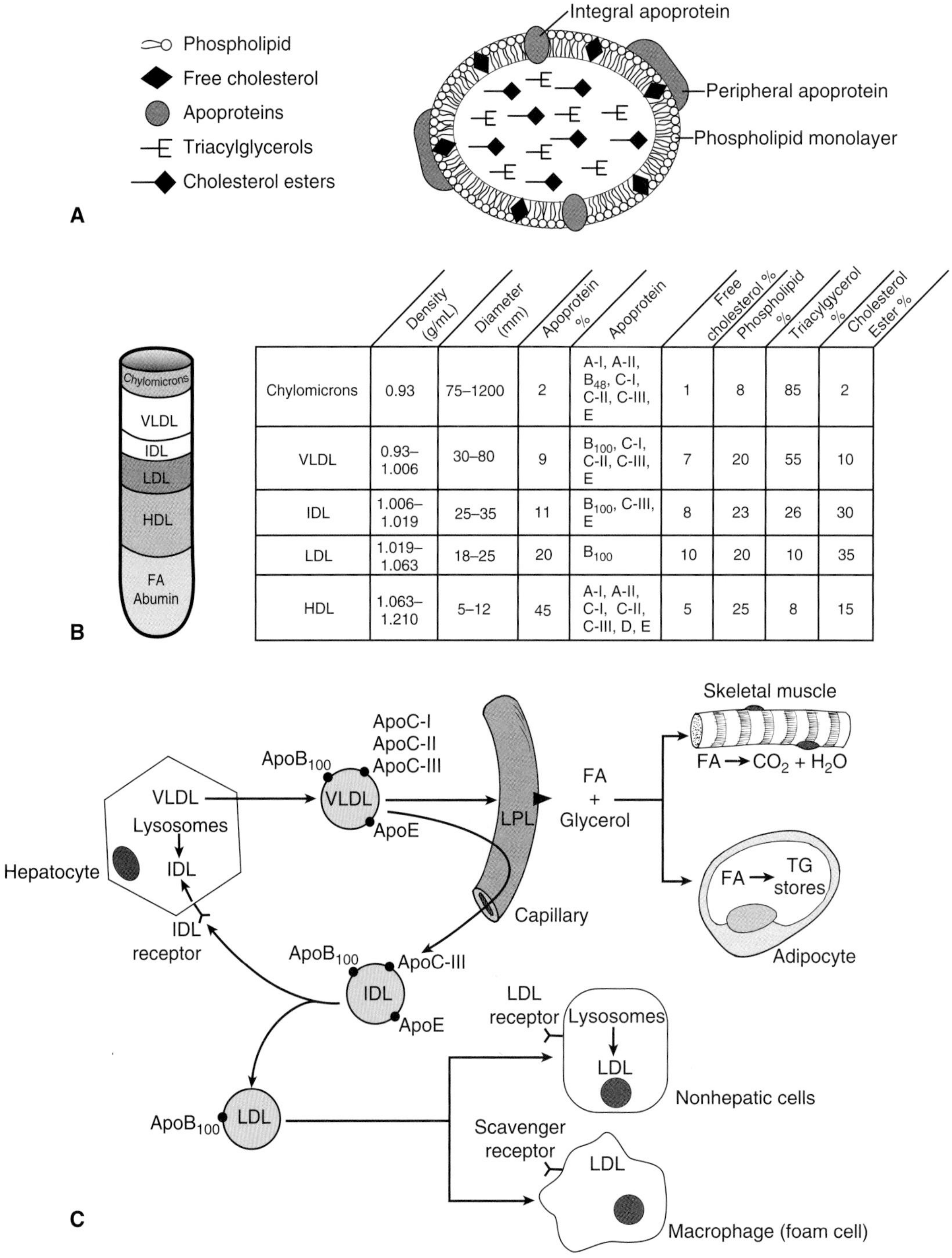

	Density (g/mL)	Diameter (mm)	Apoprotein %	Apoprotein	Free cholesterol %	Phospholipid %	Triacylglycerol %	Cholesterol Ester %
Chylomicrons	0.93	75–1200	2	A-I, A-II, B_{48}, C-I, C-II, C-III, E	1	8	85	2
VLDL	0.93–1.006	30–80	9	B_{100}, C-I, C-II, C-III, E	7	20	55	10
IDL	1.006–1.019	25–35	11	B_{100}, C-III, E	8	23	26	30
LDL	1.019–1.063	18–25	20	B_{100}	10	20	10	35
HDL	1.063–1.210	5–12	45	A-I, A-II, C-I, C-II, C-III, D, E	5	25	8	15

FIGURE 5-9. **Lipoproteins. (A)** Diagram of the contents and arrangement of a typical lipoprotein. **(B)** Composition of lipoproteins. **(C)** Metabolism of VLDL, IDL, and LDL. VLDL — very low density lipoprotein; IDL — intermediate density lipoprotein; LDL — low density lipoprotein; FA — fatty acids; TG — triacylglycerol.

4. **High density lipoprotein** (*Figure 5-10A*)
   a. Hepatocytes synthesize and release high density lipoprotein (HDL), which is relatively poor in triacylglycerols (8%), cholesterol (5%), and cholesterol esters (15%), into the plasma.
   b. HDL has various functions which include
      i. Traveling to various tissues in the body and acquiring free cholesterol with the aid of **apoprotein A-I** which is a signal transduction protein that mobilizes cholesterol esters from intracellular pools and **cholesterol**

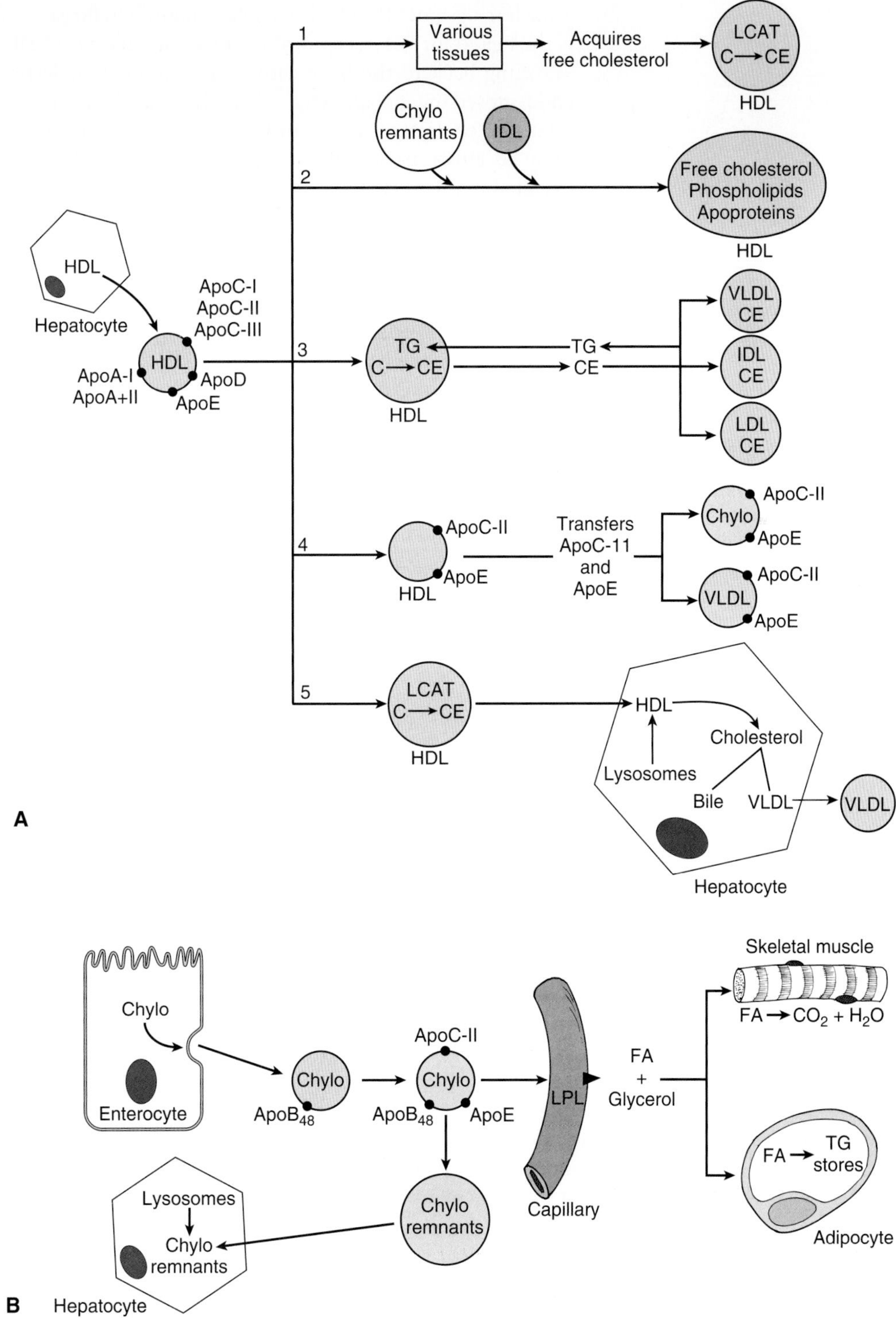

FIGURE 5-10. **Metabolism of HDL and Chylomicrons. (A)** Metabolism of HDL. **(B)** Metabolism of chylomicrons. C — cholesterol; CE — cholesterol esters; CHYLO — chylomicrons; LCAT — lecithin-cholesterol acyl transferase; FA — fatty acids; TG — triacylglycerol.

efflux regulatory protein. After diffusion of free cholesterol onto HDL, the cholesterol is re-esterified to cholesterol esters by **lecithin-cholesterol acyl transferase.**

ii. Acquiring free cholesterol, phospholipids, and apoproteins from chylomicron remnants and IDL.

iii. Transferring some of the re-esterified cholesterol esters to VLDL, IDL, and LDL using **cholesterol ester transfer protein** in exchange for triacylglycerols so that cholesterol can be delivered to various tissues for storage or steroid synthesis.

iv. Transferring apoC-II (which activates lipoprotein lipase) and apoE (which is the ligand for IDL receptors) to chylomicrons and VLDL.

v. Traveling back to the liver with its re-esterified cholesterol esters. It is endocytosed by hepatocytes where lysosomal enzymes digest the re-esterified cholesterol esters to free cholesterol. The free cholesterol can then be either packaged into VLDL and released into the plasma or excreted in the bile.

c. Since HDL facilitates the flow of excess plasma triacylglycerols and cholesterol back to the liver, HDL is called "**good cholesterol.**"

5. **Chylomicrons** (*Figure 5-10B*)
   a. Enterocytes of the small intestine synthesize and release chylomicrons which are relatively rich in triacylglycerols (85%), cholesterol esters, and phospholipids directly into the lymph which then enter the plasma.
   b. Nascent chylomicrons contain apoB$_{48}$ and then acquire apoC-II (which activates lipoprotein lipase) and apoE (which is the ligand for IDL receptors) from HDL.
   c. Chylomicrons travel to skeletal muscle and adipose tissue where the triacylglycerols are hydrolyzed by **lipoprotein lipase** (located on the endothelial cells of capillaries) to **fatty acids** and **glycerol**.
   d. The fatty acids are oxidized in skeletal muscle or stored as triacylglycerols in adipose tissue.
   e. The resulting **chylomicron remnants** travel to the liver and are endocytosed by hepatocytes where lysosomal enzymes digest the chylomicrons remnants to amino acids, fatty acids, and cholesterol which are reutilized by the hepatocytes.

VIII Degradation of Drugs

The oral bioavailability of drugs is enhanced by making drugs lipophilic. However, the lipophilic nature of drugs prevents clearance by the kidneys. Therefore, drugs must be transformed into hydrophilic compounds that are soluble in aqueous urine. Phase I and II reactions make drugs more hydrophilic. The hepatocytes metabolize drugs by biotransformation which occurs in three stages as indicated below.

A. Phase I Reactions (Oxidation)

1. The enzymes that catalyze **cytochrome P$_{450}$-dependent Phase I reactions** are **hemeprotein monooxygenases** of the **cytochrome P$_{450}$ class** (also called the **microsomal mixed function oxidases**) which catalyze the biotransformation of drugs by hydroxylation, dealkylation, oxidation, desulfuration, and epoxide formation.
2. In addition, there are **cytochrome P$_{450}$-independent Phase I reactions** which allow local hydrolysis of ester-containing and amide-containing drugs (e.g., local anesthetics) at their site of administration and allow the oxidation of amine-containing compounds (e.g., catecholamines, tyramine) using **monoamine oxidase**.

B. Phase II Reactions (Conjugation)

1. The enzymes that catalyze Phase II reactions are transfer enzymes which catalyze the biotransformation of drugs by glucuronidation (using **UDP-glucuronyl**

transferase and **UDP-glucuronic acid** as the glucuronide donor), acetylation, glycine conjugation, sulfate conjugation, glutathione conjugation, and methylation.
2. Phase II reaction metabolites are pharmacologically inactive.

C. **Phase III Reactions (Elimination).** The elimination of Phase I and II biotransformation products from hepatocytes requires active transport using transporters (i.e., ATPase pumps) that pump the products either into the blood for elimination by the kidneys or into the bile for elimination by the GI tract.

IX Degradation of Ethanol

When alchohol consumption is normal, ≈80% of the ethanol is metabolized to **acetaldehyde and NADH** by hepatocytes using **alcohol dehydrogenase.** When alcohol consumption is high, ≈20% of the ethanol is metabolized to **acetaldehyde** by hepatocytes using the **microsomal ethanol-oxidizing system.** In chronic alcoholism, much of the tissue damage is believed to result from an **excess of acetaldehyde**.

X Synthesis of Bile Salts

Bile salts are synthesized from cholesterol when an α-OH group is added to carbon 7 of cholesterol to form **7α-hydroxycholesterol** using **7α-hydroxylase** (the rate limiting step). **Chenocholic acid** can conjugate with either glycine or taurine amino acids, forming **glycochenocholic acid** or **taurochenocholic acid. Cholic acid** can also conjugate with either glycine or taurine amino acids, forming **glycocholic acid** or **taurocholic acid.** Chenocholic acid, cholic acid, and their conjugates are called **primary bile salts.**

XI Production and Composition of Bile

Bile is a green–yellow complex mixture of organic and inorganic components which are released into bile canaliculi and travel to the gallbladder by the following route: bile canaliculi → cholangioles → canals of Hering → bile ductules in the portal triad → right and left hepatic ducts → common hepatic duct → gallbladder. The liver produces ≈**700 mL of bile/day**. The components of bile include the following:

A. **Bile Salts.** Bile salts are the major component of bile and are taken up from the portal blood into hepatocytes by using the **Na^+-conjugated bile salt cotransporter, Na^+independent conjugated bile salt transporter, and anion-unconjugated bile salt exchanger**, and by **diffusion** of unconjugated bile salts. In the hepatocyte cytoplasm, bile salts are bound to **bile salt-binding proteins**, which prevents the disruption of hepatocyte organelles. The bile salts are then released into bile canaliculi using the **biliary acid transporter**.

B. **Cholesterol.** Cholesterol is released into bile canaliculi using the **MDR1 transporter** (multidrug resistance).

C. **Lecithin (Phosphatidylcholine).** Lecithin is released into bile canaliculi using the **MDR2 transporter**.

D. **Bilirubin–Glucuronide (Bile Pigment).** Bilirubin–glucuronide is released into bile canaliculi using **MOAT** (multispecific organ anionic transporter).

E. **H_2O, Na^+, Cl^-, K^+, Ca^{2+}, and HCO_3^-.** The release of H_2O and electrolytes into bile canaliculi occurs by two mechanisms.
1. **Bile salt dependent mechanism.** In this mechanism, the active transport of bile salts into bile canaliculi creates an osmotic gradient that allows H_2O to flow into bile canaliculi through the "leaky" zonula occludens whereby various electrolytes follow by solvent drag.

2. **Intrahepatic bile duct dependent mechanism**
   a. In this mechanism, the epithelial cells lining the intrahepatic bile ducts secrete an aqueous solution that makes up ≈50% of the total volume of bile. The intrahepatic bile ducts are not just merely conduits for bile.
   b. This aqueous secretion contains H_2O, Na^+, Cl^-, K^+, and HCO_3^- and is under the control of **SEC** which is secreted by enteroendocrine S cells in the crypts of Lieberkuhn of the small intestine.
   c. In addition, there appears to be a **HCO_3^-–Cl^- exchanger** located on the cell membrane of the bile canaliculi that contributes to the HCO_3^- content of bile.
   d. The intrahepatic bile ducts also absorb H_2O, Na^+, and Cl^- although secretion predominates.

F. Secretory IgA

G. **Conjugated Drugs and Steroid hormones.** Drugs and steroid hormones that have undergone Phase I and II reactions are released into bile canaliculi using unidentified ATPase pumps for elimination by the GI tract.

XII Production and Fate of Bilirubin

A. Approximately 85% of bilirubin (water insoluble) is derived from the breakdown of hemoglobin (heme moiety; i.e., senescent RBCs) by macrophages in the spleen and Kupffer cells in the liver (Heme → biliverdin → bilirubin). Approximately 15% of bilirubin is derived from the breakdown of other heme-containing proteins (e.g., myoglobin, cytochromes, and catalase).
B. Bilirubin travels in the blood as an **albumin–bilirubin complex** (Note: free bilirubin is toxic to the brain).
C. Bilirubin is endocytosed by hepatocytes and conjugated to glucuronide to form **bilirubin–glucuronide** (a water soluble bile pigment) using **UDP-glucuronyltransferase.**
D. Bilirubin–glucuronide is released into bile canaliculi using MOAT.
E. Within the distal small intestine and colon, bilirubin–glucuronide is broken down to **free bilirubin** by intestinal bacterial flora.
F. Free bilirubin is reduced to **urobilinogen** and eliminated in feces, reabsorbed, or excreted into the urine.
G. Urobilinogen is also oxidized in the urine and feces to form **urobilin** and **stercobilin** which are responsible for the color of the urine and feces.

Gallbladder

I Concentration of Bile

A. The liver produces ≈700 mL of bile/day while the gallbladder can store only ≈35 mL of bile.
B. The discrepancy between the amount of bile produced by the liver and the amount stored by the gallbladder is explained by the ability of the gallbladder to concentrate the bile 5 to 20 times through absorption of water and electrolytes by the **standing osmotic gradient mechanism**.
C. The standing osmotic gradient mechanism involves **Na^+–K^+ ATPase** located in the basolateral membrane of gallbladder epithelium near the apical end of the lateral intercellular space.
D. Na^+ is pumped from the cytoplasm into the intercellular space and Cl^- follows to preserve electroneutrality.
E. The hyperosmotic solution of NaCl near the apical end of the intercellular space causes the osmotic flow of H_2O into the lateral intercellular space from the luminal bile.

II Bile Release from Gallbladder into the Small Intestine

A. Stimulation

1. Gallbladder emptying begins several minutes after the start of a meal.
2. **During the cephalic phase of HCl secretion**, the sight, smell, taste, and conditioned reflexes involved with food begin gallbladder emptying which is mediated by **CN X (vagus nerve)** and probably **gastrin.**
3. **During the gastric phase of HCl secretion**, stomach distention also plays a role in gallbladder emptying mediated by CN X and probably gastrin.
4. **During the intestinal phase of HCl secretion, CCK** is secreted into the blood by the enteroendocrine I-cells in response to amino acids/small peptides and fatty acids/monoglycerides present in the small intestinal lumen. CCK binds to **CCK1 receptors** located on the smooth muscle cells in the wall of the gallbladder.
5. The highest rate of gallbladder emptying occurs during the intestinal phase of HCl secretion mostly in response to CCK.
6. CCK causes the contraction of smooth muscle in the wall of the gallbladder and relaxation of the smooth muscle of the sphincter of Oddi.
7. The relaxation of the smooth muscle of the sphincter of Oddi also involves the neurotransmitter **NO** released from postganglionic parasympathetic neurons.

B. Inhibition. Relaxation of the smooth muscle in the wall of the gallbladder and contraction of the smooth muscle of the sphincter of Oddi are mediated by the **sympathetic nervous system. Somatostatin** has an inhibitory effect on the gallbladder.

Exocrine Pancreas

I Pancreatic Secretion *(Figure 5-11)*

The pancreas secretes ≈**1.5 L of fluid/day** which contains digestive enzymes, cations (Na^+, K^+), anions (Cl^-, HCO_3^-), albumin, and globulins.

A. Digestive Enzymes

1. The digestive enzymes include **trypsinogen, chymotrypsinogen, proelastase, procarboxypeptidase A, procarboxypeptidase B, pancreatic lipase, colipase, cholesterol ester hydrolase, phospholipase A_2, ribonuclease, deoxyribonuclease**, and **pancreatic amylase**.
2. Several of the digestive enzymes are capable of damaging the pancreas and are therefore secreted in an inactive form (called a **proenzyme**).
3. The proenzymes are activated in the duodenum by **enterokinase** located in the glycocalyx of enterocytes which converts trypsinogen (inactive proenzyme) → trypsin (active enzyme).

B. Cl^- and HCO_3^- Secretion.

The bulk of the pancreatic juice is a **Na^+, K^+, Cl^-**, and **HCO_3^--rich juice (135 mM Na HCO_3^- at pH 8)** produced by the **duct epithelium** of the **intercalated, intralobular**, and **interlobular ducts**, which, together with the secretions from the gallbladder and intestine, serves to neutralize the gastric HCl in the duodenum. Na^+ and K^+ follow Cl^- into the pancreatic juice by moving through the zonula occludens. Cl^- and HCO_3^- are secreted into the pancreatic juice by various transporter proteins and ion channel proteins which include **Na^+–K^+ ATPase, Na^+–K^+–$2Cl^-$ Cotransporter, Na^+–HCO_3^- Cotransporter, Na^+–H^+ Exchanger, Cl^-–HCO_3^- Exchanger, Cl^- ion-channel protein (CFTR)**, and the **Cl^- ion-channel protein.**

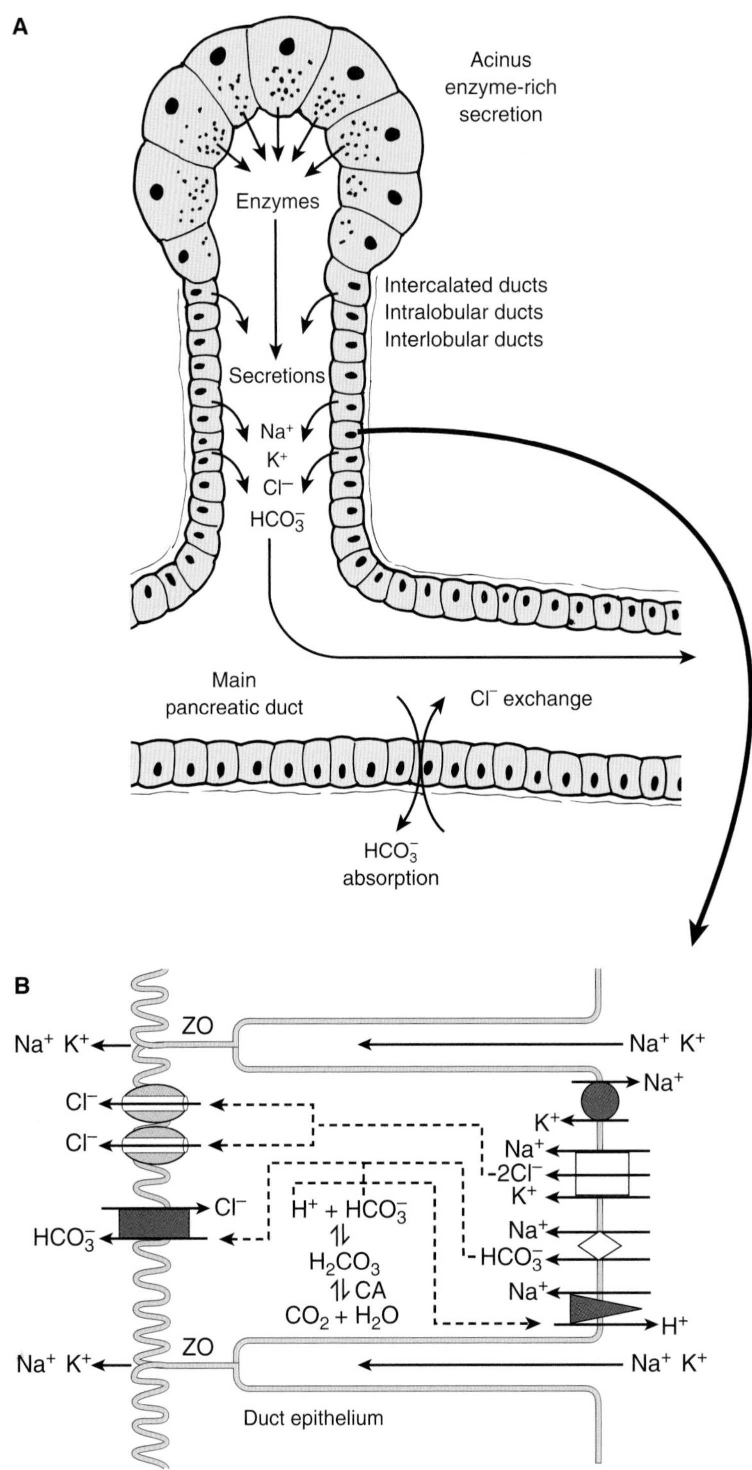

FIGURE 5-11. **Pancreatic Secretion. (A)** Diagram of an acinus and duct system shows the secretion of enzymes from the acinus and production of the aqueous component (Na^+, K^+, Cl^-, and HCO_3^-) into the duct network. **(B)** Diagram shows the mechanism of secretion of Cl^- and HCO_3^- by the duct epithelium and the flow of Na^+ and K^+ through the zonula occludens (ZO).

II Absorption of HCO_3^-

A. The HCO_3^- content of the pancreatic juice is modified by the absorption of HCO_3^- in the main pancreatic duct (duct of Wirsung).

B. HCO_3^- is absorbed into the blood by a **Cl^-–HCO_3^- Exchanger** that transports Cl^- across the basolateral membrane into the cytoplasm by countertransport with HCO_3^- into the blood.

C. In other words, Cl^- is ultimately transported into the pancreatic juice and HCO_3^- is transported out of the pancreatic juice.

III Concentration of Anions in Pancreatic Juice versus Flow *(Figure 5-12)*

The concentration of Cl^- and HCO_3^- vary with the rate of flow of the pancreatic juice.

A. Low Flow Rate (Long Contact Time)

1. When the pancreas is not stimulated by SEC, a low flow rate of pancreatic juices occurs.
2. With a low flow rate, there is more time for absorption of HCO_3^- and exchange for Cl^- by the main pancreatic duct (duct of Wirsung) to occur.
3. Therefore, the concentration of HCO_3^- will be low and the concentration of Cl^- will be high in the pancreatic juice.

B. High Flow Rate (Short Contact Time)

1. When the pancreas is stimulated by SEC, a high flow rate of pancreatic juice occurs.
2. With a high flow rate, there is less time for absorption of HCO_3^- and exchange for Cl^- by the main pancreatic duct (duct of Wirsung) to occur.
3. Therefore, the concentration of HCO_3^- will be high and the concentration of Cl^- will be low in the pancreatic juice.

IV Control of Pancreatic Secretion

A. Stimulation

1. **Cholecystokinin.** CCK increases pancreatic enzyme secretion (major role) and aqueous/HCO_3^- secretion (weak, but physiologically relevant). CCK plays a role in the intestinal phase of pancreatic secretion.
2. **Secretin.** SEC increases aqueous/HCO_3^- secretion from the duct epithelium. [illegible]C plays a role in the intestinal phase of pancreatic secretion.
3. **Parasympathetic nervous system. CN X (vagus)** enhances the rate secretion of pancreatic enzymes and aqueous components of the pancreatic juice. CN X plays a role in the cephalic and gastric phases of pancreatic secretion.

B. Inhibition

1. **Hyperglycemia** and **hyperaminoacidemia** inhibit exocrine pancreatic secretion probably through the secondary release of inhibitory hormones like **glucagon** or **somatostatin.**
2. **Presence of lipid in the colon** inhibits exocrine pancreatic secretion which may serve as physiological signal to stop pancreatic secretion after digestion and absorption are completed.
3. **Peptide YY, PP (pancreatic polypeptide)**, and **GLP-1** inhibit exocrine pancreas secretion although little is known about their mechanism except that they do not work by direct inhibition of pancreatic acinar cells.
4. **Sympathetic nervous system.** Postganglionic axons (norepinephrine) from the celiac ganglion inhibit pancreatic secretion probably by reducing the blood flow.

V Phases of Pancreatic Secretion

A. Cephalic Phase

1. The cephalic phase is initiated by **sight, smell, taste**, and **conditioned reflexes.**
2. The cephalic phase accounts for ≈25% of the total pancreatic juice secreted in response to a meal.
3. The cephalic phase is controlled by the **parasympathetic nervous system** (CN X).

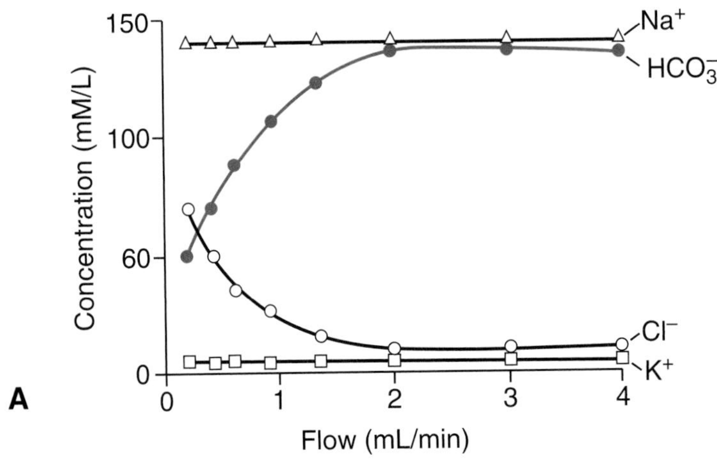

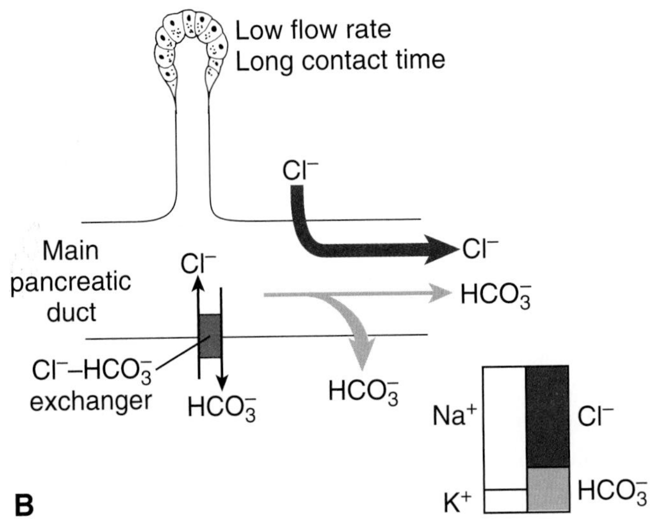

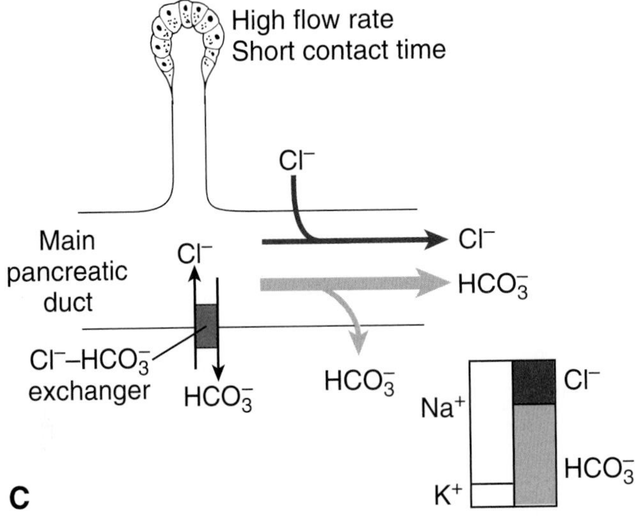

FIGURE 5-12. **Concentration of Anions in Pancreatic Juice versus Flow. (A)** Graph shows the changes in concentration of Na^+, K^+, Cl^-, and HCO_3^- in the pancreatic juice in relation to the flow rate. **(B) Low Flow Rate (Long Contact Time).** Diagram shows a relatively high Cl^- concentration and low HCO_3^- concentration of the pancreatic juice due to a Cl^-–HCO_3^- Exchanger present in the main pancreatic duct that transports Cl^- into the pancreatic juice and transports HCO_3^- out of the pancreatic juice. **(C) High Flow Rate (Short Contact Time).** Diagram shows a relatively low Cl^- concentration and high HCO_3^- concentration of the pancreatic juice because the pancreatic juice has a short contact time with the Cl^-–HCO_3^- exchanger in the main pancreatic duct.

B. Gastric Phase

1. The gastric phase is initiated by **stomach distention**.
2. The gastric phase accounts for ≈10% of the total pancreatic juice secreted in response to a meal.
3. The gastric phase is controlled by the **parasympathetic nervous system** (CN X) via a **vagovagal reflex mechanism** involving stretch receptors in the stomach wall.

C. Intestinal Phase

1. The intestinal phase is initiated by the presence of **amino acids** (**e.g., phenylalanine, valine, methionine**), **fatty acids in micelles** (**C18 > C12 > C8 order of potency**), and **monoacylglycerols** in the proximal small intestine.
2. The intestinal phase accounts for 65% of the total pancreatic juice secreted in response to a meal and is the most important phase in humans.
3. The intestinal phase is controlled by CCK and SEC.

Chapter 6

Pathology

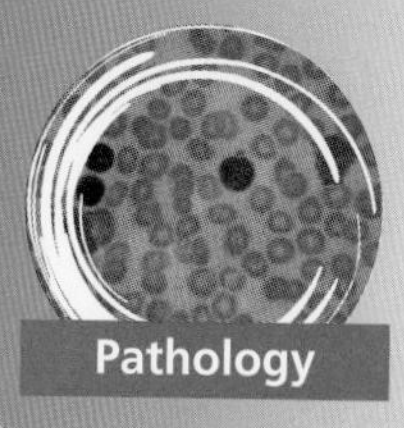

Esophagus

I Gastroesophageal Reflux Disease

A. **General Features.** Gastroesophageal reflux disease (GERD) is described as the symptoms or mucosal damage produced by the abnormal reflux of gastric contents through the lower esophageal sphincter into the esophagus.

B. **Pathological Findings.** Pathological findings include hyperemia (engorgement of blood), superficial erosions and ulcers that appear as vertical linear streaks, squamous epithelium showing hydropic changes, and increased lymphocytes, eosinophils, and neutrophils.

C. **Clinical Findings.** Clinical findings include **heartburn (or pyrosis)** which may worsen when bending or lying down, **regurgitation**, and **dysphagia (difficulty in swallowing)**. Heartburn is typically described as a retrosternal burning discomfort that radiates toward the neck most commonly experienced in the postprandial period. Regurgitation is the effortless return of gastric contents into the pharynx without nausea, retching, or abdominal contractions. Dysphagia is common in the setting of long-standing heartburn. The most dreaded cause of dysphagia is esophageal cancer (e.g., either adenocarcinoma arising from Barrett metaplasia or squamous cell carcinoma). Alcohol, chocolate, fatty foods, and cigarette smoking accentuate the reflux.

II Barrett Esophagus *(Figure 6-1)*

A. Barrett esophagus can be defined as the replacement of esophageal stratified squamous epithelium with metaplastic "intestinalized" simple columnar epithelium with Goblet cells extending **at least 3 cm** into the esophagus. This metaplastic invasion is most commonly caused by GERD. The clinical importance of this metaplastic invasion is that virtually all lower esophageal adenocarcinomas occur as a sequela.

B. The mucosal lining of the cardiac portion of the stomach **extends about 2 cm into the esophagus** such that the distal 2 cm of the esophagus is lined by a simple columnar epithelium, instead of stratified squamous epithelium. The junction where stratified squamous epithelium changes to simple columnar epithelium (or the mucosal GE junction) can be seen macroscopically as a **zigzag line** (called the **Z line**). This distinction is clinically very important especially when dealing with Barrett esophagus.

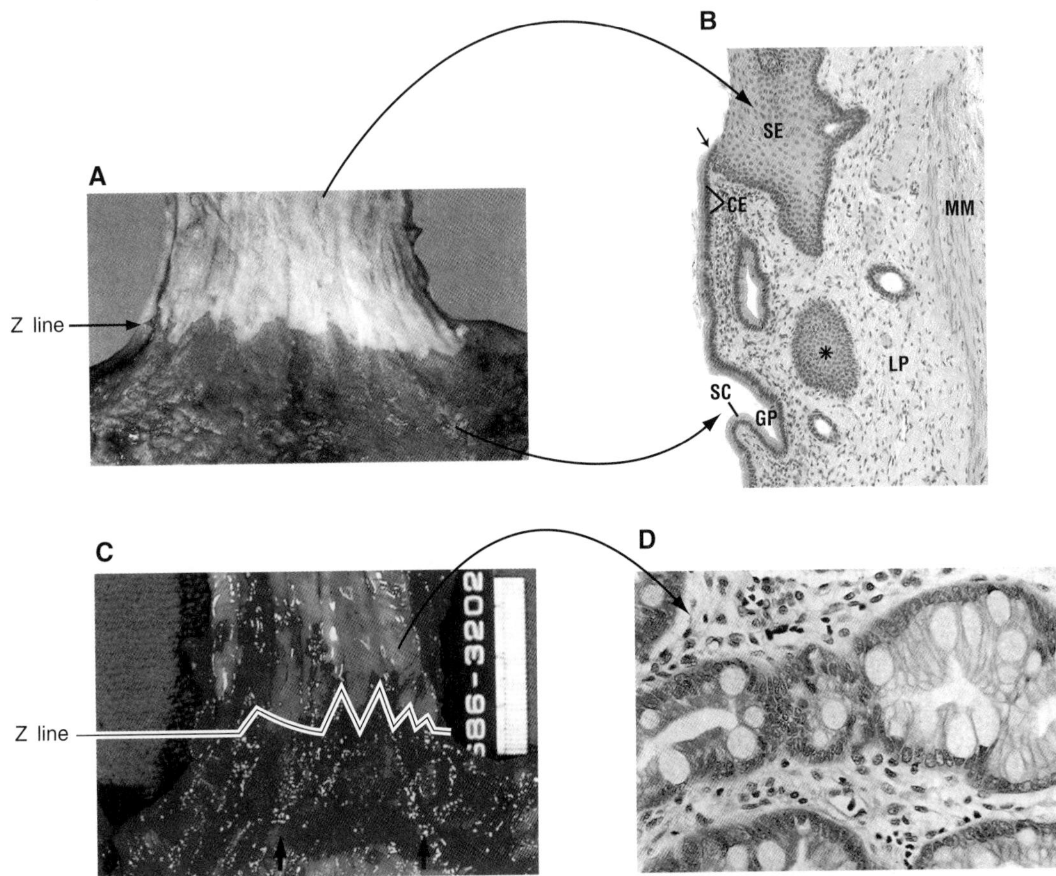

FIGURE 6-1. **(A,B) Gastroesophageal (GE) Junction. (A)** Photograph shows the Z line where the stratified squamous epithelium changes to simple columnar epithelium (or the mucosal GE junction). **(B)** LM shows the mucosal GE junction where the stratified squamous epithelium (SE) of the esophagus abruptly changes (arrow) to simple columnar epithelium (CE) similar to the stomach. **(C,D) Barrett Esophagus. (C)** Photograph shows the pathological disruption of the Z line. **(D)** LM shows the metaplastic "intestinalized" simple columnar epithelium with Goblet cells extending above the Z line.

Stomach

I Gastric Ulcers *(Figure 6-2A,B)*

A. **General Features.** Gastric ulcers most often occur within the **body of the stomach** along the **lesser curvature** above the **incisura angularis** at a histological transition zone where the gastric glands change from predominately parietal cells (HCl-producing) to G cells (gastrin-producing). They are caused by **damage to the mucosal barrier** (resulting in decreased mucus and bicarbonate production) due to smoking, salicylate or nonsteroid anti-inflammatory drugs ingestion, type B chronic atrophic gastritis, mucosal ischemia due to reduced prostaglandin E (PGE) production, or bile reflux. About 80% of patients with gastric ulcers have associated *Helicobacter pylori* infection.

B. **Clinical Findings.** Clinical findings include burning epigastric pain **soon after eating**; pain increases with food intake and is relieved by antacids; patient is afraid to eat and loses weight.

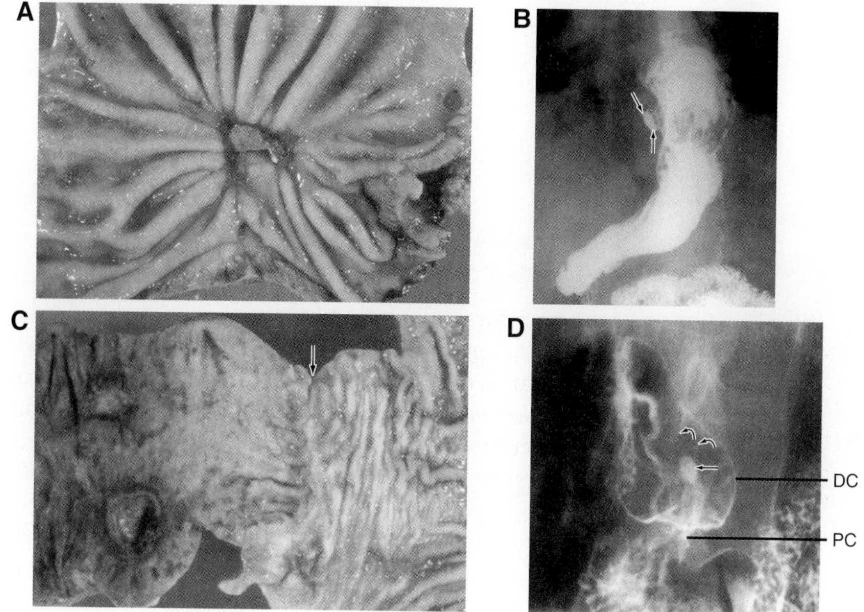

COMPARISON OF GASTRIC AND DUODENAL ULCERS

E

	Gastric Ulcer	Duodenal Ulcer
% of ulcer cases	25%	75%
Epidemiology	Male:Female ratio = 1:1 Increased risk with blood type A No association with MEN I or II COPD Renal failure	Male:Female ratio= 2:1 Increased risk with blood type O Associated with Zollinger–Ellison syndrome (MEN I) Liver cirrhosis/alcohol COPD Renal failure Hyperparathyroidism Family history with an autosomal dominant pattern
Pathogenesis	*H. pylori* infection in 80% of cases Damage to mucosal barrier due to smoking, salicylate or NSAID ingestion, type B chronic atrophic gastritis, mucosal ischemia due to reduced PGE production, or bile reflux	*H. pylori* infection in 95% of cases Damage to mucosal barrier Gastric acid hypersecretion due to increased parietal cell mass, increased secretion to stimuli, increased nocturnal secretion, or rapid gastric emptying
Location	Single ulcer within the body of the stomach along the lesser curvature above the incisura angularis	Single ulcer on the anterior wall of the first part of the duodenum (i.e., at the **duodenal cap**) most common Single ulcer on the posterior wall (danger of perforation into the pancreas)
Malignant potential	No malignant potential Cancer may be associated with a benign ulcer in 1%–3% of cases (biopsy necessary)	No malignant potential
Complications	Bleeding from left gastric artery Perforation Both are less common than seen in duodenal ulcers	Bleeding from gastroduodenal artery Perforation (air under diaphragm, pain radiates to left shoulder) Gastric outlet obstruction Pancreatitis
Clinical findings	Burning epigastric pain **soon after eating** Pain increases with food intake Pain is relieved by antacids Patient is afraid to eat and loses weight	Burning epigastric pain **1–3 h after eating** Pain decreases with food intake Pain is relieved by antacids Patient does not lose weight Patient wakes at night due to pain

COPD — chronic obstructive pulmonary disease; MEN — mulitiple endocrine neoplasia; PGE — prostaglandin E.

FIGURE 6-2. **Gastric and Duodenal Ulcers. (A,B) Gastric Ulcer. (A)** Photograph of gross specimen shows a characteristic sharp demarcation of the gastric ulcer from the surrounding mucosa with radiating folds. **(B)** Radiograph shows a gastric ulcer (arrows) along the lesser curvature of the stomach. **(C,D) Duodenal Ulcer. (C)** Photograph of gross specimen shows two sharply demarcated duodenal ulcers surrounded by an inflamed duodenal mucosa. Arrow indicates gastroduodenal junction. **(D)** Radiograph shows a duodenal ulcer (straight arrow) located in the duodenal cap (DC). The duodenal mucosal folds (curved arrows) radiate toward the ulcer crater. **(E)** Comparison table of gastric and duodenal ulcers. PC — pyloric canal.

Small Intestine

I Duodenal Ulcers *(Figure 6-2C,D)*

A. **General Features.** Duodenal ulcers most often occur on the anterior wall of the first part of the duodenum (i.e., at the **duodenal cap**) followed by the posterior wall (danger of perforation into the pancreas). They are caused by **damage to the mucosal barrier** (resulting in decreased mucus and bicarbonate production) and **gastric acid hypersecretion** due to increased parietal cell mass, increased secretion to stimuli, increased nocturnal secretion, or rapid gastric emptying. About 95% of patients have associated *H. pylori* infection.

B. **Clinical Findings.** Clinical findings include burning epigastric pain **1 to 3 h after eating**; pain decreases with food intake and is relieved by antacids; patient does not lose weight and wakes at night due to pain.

II Celiac Disease or Gluten-Sensitive Enteropathy *(Figure 6-3A,B)*

A. **General Features.** Celiac disease is a hypersensitivity to **gluten** and **gliadin** protein found in wheat, barley, and rye grains. Celiac disease is characterized by a generalized malabsorption, mucosal lesions within the small intestine, and prompt reversal of clinical symptoms when gluten-containing foods are removed from the diet.

B. **Pathological Findings.** Pathological findings include blunting or disappearance of villi; damage of mucosal epithelial cells; accumulation of a large number of lymphocytes, plasma cells, macrophages, and eosinophils within the lamina propria of the intestinal mucosa upon ingestion of gluten-containing foods; detection of gliadin antibodies in the blood; and most severe histological abnormalities are found in the duodenum and proximal jejunum.

C. **Clinical Findings.** Clinical findings include generalized malabsorption, chronic diarrhea, flatulence, weight loss, and fatigue.

III Carcinoid Tumor *(Figure 6-3E)*

A. **General Features.** Carcinoid tumors (CARs) arise from neuroendocrine cells and account for ≈50% of all malignant tumors of the small intestine. CARs are most commonly found in the **appendix** (followed by the **rectum**) where they are small and almost never metastasize. CARs may also occur in the **terminal ileum** where they are multiple and may metastasize to the liver. CARs secrete **serotonin (5-HT)** which is broken down by monoamine oxidase to **5-hydroxyindoleacetic acid (5-HIAA)**. 5-HT in the systemic circulation causes **carcinoid syndrome** which occurs mainly in patients with liver metastasis.

B. **Pathological Findings.** Pathological findings include small, round cells containing cytoplasmic granules arranged in nests, cords, or rosettes located within the submucosa; stool sample positive for heme and showing no evidence of parasites; urinalysis positive for 5-HIAA; and CT scan showing nodular masses in the duodenum and liver.

C. **Clinical Findings.** Clinical findings include auscultation revealing diffuse wheezes over both lungs and a pulmonic ejection murmur over the right sternal border at intercostal space 2, liver palpable well below the costal margin, apparent hyperactive bowel sounds, diarrhea, episodic flushing, bronchospasm, cyanosis, telangiectasia, and fibrosis of the valves on the right side of the heart.

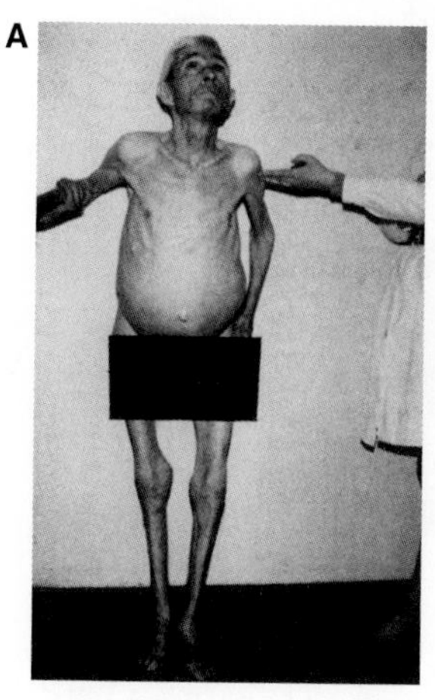

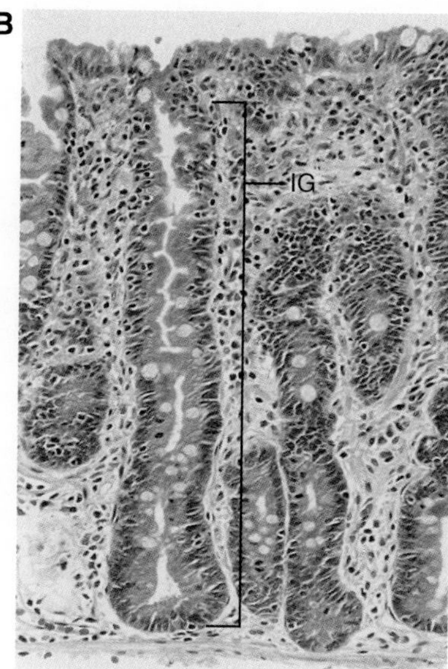

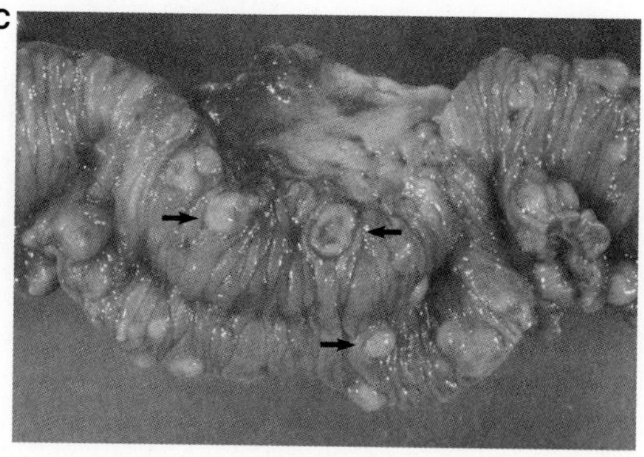

FIGURE 6-3. **(A,B) Celiac Disease or Gluten-Sensitive Enteropathy. (A)** Photograph shows an adult with long-term celiac disease. **(B) Light Micrograph of Celiac Disease.** Note the chronic inflammation of the lamina propria adjacent to intestinal glands (IG) along with the loss of villi. Inflammation is generally confined to the mucosa. A gluten-free diet will eliminate the inflammation and allow villi to return to normal. **(C) Carcinoid Tumor (CAR).** Photograph of gross specimen shows a segment of the terminal ileum with multiple CARs (arrows).

IV Crohn Disease *(Figure 6-4)*

A. **General Features.** Crohn disease (CD) is a chronic inflammatory bowel disease which usually appears in teenagers and young adults. CD most commonly affects the **ileum and the ascending right colon**. The etiology of CD is unknown although epidemiologic studies have indicated a **strong genetic predisposition** and immunological studies have indicated a role of **cytotoxic T cells** in the damage to the intestinal wall.

B. **Pathological Findings.** Pathological findings include transmural nodular lymphoid aggregates; noncaseating epithelioid granulomas; neutrophilic infiltration of the intestinal glands which ultimately destroys the glands, leading to ulcers; and coalescence of the ulcers into **long, serpentine ulcers** ("**linear ulcers**") oriented along the long axis of the bowel. A classic feature of CD is the clear demarcation between diseased bowel segments located directly next to uninvolved normal bowel and a **cobblestone appearance** that can be seen grossly and radiographically.

C. **Clinical Findings.** Clinical findings include recurrent right lower quadrant colicky abdominal pain, intermittent bouts of diarrhea, weight loss associated with malabsorption and malnutrition, recurrent fever, weakness, strictures of the intestinal lumen, formation of fistulas, and perforation.

Large Intestine

I Ulcerative Colitis *(Figure 6-4)*

A. **General Features.** Ulcerative colitis (UC) is an idiopathic inflammatory bowel disease which usually appears in teenagers and young adults. UC always involves the **rectum**

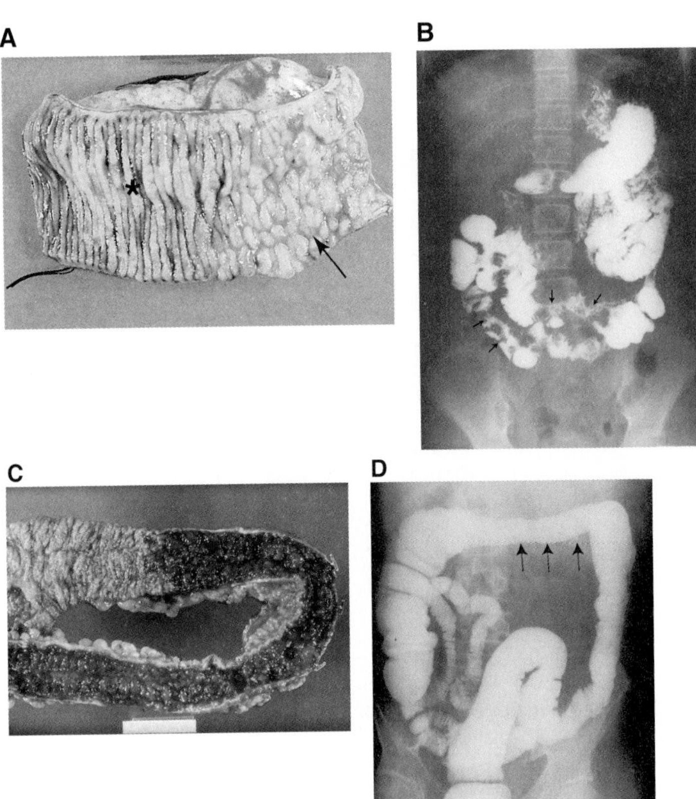

E COMPARISON OF CROHN DISEASE AND ULCERATIVE COLITIS

	Crohn Disease	Ulcerative Colitis
Epidemiology	More common in whites vs. blacks More common in Jews vs. non-Jews More common in women Affects young adults	More common in whites vs. blacks No sex predilection Affects young adults
Extent	Transmural	Mucosal and submucosal
Location	Terminal ileum alone (30%) Ileum and colon (50%) Colon alone (20%) Involves other areas of GI tract (mouth anus)	Mainly the rectum May extend into descending colon May involve entire colon Does not involve other areas of GI tract
Gross features	Thick bowel wall and narro lumen (leads to obstruction) Aphthous ulcers (early sign) Skip lesions, strictures, and fistulas Deep linear ulcers with cobblestone pattern Fat creeping around the serosa	Inflammatory pseudopolyps Areas of friable, blood residula mucosa Ulceration and hemorrhage "Collar-button" ulcers
Microscopic findings	Transmural nodular lymphoid aggregates Noncaseating granulomas Dysplasia or cancer less likely	Ulcers ad intestinal gland abscesses with neutrophils Dysplasia of cancer may be present
Clinical findings	Recurrent right lower quadrant colicky pain with diarrhea Bleeding occurs with colon or anal involvement	Recurrent left-sided abdominal cramping with bloody diarrhea and mucus
Radiology	"String" sign in terminal ileum due to luminal narrowing	"Lead pipe" appearance in chronic state
Complications	Fistulas, obstruction Calcium oxalate renal calculi Malabsorption due to bile deficiency Macrocytic anemia due to vitamin B_{12} deficiency	Toxic megacolon Primary sclerosing cholangitis Andenocarcinoma

FIGUREG. 6-4. **Crohn Disease and Ulcerative Colitis. (A,B) Crohn Disease. (A)** Photograph of a gross specimen of the ileum shows prominent cobblestoning (arrow) due to multiple transverse and linear ulcers. The other portion of the ileum is normal (*). **(B)** Radiograph shows the luminal narrowing ("string sign") and cobblestone pattern of the affected small intestines. **(C,D) Ulcerative Colitis. (C)** Photograph of a gross specimen of the colon shows inflammatory pseudopolyps and ulceration. **(D)** Radiograph shows the "lead pipe" appearance of the affected transverse and descending colon. Note the small ulcerations extending from the colon lumen (arrows). **(E)** Comparison table of Crohn disease and ulcerative colitis.

and may extend proximally for varying distances into the **descending colon**. The etiology of UC is unknown. Epidemiologic studies have not indicated a strong genetic predisposition and immunological studies have been inconclusive.

B. **Pathological Findings.** Pathological findings include raw, red, and granular mucosal surface; continuous inflammation (i.e., there are no "skip areas" as in CD); a diffuse, chronic inflammatory infiltration in the lamina propria; damage to the colorectal crypts; inflammatory pseudopolyps; areas of friable, bloody residual mucosa; "collar-button" ulcers; and "lead-pipe" appearance in the chronic state.

C. **Clinical Findings.** Clinical findings include rectal bleeding, recurrent episodes of loose bloody stools, crampy abdominal pain, low-grade fever which lasts for days or weeks, bloody diarrhea with mucus and pus, malaise, and weight loss. In severe cases, 6 to 20 bloody bowel movements/day may lead to anemia, dehydration, and electrolyte depletion. A serious complication of UC is **toxic megacolon**.

II Diverticular Disease

Diverticular disease is a term that includes both **diverticulosis** (i.e., the presence of diverticula) and **diverticulitis** (i.e., inflammation of the diverticula). Diverticular disease is **age-dependent** with a high incidence in patients >60 years of age. In Westernized societies, diverticular disease is **common and predominately left-sided.** In Asian and African societies, diverticular disease is **rare and predominately right-sided**.

A. **Diverticulosis** *(Figure 6-5A)*
1. **General features.** Diverticulosis is the presence of diverticula (abnormal pouches or sacs) which consist of the mucosa and submucosa that herniate through the muscularis externa of the colon.
2. **Pathological findings.** Pathological findings include diverticula usually arranged in parallel rows, diverticula usually developing where vasa recta penetrate the colon wall, and diverticula most commonly (95% of the cases) found in the sigmoid colon.
3. **Clinical findings.** Clinical findings include diverticulosis is generally symptom free and often an incidental finding during endoscopy. Some patients might complain of cramping, bloating, flatulence, and/or irregular defecation.

B. **Diverticulitis**
1. **General features.** Diverticulitis is inflammation of the diverticula due to a microscopic or macroscopic perforation of a diverticulum. Diverticulitis is probably caused by increased intraluminal pressure or inspissated food particles that trigger inflammation and focal necrosis.
2. **Clinical findings.** Clinical findings include pain in left lumbar region, pain that is often present for several days prior to admission, previous episodes of similar pain, palpable inflammatory mass in left lumbar region, nausea, vomiting, constipation or diarrhea, low-grade fever, mild leukocytosis, ileus, and peritonitis. Diverticulitis may lead to **diverticular bleeding** which is painless, self-limiting rectal bleeding due to progressive injury to the artery supplying that segment of the colon.

III Appendicitis *(Figure 6-5B)*

A. **General Features.** Acute appendicitis is an inflammatory disease that leads to transmural inflammation within the wall of the appendix, perforation, and peritonitis. Acute appendicitis begins with the obstruction of the appendix lumen by a fecal concretion (fecalith) in ≈30% of cases, lymphoid hyperplasia, distention of the appendix, and bacterial invasion of the wall. In many cases, the precipitating cause is unknown.

B. **Pathological Findings.** Pathological findings include a congested, tense appendix, often covered by a fibrinous exudate, purulent contents within the lumen, a fecalith that may be present (≈30% of cases), infiltration by neutrophils of the entire wall of the appendix, and perforation releasing purulent contents into the peritoneal cavity.

C. **Clinical Findings.** Clinical findings include initial pain in the umbilical or epigastric region, later pain localizes to the right lumbar region, nausea, vomiting, anorexia, low-grade fever, tenderness to palpation, and percussion in the right lumbar region. Complications may include peritonitis due to rupture of the appendix.

IV Hemorrhoids *(Figure 6-5C)*

A. Internal Hemorrhoids

1. **General features**
   a. Internal hemorrhoids are varicosities of the **superior hemorrhoidal plexus of veins** located in the submucosal layer of the anorectal region.
   b. The submucosa of the anorectal region normally has the appearance of cavernous (erectile) tissue due to the presence of sacculated veins. This vascular submucosa is especially thickened in three primary locations (left lateral, right anterior, and right posterior) which form **anal cushions**.
   c. Internal hemorrhoids are located **above the pectinate line**, are covered by a **rectal mucosa (simple columnar epithelium)**, and have a **visceral innervation** (pain receptors absent).
   d. Internal hemorrhoids are graded according to the degree of prolapse:
      i. **Grade I** hemorrhoids bulge into the lumen but do not extend below the pectinate line.
      ii. **Grade II** hemorrhoids prolapse out of anal canal upon defecation but reduce spontaneously.
      iii. **Grade III** hemorrhoids prolapse out of anal canal upon defecation but do not reduce spontaneously.
      iv. **Grade IV** hemorrhoids are irreducible and may strangulate.

B. External Hemorrhoids

1. **General features**
   a. External hemorrhoids are varicosities of the **inferior hemorrhoidal plexus of veins** located in the submucosal layer of the anorectal region.
   b. External hemorrhoids are located **below the pectinate line** near the anal verge, are covered by **skin (stratified squamous epithelium)**, and have a **somatic innervation** (pain receptors present).
   c. External hemorrhoids are not graded.
   d. Internal and external hemorrhoids communicate with one another and drain into the **internal pudendal veins** and then the **inferior vena cava (IVC)** system. Hemorrhoids do not drain into the portal system although they may exist in close proximity to rectal varices associated with portal hypertension. Hemorrhoids are not found more commonly in patients with portal hypertension.

C. **Clinical Findings.** Clinical findings of hemorrhoids include painless bleeding associated with a bowel movement, bright red blood coating the stool; dripping of blood into the toilet or staining toilet paper; hemorrhoidal bleeding that is almost always painless; anal pruritus (irritation or itching of perianal skin); pain caused by hemorrhoids is associated with a palpable lump and thrombosis; thrombosis of external hemorrhoids that is associated with excruciating pain since the overlying skin is highly innervated (pain receptors present); a thrombosed external hemorrhoid that is an easily visible, purple, elliptical mass extending from the anus to the perianal skin; and thrombosis of Grades I, II, and III internal hemorrhoids associated with some pain but to a lesser degree than external hemorrhoids; however, strangulation of Grade IV internal hemorrhoids is associated with excruciating pain.

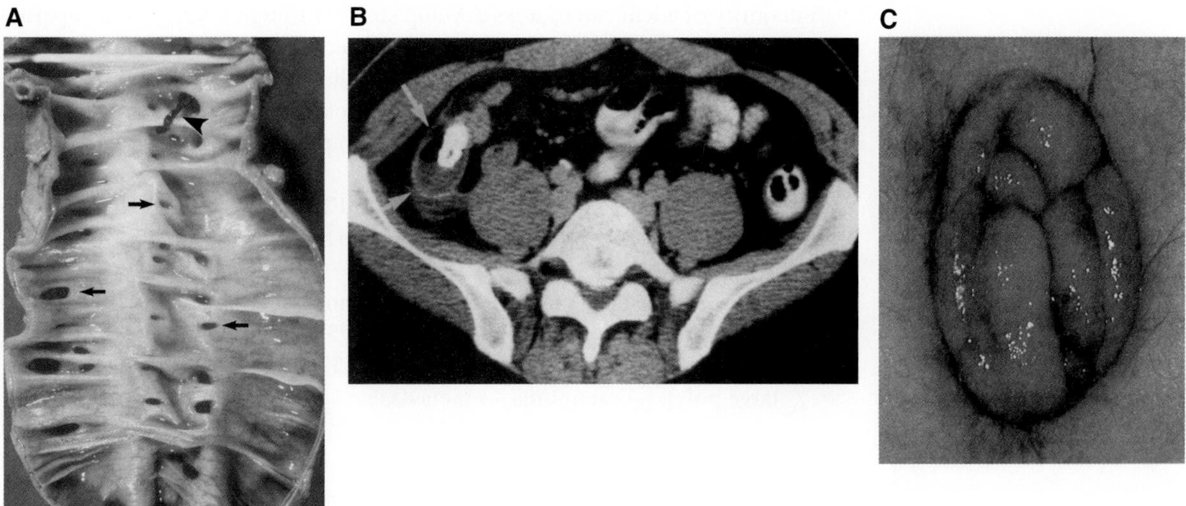

FIGURE 6-5. **Pathology of the Large Intestine. (A) Diverticulosis.** Photograph of gross specimen shows openings of numerous diverticula (arrows) arranged in parallel rows. Note the blood clot protruding from one of the diverticula (arrowhead). **(B) Appendicitis.** CT scan shows a periappendiceal abscess (arrows). The appendix contains gas, fluid, and a calcified fecalith. **(C) Hemorrhoids.** Photograph shows a Grade IV internal hemorrhoid.

V Familial Adenomatous Polyposis *(Figure 6-6A,B)*

A. General Features

1. Familial adenomatous polyposis (FAP) is an autosomal dominant genetic disorder caused by a mutation in the ***APC* tumor-suppressor gene** on **chromosome 5q21–q22** for the **adenomatous polyposis coli protein**. More than 800 different germline mutations of the *APC* gene have been identified, all of which result in a **loss-of-function mutation**. The most common germline APC mutation is a **5-bp deletion** at codon 1309.
2. APC protein binds **glycogen synthase kinase 3b (GSK-3b)** which targets **β-catenin**. APC protein maintains normal apoptosis and inhibits cell proliferation through the **Wnt signal transduction pathway** so that *APC* gene belongs to the family of **tumor-suppressor genes**.
3. **Gardner syndrome** is a variation of FAPC wherein patients demonstrate adenomatous polyps and other pathologies which include multiple osteomas (e.g., skull, long bones, and mandible), epidermoid cysts, desmoid tumors, and congenital hypertrophy of retinal pigment epithelium.
4. **Turcot syndrome** is a variation of FAPC wherein patients demonstrate adenomatous polyps and other pathologies which include gliomas and medulloblastomas.

B. Clinical Findings.

Clinical findings include colorectal adenomatous polyps appearing at 7 to 35 years of age inevitably leading to colon cancer by ≈40 years of age, thousands of polyps observed in the colon, and gastric polyps that may be present.

VI Adenocarcinoma of the Colon *(Figure 6-6C,D)*

A. General Features

1. Adenocarcinoma of the colon will inevitably develop in patients with FAP and accounts for 98% of all colorectal cancers, i.e., the vast majority of colorectal cancers are adenocarcinoma.

2. A majority of adenocarcinomas develop slowly through a series of histopathological changes each of which has been associated with mutations of specific proto-oncogenes and tumor-suppressor genes as follows:
   a. *APC* **tumor-suppressor gene** on **chromosome** 5q21–q22 for the **adenomatous polyposis coli protein** is involved in the transition of normal epithelium → a small polyp.
   b. *KRAS* **proto-oncogene** on **chromosome 12p12.1** for the **Kirsten rat sarcoma 2 viral oncogene homolog** (a G protein) is involved in the transition of a small polyp → large polyp.
   c. *DCC* **tumor-suppressor gene** on **chromosome 18q21.1** for the **deleted in colorectal carcinoma protein** and the *TP53* **tumor-suppressor gene** on **chromosome 17p13.1** for the **tumor protein 53** are involved in the transition of a large polyp → carcinoma → metastasis.

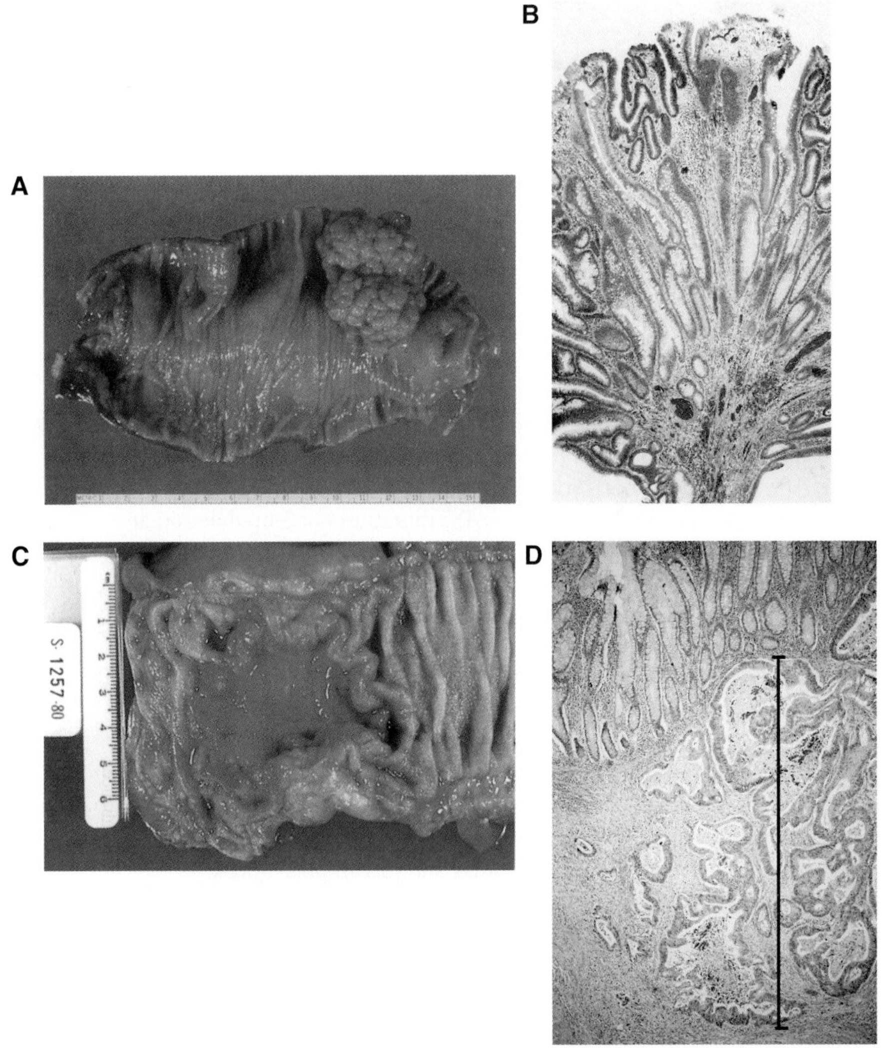

FIGURE 6-6. **(A,B) Familial Adenomatous Polyposis. (A)** Photograph of a gross specimen of the colon shows a tubulovillous adenoma with a prominent villous architecture. The lesion has a sessile nature, a smooth surface, and a lobulated appearance. **(B)** Light micrograph shows a convoluted, irregular arrangement of the intestinal glands with the basement membrane intact and an epithelium that is transformed into a pseudostratified epithelium with mitotic figures apparent. A polyp is a tumorous mass that extends into the lumen of the colon. **(C,D) Adenocarcinoma of the Colon. (C)** Photograph of a gross specimen of the colon shows the ulcerated center of the cancerous lesion with heaped up edges. **(D)** Light micrograph shows the convoluted, irregular arrangement of the intestinal glands that have breached the basement membrane to extend deep into the submucosa and/or muscularis externa (bracket). The epithelium is transformed into a pseudostratified epithelium that grows in a disorderly pattern extending into the lumen of the gland.

B. Pathological Findings. Pathological findings include malignant polyps that are irregular in shape, sessile, >2 cm in diameter, exhibit sudden growth, and have a base broader than height; and ulcerating or infiltrative adenocarcinoma.

C. Clinical Findings. Clinical findings include fatigue, weakness, change in bowel habits, and weight loss. Right-sided tumors are associated with iron-deficiency anemia. Left-sided tumors are associated with obstruction and bloody stools. It is a clinical maxim that iron-deficiency anemia in an older man means adenocarcinoma of the colon until shown otherwise. Metastasis occurs most commonly to the **liver** since the sigmoid veins and superior rectal veins drain into the hepatic portal system. A posterior metastasis may involve the **sacral nerve plexus** causing sciatica.

Liver

I Cholestasis

A. General Features

1. Cholestasis is caused by a defect in the **transport of bile** from the hepatocyte cytoplasm into the bile canaliculus lumen.
2. Cholestasis results in a **reduced bile flow** through the bile canaliculi and a **reduced transport of H_2O, bilirubin**, and **bile salts** from the hepatocyte cytoplasm into the bile canaliculus lumen.
3. Cholestasis that occurs as a result of intrahepatic liver disease (e.g., primary biliary cirrhosis) is called **intrahepatic cholestasis**.
4. Cholestasis that occurs as a result of obstruction of large bile ducts (e.g., gallstones, bile duct cancer or surrounding tissues, external compression by enlarged lymph nodes, benign strictures, or congenital biliary atresia) is called **extrahepatic cholestasis**.

A. Pathological Findings

1. Pathological findings in general include brown bile pigment within hepatocytes and dilated canaliculi, early cholestasis involving the central zone of the liver lobule (or Zone 3 of the liver acinus), and chronic cholestasis involving the peripheral zone of the liver lobule (or Zone 1 of the liver acinus).
2. Pathological findings in extrahepatic cholestasis include swollen and bile-stained liver, colorless bile ("white bile"), inflammation within the portal triads, tortuous and distended bile ductules, damaged hepatocytes showing **feathery degeneration** (i.e., hydropic swelling, contains brown bile pigment and a reticulated appearance), and bile ducts that may rupture and form **bile lakes**.

B. Clinical Findings. Clinical findings include jaundice; severe, intractable itching (pruritus); xanthomas; and elevated serum and hepatocellular bile salt concentration.

II Hereditary Diseases Associated with Cirrhosis

A. α1-Antitrypsin Deficiency

1. **General features**
   a. α1-Antitrypsin deficiency (AATD) is an autosomal recessive genetic disorder caused by a mutation in the ***SERPINA1* gene** on **chromosome 14q32.1** for **α1-antitrypsin** which is a major serum protease inhibitor A1 (or PI) that inhibits tissue elastase.
   b. AATD is most commonly (95% of cases) caused by a missense mutation which results in a **normal glutamic acid → lysine** substitution at position 342 (E342K) which is called the PI*Z allele.

c. Individuals who are **PI ZZ** (i.e., homozygous for the PI*Z allele) account for 95% of all AATD cases. PIZZ results in an ≈82% reduction in α1-antitrypsin.
d. PI Z variant protein self-aggregates and polymerizes.
e. The prevalence of AATD is ≈1/6,000 in the Caucasian population.

2. **Pathological findings.** Pathological findings include inclusions within hepatocytes and bile duct epithelium that appear as bright pink globules of various sizes using periodic-Schiff stain following diastase treatment, intrahepatic cholestasis, hepatocellular injury due to the aggregation of the PI Z variant protein, moderate fibrosis, and inflammatory cells within the portal area.
3. **Clinical findings.** Clinical findings include chronic obstructive pulmonary disease (specifically emphysema) in adults; jaundice, hyperbilirubinemia, and increased serum aminotransferase levels in the early neonatal period; cirrhosis, fibrosis, and rapid destruction of the liver in adults; and liver involvement associated mainly with the PI ZZ genotype.

III HFE-Associated Hereditary Hemochromatosis *(Figure 6-7A)*

A. General Features

1. HFE-associated hereditary hemochromatosis (HHH) is an autosomal recessive genetic disorder caused by ≈28 different mutations in the ***HFE* gene** on **chromosome 6p21.3** for **hereditary hemochromatosis protein** which is a cell surface protein expressed as a heterodimer with β_2-microglobulin, binds the transferrin receptor 1, and reduces cellular iron uptake although the exact mechanism is unknown.
2. HHH is most commonly caused by two missense mutations which result in a **normal cysteine → tyrosine** substitution at position 282 (C282Y) causing a decreased cell surface expression or a **normal histidine → asparagine** substitution at position 63 (H63D), causing pH changes that affect binding to the transferrin receptor 1.
3. Approximately 87% of HHH affected individuals in the European population are homozygous for the C282Y mutation or are **compound heterozygous** (i.e., two different mutations at the same gene locus) for the C282Y and H63D mutations.
4. The prevalence of HHH is 1/200–500 births in European populations.

B. Pathological Findings.
Pathological findings include hepatic iron overload in hepatocytes and bile duct epithelium assessed by Prussian blue staining of a liver biopsy, enlarged, reddish-brown liver; micronodular cirrhosis; and fibrotic, rust-colored pancreas.

C. Clinical Findings.
Clinical findings include excessive storage of iron in the liver, heart (fatigue), skin (bronzing), pancreas, joints (arthralgia), ovaries (amenorrhea), and testes (subfertility and loss of libido); abdominal pain, weakness, lethargy, weight loss, hepatic fibrosis. Pigmented skin and glucose intolerance are called **bronze diabetes.** Hepatocellular carcinoma is a late complication. Plasma iron concentration is ≈160 to 200 g/dL (normal value = 80 to 100 g/dL), and elevated transferrin-iron saturation and elevated serum ferritin concentration are noted. Without therapy, symptoms appear in males at 40 to 60 years of age and in females after menopause.

IV Alcoholic Liver Disease *(Figure 6-7B,C)*

The spectrum of alcoholic liver disease ranges from a fatty liver to alcoholic hepatitis and cirrhosis.

A. Fatty Liver

1. General features
   a. Virtually all chronic alcoholics accumulate fat within hepatocytes (i.e., steatosis), which varies from lipid droplets scattered throughout the cytoplasm

to a distention of the cytoplasm by a single lipid droplet resembling an adipocyte.

b. The effects of ethanol within the hepatocyte include increased fatty acid synthesis, decreased mitochondrial oxidation of fatty acids, increased production of triglycerides, and reduced release of lipoproteins. In the alcoholic, the liver becomes yellow and may massively enlarge to as much as three times the normal weight. The pathogenesis of fat accumulation is not precisely understood. An alcoholic fatty liver is reversible and does not necessarily progress toward more severe disease like cirrhosis. A fatty liver is also observed in obesity, uncontrolled diabetes, kwashiorkor, and prolonged administration of corticosteroids.

2. **Pathological findings.** Pathological findings include enlarged, yellow liver; liver that may enlarge to as much as three times the normal weight; fat accumulation within hepatocytes that varies from small, scattered lipid droplets within the cytoplasm to total fat accumulation so that the hepatocyte resembles an adipocyte; bizarre, giant mitochondria; and proliferation of smooth endoplasmic reticulum.
3. **Clinical findings.** Clinical findings include: Patients have few symptoms; an alcoholic fatty liver is reversible; alcoholic fatty liver does not necessarily progress toward more severe disease like cirrhosis; a fatty liver may also be observed in obesity, uncontrolled diabetes, kwashiorkor, and prolonged administration of corticosteroids.

B. Alcoholic Hepatitis

1. **General features.** Alcoholic hepatitis is an acute necrotizing lesion of the liver that may suddenly occur in patients who have had a fatty liver for many years.
2. **Pathological findings.** Pathological findings include isolated or clusters of necrotic hepatocytes predominately in the central zone of the liver lobule (or Zone 3 of the liver acinus), hepatocytes contain eosinophilic Mallory bodies (alcoholic hyaline) composed of intermediate filaments; collagen deposition around the central vein, and inflammation characterized by neutrophil infiltration.
3. **Clinical findings.** Clinical findings include malaise, anorexia, fever, right upper quadrant pain, jaundice, and a mild leukocytosis. The prognosis in patients with alcoholic hepatitis correlates with the severity of the hepatocyte injury. In some patients, alcoholic hepatitis progresses rapidly to liver failure and death. As a group, alcoholics with alcoholic hepatitis are at a very high risk of permanent liver disease whereby ≈70% may develop liver cirrhosis.

C. Alcoholic Cirrhosis

1. **General features**
   a. Cirrhosis is the end-stage of chronic liver disease including alcoholism.
   b. In alcoholic cirrhosis, pathological findings of fatty liver and alcoholic hepatitis are often seen in conjunction with cirrhosis.
   c. All advanced cases of cirrhosis have the same appearance no matter the cause.
   d. Alcoholic cirrhosis is the most common cause of liver transplantation among adults in the United States.
   e. The prognosis in patients with alcoholic cirrhosis is better if the patient refrains from further drinking.
2. **Pathological findings.** Pathological findings include hepatocyte necrosis, fibrous septae surround regenerative nodules, **micronodular cirrhosis** showing nodules <3 mm in diameter with the destruction of normal liver lobule architecture and thin fibrous septae, and **macronodular cirrhosis** showing large nodules, thick fibrous septae containing portal triads, inflammatory cells, and proliferating bile ductules.
3. **Clinical findings.** Clinical findings include testicular atrophy, impotence, and loss of libido in chronic male alcoholics; and ovarian atrophy, oligomenorrhea, amenorrhea,

and loss of secondary sex characteristics in chronic female alcoholics. Many alcoholics with alcoholic cirrhosis progress to end-stage liver disease. Causes of cirrhosis include alcoholic liver disease, chronic viral hepatitis, biliary disease, various metabolic diseases (e.g. hemochromatosis, Wilson disease, cystic fibrosis, AATD), and cryptogenic causes.

V Toxic Liver Injury *(Table 6-1, Figure 6-7E)*

A. In general, toxic liver injury is due to the metabolism of a compound by **cytochrome P_{450} mono-oxygenase system (or microsomal mixed-function oxidase system)**, which produces free radicals and other reactive metabolites.

B. Some hepatotoxins invariably produce hepatocyte necrosis in a **predictable fashion.** The hallmarks of these classic hepatotoxins include high doses always causing hepatocyte necrosis; high doses causing the same pattern of hepatocyte necrosis in different animal models; high doses causing a zonal pattern of hepatocyte necrosis, often in the central zone of the liver lobule (or Zone 3 of the liver acinus); high doses causing hepatocyte necrosis in brief period of time; and dose-dependency.

C. Some therapeutic drugs produced hepatocyte necrosis in an **unpredictable fashion.** The hallmarks of these therapeutic drugs include a predisposition to an idiosyncratic reaction by a sensitive person, a genetic variation in the cytochrome P_{450} mono-oxygenase system, and a dose-dependency side effect.

TABLE 6-1 VARIOUS TYPES OF LIVER DAMAGE DUE TO DRUGS/CHEMICALS

Morphological Appearance	Drug/Chemical
Acute hepatitis	Isoniazid (10%–20% liver damage; acetyl hydrazine is the active metabolite); salicylate, halothane (symptoms occur after 1 week, fever precedes jaundice, and metabolites form via action of P_{450} system); methyldopa (positive Coombs test), phenytoin, acetaminophen, and ketoconazole
Chronic active hepatitis	Methyldopa, acetaminophen (e.g., Tylenol), aspirin, isoniazid, nitrofurantoin, and halothane
Zonal necrosis	**Zone 1**: Undergoes necrosis due to poisoning by yellow phosphorus, manganese, ferrous sulphate, allyl alcohol, and endotoxin of *Proteus vulgaris* Undergoes necrosis due to chronic hepatitis, primary biliary cirrhosis, bile duct occlusion, and preeclampsia/eclampsia (Note: Hepatic disease is very common in preeclamptic women and monitoring of platelet count and serum liver enzymes is standard practice.) Is exposed to blood high in nutrients and oxygen; synthesizes glycogen and plasma proteins actively **Zone 2:** Undergoes necrosis due to yellow fever Is exposed to blood intermediate in nutrients and oxygen **Zone 3**: Undergoes necrosis due to poisoning by carbon tetrachloride, chloroform, L-amanitine, pyrrolizidine alkaloids (bush tea), tannic acid, copper, acetaminophen (free radicals formed; acetylcysteine therapy replaces glutathione to neutralize free radicals) Undergoes necrosis due to ischemic injury, right-sided cardiac failure, Budd–Chiari syndrome, hepatic veno-occlusive disease, and bone marrow transplantation Is exposed to blood low in nutrients and oxygen
Intrahepatic cholestasis	**Noninflammatory:** oral contraceptives and anabolic steroids **Inflammatory:** erythromycin estolate, amoxicillin–clavulanic acid, chlorpromazine, and thiazides
Fatty change	**Macrovesicular (single droplet)**: ethanol, corticosteroids, amiodarone (looks like alcoholic hepatitis), and methotrexate **Microvesicular**: tetracycline, valproic acid, Reye Syndrome, fatty liver of pregnancy, and phospholipidosis due to amiodarone

(Continued)

TABLE 6-1 CONTINUED

Morphological Appearance	Drug/Chemical
Fibrosis	Methotrexate, hypervitaminosis A, retinoic acid, and amiodarone
Vascular lesions	**Budd–Chiari syndrome**: oral contraceptives **Hepatic veno-occlusive disease**: pyrrolizidine alkaloids (bush tea) **Peliosis hepatis**: oral contraceptives, anabolic steroids, and tamoxifen **Angiosarcoma**: vinyl chloride, arsenic, and thorium dioxide (radioactive contrast material; Thorotrast)
Tumors	**Nodular hyperplasia**: azathioprine, anticancer agents **Benign tumors**: oral contraceptives **Malignant tumors**: oral contraceptives **Cholangiocarcinoma**: thorium dioxide (radioactive contrast material; Thorotrast) **Hepatocellular carcinoma**: vinyl chloride, aflatoxin B_1 (from *Aspergillus* mold)
Granulomatous hepatitis	Allopurinol, hydralazine, sulfonamides, and phenylbutazone

VI Portal Hypertension

Portal hypertension is characterized by a sustained increase in portal venous pressure due to obstruction of portal blood flow. Obstruction of portal blood flow may be in either a **prehepatic, intrahepatic**, or **posthepatic (beyond the liver lobules)** location.

A. Prehepatic Portal Hypertension

1. Prehepatic portal hypertension is usually caused by **portal vein thrombosis**.
2. Portal vein thrombosis may occur as a result of cirrhosis, tumors, hypercoagulability states, pancreatitis, or surgical trauma.

B. Intrahepatic Portal Hypertension

1. Intrahepatic portal hypertension is usually caused by **cirrhosis,** which results in the following changes: regenerative nodules narrowing hepatic veins, and fibrosis narrowing portal venules, central veins, and sinusoids.
2. Intrahepatic portal hypertension may also be caused by schistosomiasis (i.e., *Schistosoma mansoni, S. japonicum*), sarcoidosis, primary biliary cirrhosis, congenital hepatic fibrosis, arsenic poisoning, and idiopathic portal hypertension.

C. Posthepatic Portal Hypertension

1. General features
   a. Posthepatic portal hypertension is caused by **Budd–Chiari syndrome** which results in the **thrombosis of hepatic veins**. Budd–Chiari syndrome may occur as a result of polycythemia vera and other myeloproliferative disorders, hypercoagulability states, oral contraceptives, pregnancy, bacterial infections, tumors, or surgical trauma.
   b. Posthepatic portal hypertension is also caused by **hepatic veno-occlusive disease** (a variant of Budd–Chiari syndrome) which results in the **thrombosis of central veins and small tributaries of the hepatic veins.** Hepatic veno-occlusive disease may occur as a result of ingestion of pyrrolizidine alkaloids (bush tea), chemotherapy, or radiation therapy.
2. Pathological findings
   a. Pathological findings in the acute stage include swollen, tense liver; cut surface has a mottled appearance and oozes blood; sinusoids in the central zone of the liver lobule (or Zone 3 of the liver acinus) are dilated and packed with RBCs; and necrotic hepatocytes predominately in the central zone of the liver lobule (or Zone 3 of the liver acinus).

b. Pathological findings in the chronic stage include firm liver due to fibrosis; pale cut surface due to fibrosis; recent and well-organized thrombi within hepatic veins; fibrosis in the central zone of the liver lobule (or Zone 3 of the liver acinus); dilated sinusoids; pressure atrophic hepatocytes predominately in the central zone of the liver lobule (or Zone 3 of the liver acinus) and midportion of the liver lobule (or Zone 2 of the liver acinus); and fibrosis links adjacent central zones of the liver lobule (or Zone 3 of the liver acinus).

3. **Clinical findings.** Clinical findings include enlarged liver, abdominal pain, mild jaundice, severe ascites, splenomegaly, a protracted course from months → a few years, hepatic failure, and death.

D. **Portal Hypertension Complications.** All types of portal hypertension may lead to the following complications which include:

1. **Esophageal varices**
   a. Esophageal varices are characterized by a reversal of blood flow in a portal–IVC (caval) anastomosis in order to decrease portal venous pressure.
   b. The most important clinical anastomosis involves the **left gastric (coronary) vein** of the portal system and the **esophageal vein** of the caval system located around the lower esophagus and upper stomach.
   c. Bleeding esophageal varices have a very poor prognosis and exsanguination is a common cause of death.
2. **Caput medusae**
   a. Caput medusae are characterized by a reversal of blood flow in a portal–IVC (caval) anastomosis in order to decrease portal venous pressure.
   b. The anastomosis involves the **paraumbilical vein** of the portal system and the **superficial and inferior epigastric veins** of the caval system located around the umbilicus.
3. **Anorectal varices**
   a. Anorectal varices are characterized by a reversal of blood flow in a portal–IVC (caval) anastomosis in order to decrease portal venous pressure.
   b. The anastomosis involves the **superior rectal vein** of the portal system and the **middle and inferior rectal veins** of the caval system located around the rectum.

VII Familial Hypercholesterolemia

A. General Features

1. Familial hypercholesterolemia is an autosomal dominant genetic disorder caused by >400 different loss-of-function mutations in the ***LDLR* gene** on **chromosome 19p13.1–p13.3** for the **low-density lipoprotein (LDL) receptor** which binds LDL and delivers LDL into the cell cytoplasm.
2. The LDL receptor has an extracellular portion that consists of one domain with seven cysteine-rich areas called **LDL-binding region**, a second domain with epidermal growth factor homology, and a third domain with serine and threonine-rich areas linked to oligosaccharides. When LDL (the principal carrier of serum cholesterol) binds to the LDL receptor, **receptor-mediated endocytosis** occurs.
3. Most cases of hypercholesterolemia and hyperlipoproteinemia in the general population are of multifactorial origin.
4. Mutations in the *LDLR* gene are grouped into six classes:
   a. **Class 1** mutations prevent LDLR synthesis.
   b. **Class 2** mutations prevent LDLR transport to the cell membrane.
   c. **Class 3** mutations prevent LDL binding to LDLR.
   d. **Class 4** mutations prevent LDL internalization into the cell cytoplasm by coated pits.

e. **Class 5** mutations prevent LDLR recycling back to the cell membrane after LDL + LDLR dissociation.

f. **Class 6** mutations prevent LDLR targeting to the apical membrane adjacent to the blood capillaries.

B. Pathological Findings. Pathological findings include: Atherosclerosis is considered an **intimal disease** with the presence of an atheromatous plaque (tunica intima thickening); an atheromatous plaque has a fibrous cap composed of smooth muscle cells, a few leukocytes, and a relatively dense deposition of collagen; an atheromatous plaque has a deeper necrotic core composed of a disorganized mass of lipid material, cholesterol crystals, cell debris, and foam cells (macrophages digesting modified LDL) of the fatty streak; an atheromatous plaque may undergo many histologic changes, such as:

1. **Plaque calcification** that turns arteries into brittle pipes.
2. **Hemorrhage into the plaque** that induces focal rupture or ulceration.
3. **Focal plaque rupture** at the luminal surface that results in **thrombus formation**, whereby the thrombus may partially or completely occlude the lumen, leading to ≈90% of all myocardial infarctions.

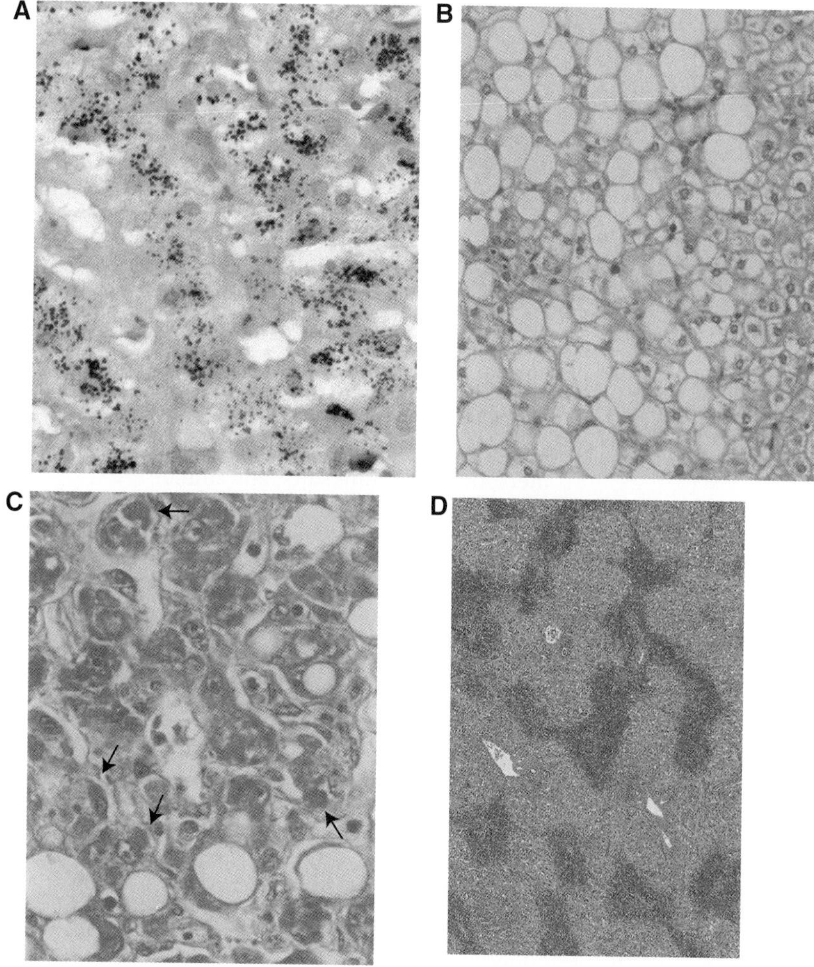

FIGURE 6-7. **Liver Pathology. (A) Hereditary Hemochromatosis.** Light micrograph shows iron overload within the hepatocytes assessed by Prussian blue staining. **(B) Fatty Liver.** Light micrograph shows fat accumulation within hepatocytes that varies from small, scattered lipid droplets within the cytoplasm to total fat accumulation so that the hepatocytes resemble adipocytes. **(C) Alcoholic Hepatitis.** Light micrograph shows hepatocytes that contain eosinophilic Mallory bodies (arrows) composed of intermediate filaments. **(D) Acetaminophen Liver Injury.** Light micrograph shows hemorrhagic necrosis in the central zone of the liver lobule (or Zone 3 of the liver acinus) due to acetaminophen (e.g., Tylenol) overdose.

C. **Clinical Findings.** Clinical findings include increased serum LDL cholesterol levels; premature heart disease as a result of atheromas (deposits of LDL-derived cholesterol in the coronary arteries); accelerated atherosclerosis; xanthomas (cholesterol deposits in the skin and tendons); arcus lipoides (deposits of cholesterol around the cornea of the eye); homozygotes develop severe symptoms early in life and rarely live past 30 years of age; and heterozygotes have plasma cholesterol level twice that of normal.

Gallbladder

 I Cholelithiasis *(Figure 6-8)*

A. General Features

1. Cholelithiasis is characterized by the presence or formation of gallstones either in the gallbladder (called **cholecystolithiasis**) or in common bile duct (called **choledocholithiasis**).
2. Gallstones form when bile salts and lecithin are overwhelmed by cholesterol. Most stones consist of **cholesterol (major component)**, **bilirubin**, and **calcium**. There are three main types of gallstones:
   a. **Cholesterol stones**
      i. These stones are yellow → tan, round or faceted, smooth, and single or multiple.
      ii. These stones are composed mainly of cholesterol.
      iii. These stones are associated with obesity, CD, cystic fibrosis, clofibrate, estrogen levels in premenopausal women, oral contraceptives, rapid weight loss, and the US or Native American (e.g., Pima Indian women) population, and the 4F's: female, fat, fertile, over forty.
   b. **Black pigment stones**
      i. These stones are black, irregular, glassy upon cross-section, and <1 cm in diameter.
      ii. These stones are composed mainly of calcium bilirubinate, bilirubin polymers, other calcium salts, and mucin.
      iii. These stones are associated with the elderly, undernourishment, chronic RBC hemolysis (e.g., sickle cell anemia or spherocytosis), alcoholic cirrhosis, biliary infection, and the Asian population. In most cases, no predisposing factor is apparent.
   c. **Brown pigment stones**
      i. These stones are brown, spongy, and laminated.
      ii. These stones are composed mainly of calcium bilirubinate, cholesterol, and calcium soaps of fatty acids.
      iii. These stones are found predominately within the intrahepatic and extrahepatic bile ducts.
      iv. These stones are associated with: *E. coli* bacterial cholangitis, *Ascaris lumbricoides* and *Clonorchis sinensis* helminth infection, and chronic obstruction to bile flow.
3. **Gallstone obstruction.** There are three clinically important sites of gallstone obstruction as follows:
   a. **Within the cystic duct.** A stone may transiently lodge within the cystic duct and cause pain (**biliary colic**) within the epigastric region due to the distention of the duct. If a stone becomes entrapped within the cystic duct, bile flow from the gallbladder will be obstructed resulting in inflammation of the gallbladder (**acute cholecystitis**), and pain will shift to the right hypochon-

driac region. Bile becomes concentrated and precipitates in the gallbladder forming a layer of high-density material called **"milk of calcium" bile** due to large amount of calcium carbonate. Bile flow from the liver remains open (i.e., **no jaundice**). This may lead to **Mirizzi syndrome** where impaction of a large gallstone in the cystic duct extrinsically obstructs the nearby common hepatic duct.

b. **Within the common bile duct.** If a stone becomes entrapped within the common bile duct, bile flow from both the gallbladder and liver will be obstructed, resulting in inflammation of the gallbladder and liver. **Jaundice** is frequently observed and is first observed clinically **under the tongue**. The jaundice is moderate and fluctuates since a stone rarely causes complete blockage of the lumen.

c. **At the hepatopancreatic ampulla**. If a stone becomes entrapped at the ampulla, bile flow from both the gallbladder and liver will be obstructed. In addition, the pancreatic duct may be blocked. In this case, **jaundice** and **pancreatitis** are frequently observed.

B. **Clinical Findings.** Clinical findings include many gallstones remaining silent for many years, severe biliary colic, acute cholecystitis, obstructive jaundice, pancreatitis, gallstone ileus, and hydrops of the gallbladder.

II Acute Cholecystitis *(Figure 6-8)*

A. General Features

1. Acute cholecystitis is characterized by diffuse inflammation of the gallbladder.
2. Approximately 90% of acute cholecystitis cases are due to gallstone obstruction. The remaining ≈10% of cases (called acalculous cholecystitis) are due to sepsis, severe trauma, *Salmonella typhosa* bacterial infection, or polyarteritis nodosa.

B. **Pathological Findings.** Pathological findings include outer surface of the gallbladder being covered by a fibrinous exudate, gallbladder wall thickened by edema and hemorrhage, gallbladder wall that may perforate leading to bile peritonitis, and gallbladder mucosa being fiery red or purple with focal ulceration or widespread necrosis.

C. **Clinical Findings.** Clinical findings include right upper quadrant abdominal pain, biliary colic, mild jaundice, persistent pain, fever, leukocytosis, and shaking chills indicating the need for a cholecystectomy.

III Chronic Cholecystitis *(Figure 6-8)*

A. General Features

1. Chronic cholecystitis is characterized by persistent inflammation of the gallbladder.
2. Approximately 99% of chronic cholecystitis cases are due to gallstone obstruction. The remaining ≈1% of cases are due to repeated attacks of acute cholecystitis involving chronic irritation and/or chemical injury to the gallbladder.
3. Chronic cholecystitis is the most common gallbladder disease.

B. **Pathological Findings.** Pathological findings include outer surface of the gallbladder having fibrous adhesions, thickened gallbladder wall that is fibrotic and penetrated by Rokitansky–Aschoff sinuses, ulcerated and atrophic gallbladder mucosa, widespread inflammation throughout the gallbladder, and gall stones in gallbladder.

C. **Clinical Findings.** Clinical findings include nonspecific abdominal symptoms and episodic right upper quadrant pain.

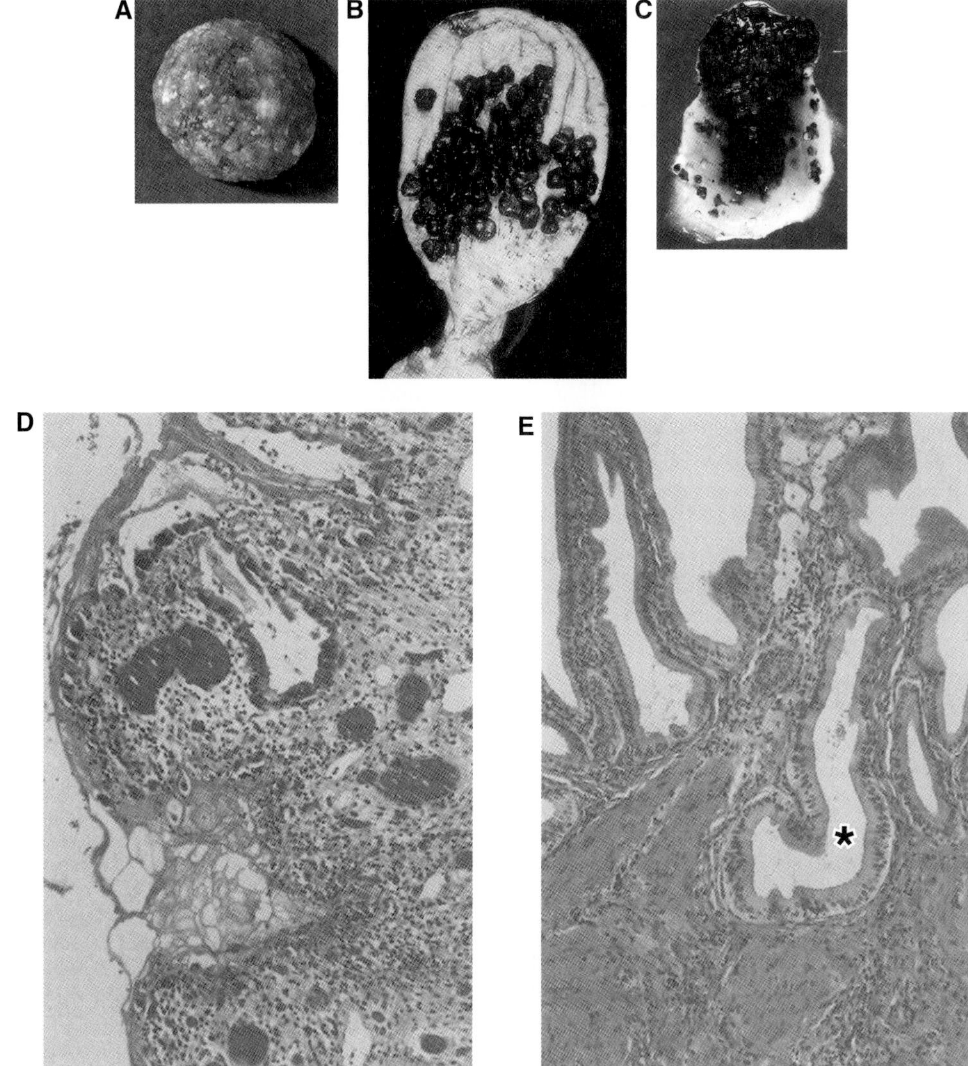

FIGURE 6-8. **Gallbladder. (A)** Photograph shows a solitary cholesterol gallstone. **(B)** Photograph shows the inner lumen of the gallbladder containing pigment gallstones. **(C)** Photograph shows a pigment gallstone embedded in a mucus gel. **(D) Acute Cholecystitis.** Light micrograph shows a mucosa that is congested, edematous, and infiltrated with neutrophils. The surface epithelium demonstrates focal necrosis and is covered with a fibrinous exudate. **(E) Chronic Cholecystitis.** Light micrograph shows a Rokitansky–Aschoff sinus (*) that extends into the smooth muscle layer.

Pancreas

 Acute Pancreatitis *(Figure 6-9)*

A. General Features

1. Acute pancreatitis is characterized by inflammation of the exocrine pancreas due to acinar cell injury.
2. The three main causes of acute pancreatitis include:
   a. **Inappropriate activation of pancreatic proenzymes by trypsin.** This leads to acinar cell injury, enzymatic fat necrosis, and elastic fiber destruction within blood vessels (hemorrhage).
   b. **Pancreatic duct obstruction.** Pancreatic duct obstruction due to **gallstones**. Approximately 50% of patients with acute pancreatitis have cholelithiasis.
   c. **Alcohol abuse.** Approximately 30% of patients with acute pancreatitis are alcoholics.

B. Pathological Findings. Pathological findings of the most severe form of acute pancreatitis (known as **acute hemorrhagic pancreatitis**) include edema and hyperemia of the pancreas, appearance of pale, gray foci, foci that grow to form a large retroperitoneal hematoma, yellow-white areas of fat necrosis near the mesentery, and pancreatic calcifications (pathognomonic) that are frequently diagnosed by imaging procedures.

C. Clinical Findings. Clinical findings include pain in the epigastric region that radiates to the back, nausea, vomiting, elevated amylase or lipase levels within 24 to 72 h, neuromuscular irritability due to hypocalcemia, and retroperitoneal hemorrhage that may lead to flank ecchymosis (Turner sign) or periumbilical ecchymosis (Cullen sign).

II Chronic Pancreatitis *(Figure 6-9)*

A. General Features

1. Chronic pancreatitis is characterized by chronic inflammation and fibrosis, which leads to the destruction of the exocrine pancreas.
2. The most common type of chronic pancreatitis is **chronic calcifying pancreatitis**.
3. The main causes of chronic pancreatitis include:
   a. **Pancreatic duct obstruction.** Pancreatic duct obstruction due to **pancreas divisum** or **mechanical blockage** by cancer or mucus (e.g., cystic fibrosis) may lead to chronic pancreatitis. Gallstone obstruction does not seem to be involved.
   b. **Alcohol abuse.** Approximately 66% of patients with chronic pancreatitis are alcoholics. More than 90% of patients with chronic calcifying pancreatitis are alcoholics. An early sign of chronic pancreatitis in alcoholics is the precipitation of protein (i.e., pancreatic enzymes) within the pancreatic duct which provides a nidus for the formation of calculi.
   c. **Autoimmunity.** Autoimmune chronic pancreatitis may occur in association with other autoimmune disorders (e.g., Sjogren syndrome, ulcerative colitis, CD).
   d. **Hereditary pancreatitis.** Hereditary pancreatitis is an autosomal dominant genetic disorder caused by point mutations in either the ***PRSS1* gene** on **chromosome** 7q34 for the **protease serine 1** protein or in the ***SPINK1* gene** on **chromosome** 5q32 for the **serine peptidase inhibitor Kazal 1** protein.

B. Pathological Findings. Pathological findings include firm pancreas, dilated pancreatic duct and tributaries, calcified proteinaceous plugs, ductal strictures, irregular areas of fibrosis; infiltration of lymphocytes, plasma cells, and macrophages; and destruction of endocrine islet tissue.

C. Clinical Findings. Clinical findings include recurrent or persisting abdominal pain that radiates to the back and may be crippling, exocrine pancreas insufficiency, endocrine pancreas insufficiency, intermittent acute attacks followed by quiet periods, diabetes, and malabsorption.

III Pancreatic Ductal Adenocarcinoma *(Figure 6-9)*

A. General Features

1. Pancreatic ductal adenocarcinoma accounts for ≈90% of all pancreatic cancers.
2. Pancreatic ductal adenocarcinoma is a very aggressive malignant tumor that usually occurs within the head of the pancreas.
3. A majority of pancreatic ductal adenocarcinomas have been associated with mutations of specific proto-oncogenes, tumor-suppressor genes, and transcription factor genes as follows:
   a. ***KRAS* proto-oncogene** on **chromosome 12p12.1** for the **Kirsten rat sarcoma 2 viral oncogene homolog** (a G protein). A mutation of the *KRAS* gene appears to be an early event in the development of pancreatic ductal adenocarcinoma.

b. *TP53* **tumor-supressor gene** on **chromosome 17p13.1** for **tumor protein 53.**
c. *CDKN2A* (or *p16*) **tumor-suppressor gene** on **chromosome 9p21** for the **cyclin-dependent kinase inhibitor 2A (or p16INK4a)** protein.
d. *SMAD4* **transcription factor gene** on **chromosome 18q21.1** for **small mothers against decapentaplegic** proteins which modulate the activity of TGF-β (transforming growth factor) receptors.

B. Pathological Findings. Pathological findings include firm, gray, multinodular mass within the pancreas that is poorly demarcated, blockage of the common bile duct and the main pancreatic duct, and metastasis to regional lymph nodes and the liver.

C. Clinical Findings. Clinical findings include: Common in men 60 to 80 years of age; midgastric pain that radiates to the back and worsens upon lying down, weight loss, obstructive jaundice, clay-colored stools, hepatomegaly, glucose intolerance, palpable gallbladder (Courvoisier sign), elevated CA19-9 levels (the gold standard marker), a poor prognosis with a 5 year survival rate of <5%. It usually has already metastasized upon presentation. A pancreaticoduodenectomy (**Whipple procedure**) that removes the head of the pancreas, duodenum, distal common bile duct, gallbladder, and distal stomach may be a surgical treatment.

IV Gastrinoma (Zollinger–Ellison Syndrome)

A. General Features

1. A gastrinoma is a tumor of the endocrine pancreas consisting of **G cells** which secrete **gastrin** even though G cells are not normally found within the endocrine pancreas.
2. A gastrinoma secretes excess gastrin which stimulates **parietal cells** (which produce HCl) and **enterochromaffin cells** (which secrete histamine).
3. Gastrin stimulates the release of HCl from parietal cells largely via histamine action (which stimulates HCl release from parietal cells), thereby producing **hyperacidity** and **peptic ulcer disease**.
4. In most cases, a single peptic ulcer is observed but multiple peptic ulcers may also occur. A gastrinoma should always be suspected if a peptic ulcer is found in an unusual site.
5. A gastrinoma is generally malignant (70% to 90% of cases).
6. A gastrinoma may be a solitary tumor or multiple tumors. Multiple gastrinoma tumors are usually associated with the **MEN I syndrome** (multiple endocrine neoplasia-type 1).

B. Pathological Findings. Pathological findings include neoplastic cells being well differentiated and containing secretory granules, gastrinomas resembling other pancreatic endocrine tumors, degree of malignancy that cannot be determined by histological appearance, and metastasis to regional lymph nodes and the liver.

C. Clinical Findings. Clinical findings include: Most commonly occurs in persons 30 to 50 years of age, Zollinger–Ellison syndrome which is characterized by intractable gastric hypersecretion, severe peptic ulcers in the duodenum and jejunum, high serum levels of gastrin, abdominal pain caused by peptic ulcer, diarrhea (malabsorption since enzymes cannot work in an acid pH), markedly increased basal acid output test, confirmatory secretin test (secretin administration results in an elevation of gastrin levels in patients with a gastrinoma), and serum gastrin levels >600 pg/mL. Other causes of elevated serum gastrin levels include use of H_2 blockers (e.g., Tagamet, Zantac, etc.) which decreases HCl production and thereby elevates gastrin, and atrophic gastritis which decreases HCl production (by destruction of parietal cells) and thereby elevates gastrin.

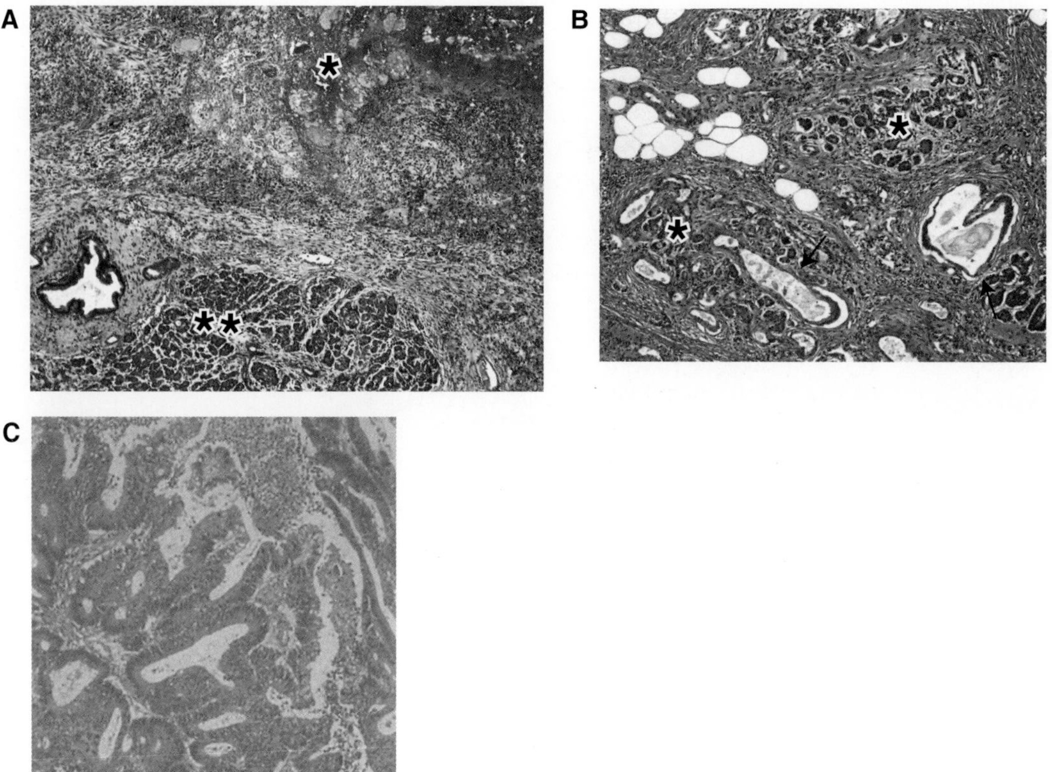

FIGURE 6-9. **Pancreas. (A) Acute Hemorrhagic Pancreatitis.** Light micrograph shows acinar cell necrosis, fat necrosis, and hemorrhage (*) along with an intact pancreatic lobule (**). **(B) Chronic Calcifying Pancreatitis**. Light micrograph shows atropic pancreatic lobules (*) that are surrounded by irregular areas of fibrosis infiltrated by inflammatory cells. The pancreatic ducts are dilated and contain proteinaceous plugs (arrows). **(C)** Light micrograph shows a well-differentiated ductal adenocarcinoma with numerous neoplastic ducts invading the pancreatic parenchyma.

Chapter 7

Microbiology

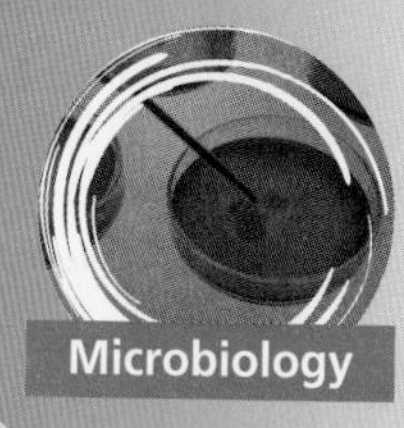

Stomach (Table 7-1)

I Peptic Ulcer Disease (Figure 7-1)

A. **General Features.** Peptic ulcer disease is a general term that refers to the focal destruction of the distal gastric mucosa (i.e., gastric ulcers; see Chapter 6, Stomach I) or proximal duodenal mucosa (i.e., duodenal ulcers; see Chapter 6, Small Intestine I). There is a variety of factors implicated in peptic ulcer disease one of which is *Helicobacter pylori* infection. *H. pylori* infection is associated with ≈80% of the gastric ulcers and ≈95% of the duodenal ulcers.

B. **Causative Agent (*H. pylori*).** The genus ***Helicobacter*** is a **Gram-negative bacillus** that does not ferment carbohydrates and grows only in a reduced level of oxygen (i.e., microaerophilic). *H. pylori* is a Gram-negative bacillus, does not ferment glucose, and is microaerophilic, flagellated, highly motile, spiral shaped, oxidase positive, and urease positive.

C. **Reservoir.** *H. pylori* is found only in humans (i.e., humans are the primary reservoir). In developing countries, ≈100% of the population is colonized by 40 years of age (many are colonized before 10 years of age). In developed countries, ≈30% of the population is colonized by 40 years of age. *H. pylori* is transmitted by the fecal–oral route, possibly during diarrheal episodes.

D. **Virulence Factors**

1. *H. pylori* produces **mucinase** and **phospholipase** that break down the mucus layer and allow *H. pylori* to penetrate the mucus layer (along with the corkscrew motility of *H. pylori*) and bind to Lewis blood group antigens on gastric epithelial cells.
2. *H. pylori* produces **urease** that cleaves urea into ammonium (NH_4^-) and bicarbonate (HCO_3^-), both of which provide an alkaline microenvironment that allows *H. pylori* to survive the acid pH (i.e., gastric HCl acid) of the stomach lumen.
3. *H. pylori* produces **HspB (heat shock protein)** that enhances the activity of urease.
4. *H. pylori* injects **VacA (vacuolating toxin)** into gastric epithelial cells which induces apoptosis.
5. *H. pylori* produces **superoxide dismutase** and **catalase** that prevent phagocytosis and intracellular killing.

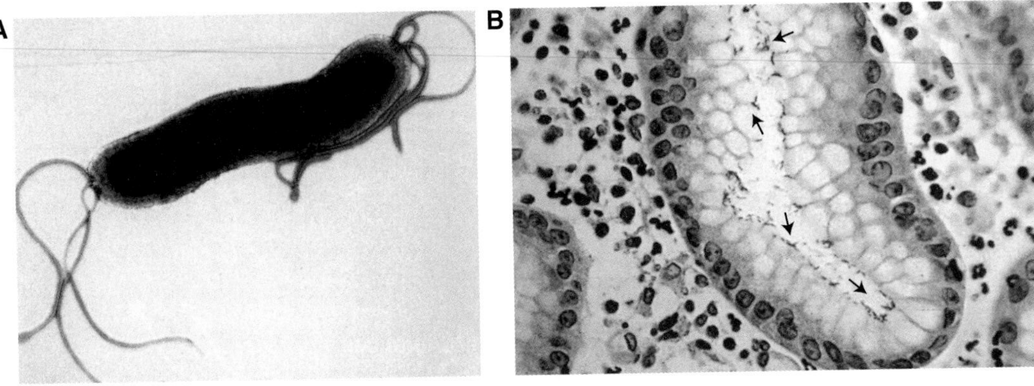

FIGURE 7-1. **Microbiology of the Stomach. (A,B) *Helicobacter pylori*. (A)** Light micrograph shows the Gram-negative, flagellated, spiral-shaped bacillus called *Helicobacter pylori*. **(B)** Light micrograph of a stomach biopsy shows *H. pylori* within the lumen of the gastric gland (arrows) in association with the gastric mucosa. The visualization of *H. pylori* is enhanced in this light micrograph by the use of special silver staining.

Small Intestine *(Table 7-1)*

I Viral Gastroenteritis Caused by Rotavirus Infection

A. **General Features.** Rotavirus Type A is the leading cause of viral gastroenteritis worldwide. Almost every child develops rotavirus gastroenteritis by 3 years of age. Clinical findings include watery, nonbloody diarrhea, fever, vomiting (may be predominant), and dehydration in children at 6 to 24 months of age; incubation period that is <48 h; fall/winter is the predominant season of infection; and duration of illness is 5 to 7 days.

B. **Causative Agent (Rotavirus Type A).** Rotavirus belonging to the **Reoviridae family** is a **segmented (11 segments), double-stranded RNA virus**. The virion is a **naked** (nonenveloped) icosahedron. The capsid consists of a double-layered protein capsid. The outer capsid layer consists of structural proteins (e.g., **VP4** and **VP7**). The inner capsid layer consists of a complete transcription system (e.g., **VP1, VP2, VP3, and VP6**).

C. **Reservoir.** Rotavirus is transmitted by the fecal–oral route since it is shed in large quantities in the feces. During the disease, 10^{10} virions/g of stool may be present.

D. **Virulence Factor.** The protein **nsP4** acts as a viral enterotoxin.

II Viral Gastroenteritis Caused by Adenovirus Infection

A. **General Features.** Enteric adenovirus (serotypes 40 and 41) causes 3% to 10% of endemic pediatric gastroenteritis. Pathological findings include cells that contain both eosinophilic nuclear inclusion bodies (similar to herpes infections) and indistinct, basophilic nuclear inclusion bodies (called **smudge cells**). Clinical findings include watery diarrhea in children <2 years of age, which may be accompanied by fever, vomiting, and dehydration; incubation period is 8 to 10 days; summer is the predominant season of infection; and duration of illness is 6 to 9 days.

B. **Causative Agent (Adenovirus).** Adenoviruses (42 different serotypes) belonging to the **Adenovirus family** are **linear, double-stranded DNA viruses** with **terminal**

proteins located at the 5′ end. The virions are **naked** (nonenveloped) **icosahedrons** with a **capsid**. The capsid is associated with **fibers** that serve as **viral attachment proteins** and also carry **type-specific antigens**.

C. **Reservoir.** Adenovirus is transmitted by respiratory droplets or the fecal–oral route promoted by close human contact (e.g., classrooms, day care centers, and military barracks). Adenovirus is resistant to drying, detergents, GI secretion, and mild chlorine treatment. Serotypes 1 to 7 are the most prevalent.

III Viral Gastroenteritis Caused by Norovirus (Norwalk Agent) Infection

A. **General Features.** Norwalk agent is a major cause of viral gastroenteritis in the United States with outbreaks reported in hospitals, resorts, cruise ships, and nursing homes. Pathological findings include jejunal biopsies showing epithelial cells with blunted villi and cytoplasmic vacuolation and presence of inflammatory cells. Clinical findings include watery diarrhea, low-grade fever, and vomiting in older children and adults; incubation period is 1 to 2 days; no predominant season of infection (small peaks in winter months have been reported); and duration of illness is 1 to 4 days.

B. **Causative Agent (Norwalk Agent).** Norwalk agent belonging to the **Caliciviridae family** is a **nonsegmented positive sense RNA virus [(+)RNA]**. The virion is naked (nonenveloped) icosahedron. The capsid contains one 60 kDa protein.

C. **Reservoir.** Norwalk agent is transmitted by the fecal–oral route or contaminated shellfish. Norwalk agent is shed in the feces for up to 2 weeks after infection. Norwalk agent is highly transmissible as only 10 to 100 virions are required for infection.

IV Cholera *(Figure 7-2A,B)*

A. **General Features.** *Vibrio cholerae* (O1 or O139 strains of the El Tor biotype) causes cholera. Clinical findings include sudden onset of profuse watery diarrhea with mucus flecks but no blood ("rice-water stools"); no fever; there may be vomiting; hypovolemic shock will occur (fatal within 8 h) if electrolytes and fluid are not replaced; incubation period is 2 to 3 days; and a long-lasting immunity to the serotype occurs.

B. **Causative Agent (*V. cholerae*).** The genus ***Vibrio*** is a **Gram-negative bacillus** *V. cholerae* is a Gram-negative bacillus, facultative anaerobic, oxidase positive, a slow lactose fermenter, does not produce H_2S gas, prefers an alkaline environment, has a single flagellum, and is comma shaped.

C. **Reservoir.** *V. cholerae* is transmitted by contaminated food and water. There are no known animal reservoirs or vectors. Human fecal contamination of coastal sea waters has caused epidemics associated with eating raw or undercooked sea food.

D. **Virulence Factors**

1. *V. cholerae* does not enter enterocytes but instead remains in the intestinal lumen and secretes an enterotoxin called **cholera toxin (choleragen)**. Cholera toxin consists of **one A subunit (with A1 and A2 component)** and **five B subunits (an A–B component toxin)**. The B subunits bind to the **GM_1 ganglioside** on the cell membrane. The A2 component facilitates entry into the cell membrane. The A1 component (an ADP-ribosyl transferase) ADP-ribosylates a G protein (called G_s) which in turn stimulates adenylate cyclase. ADP-ribosylated G_s protein remains permanently in an active GTP-bound state resulting in persistent activation of **adenylate cyclase** and **↑cAMP levels.** The ↑cAMP levels keep Cl^- ion channel proteins permanently open resulting in the diffusion of Cl^- into the small intestinal lumen; Na^+ and H_2O follow.

2. *V. cholerae* produces ToxR that acts as an upregulator for cholera toxin.
3. *V. cholerae* produces **toxin coregulated pili**.

V Diarrhea Caused by Enterotoxigenic *Escherichia coli* (*Figure 7-2C,D*)

A. **General Features.** Enterotoxigenic *E. coli* causes "traveler's diarrhea" (Turista) and infant diarrhea in developing countries. Clinical findings include watery diarrhea; vomiting; abdominal cramps; incubation period is 24 to 48 h; duration of illness is 1 to 2 days; and hypovolemic shock will occur if electrolytes and fluids are not replaced.

B. **Causative Agent (Enterotoxigenic *E. coli*).** **Enterobacteriaceae** are ubiquitous bacteria found in the soil, water, vegetation, and normal intestinal flora. All members of this family are Gram-negative bacilli, facultative anaerobic, catalase positive, oxidase negative, ferment glucose, and reduce nitrites to nitrates. Some members of this family are lactose-fermenting bacilli (i.e., *Escherichia, Klebsiella, Enterobacter, Serratia,* and *Citrobacter*). Other members of this family are nonlactose-fermenting bacilli (i.e., *Proteus, Salmonella, Shigella,* and *Yersinia*). MacConkey and eosin methylene blue agar are two commonly used selective primary isolation media for the differentiation of lactose-fermenting versus nonlactose-fermenting members of Enterobacteriaceae. The heat-stable **lipopolysaccharide** (**LPS**) is the major cell wall antigen and consists of the **somatic O polysaccharide**, a **polysaccharide core (common antigen)**, and **Lipid A**. The serologic classification of members of the Enterobacteriaceae family is based on three major groups of antigens which are detected by specific antibodies **somatic O polysaccharides (O antigens)**, **flagellar H proteins (H antigens)**, and **capsular K antigens (K antigens)**.

The genus *Escherichia* belonging to the **Enterobacteriaceae family (Gram-negative facultative anaerobic bacilli)** is a Gram-negative bacillus, facultative anaerobic, motile, catalase positive, oxidase negative, ferments glucose, ferments lactose, phenylalanine positive (produces indole), and reduces nitrites to nitrates. *E. coli* is the most common species.

C. **Reservoir.** *E. coli* normally colonizes the human intestinal tract. Enterotoxigenic *E. coli* is transmitted by contaminated food and water through poor sanitation and the use of human feces as fertilizer.

D. **Virulence Factors**

1. Enterotoxigenic *E. coli* does not enter enterocytes but instead remains in the intestinal lumen and secretes an enterotoxin called **heat labile toxin** (**LT** is similar to cholera toxin). LT is composed of two subunits. **Subunit B** binds to the cell membrane. **Subunit A** ADP-ribosylates a G protein (called G_s) which in turn stimulates adenylate cyclase. ADP-ribosylated G_s protein remains permanently in an active GTP-bound state, resulting in persistent activation of **adenylate cyclase** and **↑cAMP levels.** The ↑cAMP levels keep Cl^- ion channel proteins permanently open, resulting in the diffusion of Cl^- into the small intestinal lumen; Na^+ and H_2O follow.
2. Enterotoxigenic *E. coli* produces **heat stabile toxin (ST)** that stimulates **guanylate cyclase** and **↑cGMP levels** causing a similar reaction as LT.
3. **Other virulence factors common to all members of Enterobacteriaceae**. See Small Intestine V B above.

VI Diarrhea Caused by Enteropathogenic *E. coli* (*Figure 7-2C,D*)

A. **General Features.** Enteropathogenic *E. coli* causes chronic infant diarrhea in developing countries and is the reason many infants fail to thrive. Pathological findings include enterocytes show microvillus damage and surface effacement (i.e., **A/E histopathology**). Clinical findings include watery diarrhea with mucus, vomiting, fever, and malaise.

B. **Causative Agent (Enteropathogenic *E. coli*).** The genus *Escherichia* belonging to the **Enterobacteriaceae family (Gram-negative facultative anaerobic bacilli**; see Small Intestine V B) is a Gram-negative bacillus, facultative anaerobic, motile, catalase positive, oxidase negative, ferments glucose, ferments lactose, phenylalanine positive (produce indole), and reduces nitrites to nitrates. *E. coli* is the most common species.

C. **Reservoir.** *E. coli* normally colonizes the human intestinal tract. Enteropathogenic *E. coli* is transmitted by contaminated food and water through poor sanitation.

D. **Virulence Factors**
1. Enteropathogenic *E. coli* does not enter enterocytes but instead remains in the intestinal lumen and binds to epithelial cells through **bundle-forming pili (Bfp).**
2. Binding is followed by active secretion of bacterial proteins (a **bacterial Type III secretion system**) into the host epithelial cell cytoplasm. One of these proteins called **translocated intimin receptor (TIR)** is inserted into the epithelial cell membrane and serves as a receptor for the bacterial adhesin called **intimin**. This leads to actin rearrangement within the epithelial cell and microvillus damage.
3. **Other virulence factors common to all members of Enterobacteriaceae**. See Small Intestine V B above.

VII Food Poisoning Caused by *Staphylococcus aureus* (Figure 7-2E)

A. **General Features.** *S. aureus* causes food poisoning associated with foods (e.g., dairy produce, canned or salted meats, eggs, and salads) contaminated by a food handler and stored in a room temperature where bacteria can multiply and enterotoxin levels can increase. Staphylococcal-contaminated foods look and taste normal. Cooking does not destroy either the bacteria or the enterotoxin. Both the bacteria and the enterotoxin proliferate at 68 °F to 99 °F. Clinical findings include watery diarrhea; vomiting; nausea; abdominal cramps; incubation period is 1 to 6 h after ingestion of preformed toxin; and duration of illness is 24 h.

B. **Causative Agent (*S. aureus*).** The genus *Staphylococcus* is a Gram-positive coccus that tends to grow in clusters and is catalase positive. *S. aureus* is a Gram-positive coccus, aerobic or facultative anaerobic, catalase positive, coagulase positive (initiates the formation of a fibrin clot), β-hemolytic (a clear zone surrounding a bacterial colony grown on blood-agar medium), salt tolerant (haloduric), contains protein A (binds to Fc fragment of IgG and inhibits phagocytosis), produces a yellow pigment, and may produce exotoxins.

C. **Reservoir.** *S. aureus* normally colonizes the nasopharyngeal mucosa and resides on the skin. *S. aureus* is transmitted by sneezing, skin lesions, and touch with the hands.

D. **Drug Resistance.** Methicillin resisitance of Methicillin-resistant *S. aureus* (MRSA) is due to the acquisition of the *mec*A gene that codes for an abnormal penicillin-binding protein (PBP2′) that does not bind penicillins. Expression of PBP2′ renders bacteria resistant to all β-lactam antibiotics (including cephalosporins and carbapenems). Most MRSA strains also have plasmid-mediated resistance to other drugs except glycopeptides (e.g., vancomycin).

E. **Virulence Factors**
1. *S. aureus* contains **Protein A** on the cell surface which binds the Fc portion of IgG and prevents antibody-mediated clearance of the bacteria.
2. *S. aureus* produces five cytolytic toxins (α, β, δ, γ, and Panton–Valentine leukocidin). **α toxin** is a 33,000d protein that integrates into the host cell

membrane (e.g., RBCs, leukocytes, hepatocytes, platelets, and smooth muscle cells) forming 1 to 2 nm pores that lead to osmotic swelling and cell lysis. **β toxin** (sphingomyelinase C) is a 35,000d protein that catalyzes the hydrolysis of phospholipids in the host cell membrane (e.g., RBCs, leukocytes, macrophages, and fibroblasts) proportional to the amount of sphingomyelin exposed on the cell surface. **δ toxin** is a 3,000d polypeptide that disrupts the cell membrane and intracellular membranes by a detergent like action. **γ toxin** and **Panton–Valentine leukocidin** are bicomponent toxins (composed of two polypeptide chains The S [slow-eluting] component and the F [fast-eluting] component) that integrate into the host cell membrane (e.g., RBCs, neutrophils, and macrophages) forming 1 to 2 nm pores that lead to osmotic swelling and cell lysis.

3. *S. aureus* produces two exfoliative toxins (ETA and ETB). **ETA** is a heat-stable serine protease whose gene is chromosomal. **ETB** is a heat-labile serine protease and is plasmid mediated. ETA and ETB promote the splitting of desmosomes within the stratum granulosum of the skin epidermis.
4. *S. aureus* produces **eight enterotoxins (A–E, G–I)**. All the enterotoxins are heat stable (heating to 100 °C for 30 min) and hydrolysis resistant to gastric and jejunal enzymes. The precise mechanism of action is not known; however, these enterotoxins are superantigens that activate T cells causing the release of cytokines and mast cells causing the release of inflammatory mediators.
5. *S. aureus* produces **toxic shock syndrome toxin-1 (TSST-1)**. TSST-1 is a 22,000d heat-stable, proteolysis-resistant protein whose gene is chromosomal. TSST-1 is a superantigen that activates T cells and macrophages causing release of cytokines and reduces normal liver clearance of endogenous endotoxin.

VIII Food Poisoning Caused by *Clostridium perfringens* (Figure 7-2F,G)

A. **General Features.** *C. perfringens* causes food poisoning associated with heavily contaminated meats usually prepared in large quantities and kept warm (not hot) for an extended period of time. The primary contamination of the meat with spores is common when food is allowed to stand at 80 °F to 120 °F. The enterotoxin is produced after the spores are ingested and germinate in the small intestine. Clinical findings include watery diarrhea; acute midgastric cramping; incubation period is 8 to 24 h; and duration of illness is 24 h.

B. **Causative Agent (*C. perfringens*).** The genus *Clostridium* is a large, Gram-positive bacillus, spore forming, and anaerobic. *C. perfringens* is a large, rectangular, Gram-positive bacillus, spore forming (although spores are rarely seen in clinical specimens or culture), obligate anaerobic, hemolytic (a "double zone" is seen on blood agar), grows rapidly in tissues and cultures, and nonmotile.

C. **Reservoir.** *C. perfringens* normally colonizes the colon of humans and animals. *C. perfringens* spores are found in the soil and dust contaminated by feces. Spores are formed under adverse environmental conditions and survive for prolonged periods.

D. **Virulence Factors**

1. *C. perfringens* Type A produces an **enterotoxin** that is heat-labile, produced during the transition from vegetative bacteria to spores, and released when the bacteria undergo lysis. The alkaline conditions of the small intestines provoke sporulation. The enterotoxin binds to epithelial cells and disrupts the microvillus border, both of which disrupt ion transport.
2. *C. perfringens* Type A produces lethal **α toxin**, known as **phospholipase C (a lecithinase)**, which lyses RBCs, platelets, and WBCs. This results in massive hemolysis, myonecrosis, hepatic toxicity, and myocardial dysfunction.

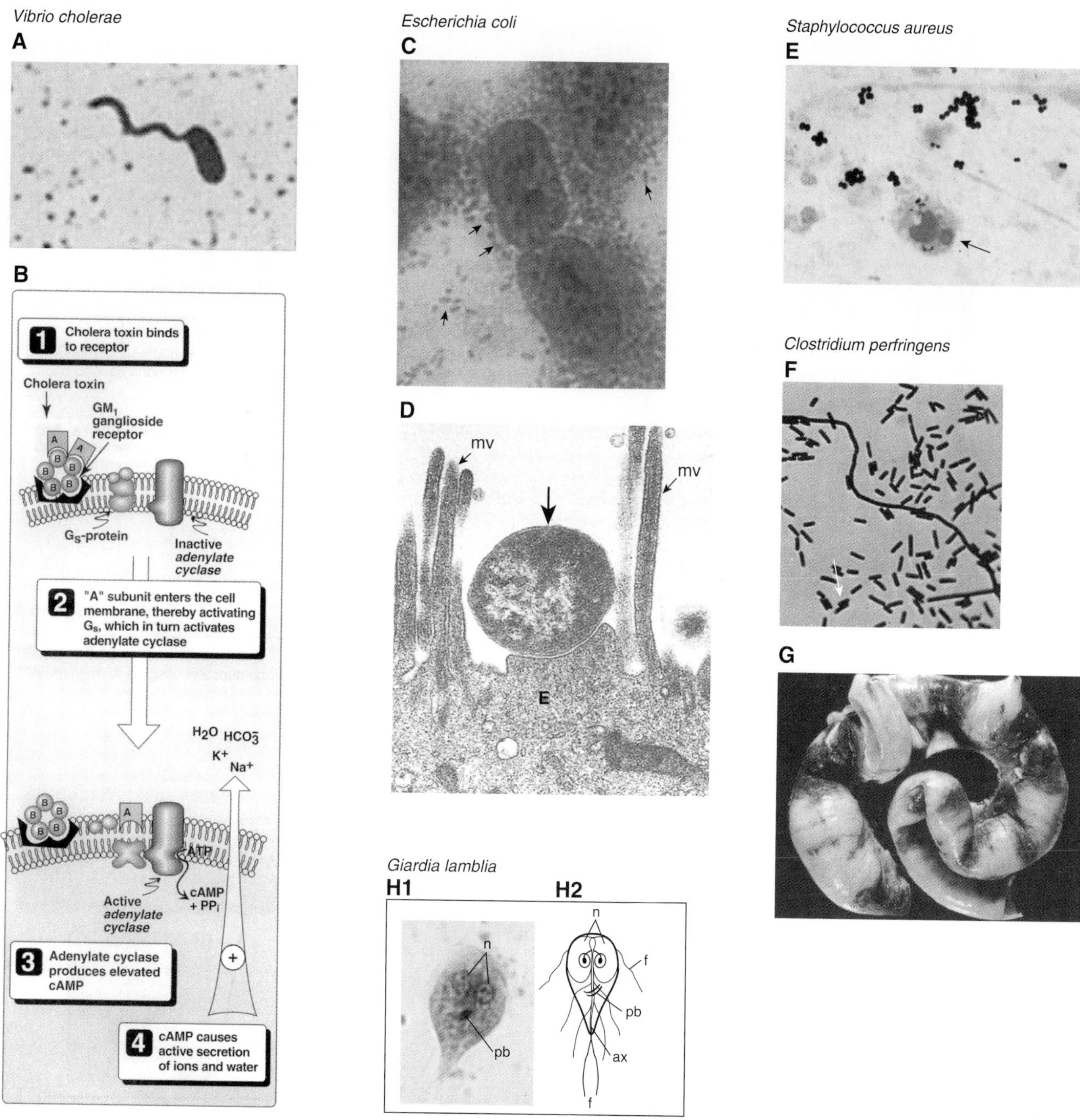

FIGURE 7-2. **Microbiology of the Small Intestine. (A,B)** ***Vibrio cholerae.*** **(A)** Light micrograph shows the Gram-negative, single-flagellated, comma-shaped bacillus called *Vibrio cholerae*. **(B)** Diagram shows the mechanism of action of cholera toxin (choleragen). **(C,D) Enterotoxigenic and Enteropathogenic** ***Escherichia coli.*** **(C)** Light micrograph shows enterotoxigenic or enteropathogenic *E. coli* (arrows) within the intestinal lumen some of which are bound to the surface of epithelial cells. **(D)** Electron micrograph shows enterotoxigenic or enteropathogenic *E. coli* (arrow) bound to the surface of an intestinal epithelial cell (E). **(E)** ***Staphylococcus aureus.*** LM shows Gram-positive grapelike clusters of staphylococci in a Gram-stained smear of a purulent sputum. Note that a neutrophil (arrow) can also be seen. **(F,G)** ***Clostridium perfringens.*** **(F)** Light micrograph shows Gram-positive, large, rectangular bacilli called *Clostridium perfringens* after a 24-h growth in broth culture. **(G) Pig Bel due to** ***C. perfringens*** **Infection.** Photograph of gross specimen shows patchy, segmental necrosis of the small intestine. The necrosis starts at the tips of the villi and progresses toward the base of the villi. There is a clear transition zone observed between the necrotic mucosa and the submucosa. The blood vessels at this transitional zone are thrombosed. **(H)** ***Giardia lamblia.*** **(H1)** Light micrograph shows a *G. lamblia* trophozoite with its distinctive pear-shaped appearance, two nuclei (n), and a parabasal body (pb). **(H2)** Diagram shows a *G. lamblia* trophozoite. Trophozoites are bilaterally symmetrical, pear-shaped, have two nuclei (n) with large central karyosomes, two oblong parabasal bodies (pb) located below the nucleus, four pairs of flagella (f), a rodlike axostyle (ax) that runs the length of the organism, and a ventral sucking disc (not shown). mv — microvilli.

TABLE 7-1 SUMMARY TABLE OF MICROBIOLOGIC DISEASES ASSOCIATED WITH THE ESOPHAGUS, STOMACH, AND SMALL INTESTINE

Disease	Causative Agent	Reservoir	Virulence Factors	Clinical Findings
Stomach				
Peptic ulcer disease	*H. pylori* Gram-negative bacilli	Found only in humans Transmitted by fecal–oral route	Mucinase Phospholipase Urease HspB VacA Superoxide dismutase Catalase	**Gastric ulcers:** Burning epigastric pain soon after eating; pain increases with food intake; pain is relieved by antacids; patient is afraid to eat and loses weight **Duodenal ulcers:** Burning epigastric pain 1–3 h after eating; pain decreases with food intake; pain is relieved by antacids; patient does not lose weight; patient wakes up at night due to pain
Small intestine				
Viral gastroenteritis	Rotavirus Type A Segmented double-stranded RNA virus	Transmitted by the fecal–oral route	nsP4	Watery, nonbloody diarrhea, fever, vomiting (may be predominant), and dehydration in children 6–24 months of age; incubation period is <48 h; fall/winter is the predominant season of infection; and duration of illness is 5–7 days
Viral gastroenteritis	Adenovirus Linear double-stranded DNA virus	Transmitted by respiratory droplets or fecal–oral route		Watery diarrhea in children <2 years of age, which may be accompanied by fever, vomiting, and dehydration; incubation period is 8–10 days; summer is the predominant season of infection; and duration of illness is 6–9 days
Viral gastroenteritis	Norwalk agent Nonsegmented + sense RNA virus	Transmitted by fecal–oral route or by shellfish		Watery diarrhea, low-grade fever, and vomiting in older children and adults; incubation period is 1–2 days; no predominant season of infection (small peaks in winter months have been reported); and duration of illness is 1–4 days
Cholera	*V. cholerae* O1 or O139 strains of the E1 Tor biotype Gram-negative bacilli	Transmitted by contaminated food and water; associated with eating of raw or undercooked seafood	Cholera toxin with which ADP-ribosylates a G protein ToxR upregulates cholera toxin Toxin coregulated pili	Sudden onset of profuse watery diarrhea with mucus flecks but no blood (rice-water stools); no fever; there may be vomiting; hypovolemic shock will occur (fatal within 8 h) if electrolytes and fluids are not replaced; incubation period is 2–3 days; and a long-lasting immunity to the serotype occurs
Diarrhea (Traveler's diarrhea)	Enterotoxigenic *E. coli* Gram-negative bacilli Facultative anaerobe Motile	Transmitted by contaminated food or water through poor sanitation and the use of human feces as fertilizer	LT (similar to cholera toxin) ST Endotoxin (LPS) Capsular antigens Antigenic phase variation (H&K antigens) Enterobactin Resistance to serum killing Resistance to antibiotics	Watery diarrhea; vomiting; abdominal cramps; incubation period is 24–48 h; duration of illness is 1–2 days; and hypovolemic shock will occur if electrolytes and fluids are not replaced.

Diarrhea	Enteropathogenic *E. coli* Gram-negative bacilli Facultative anaerobe Motile	Transmitted by contaminated food or water through poor sanitation and the use of human feces as fertilizer	Bfp TIR Intimin Bacterial Type III secretion system Endotoxin (LPS) Capsular antigens Antigenic phase variation (H&K antigens) Enterobactin Resistance to serum killing Resistance to antibiotics	Watery diarrhea with mucus; vomiting; fever; and malaise
Food poisoning	*S. aureus* Gram-positive cocci Aerobic or facultative anaerobe	Normally colonizes the nasopharynx and resides on the skin Transmitted by sneezing, skin lesions, and touch with hands Food (dairy, produce, canned or salted meats, eggs, and salads) contaminated by food handler and stored at room temperature	Protein A α toxin β toxin δ toxin γ toxin Panton–Valentine leukocidin ETA and ETB Enterotoxins A–E, G–I TSST-1	Watery diarrhea; vomiting; nausea; abdominal cramps; incubation period is 1–6 h after ingestion of preformed toxin; and duration of illness is 24 h
Food poisoning	*C. perfringens* Gram-positive bacilli Spore-forming Obligate anaerobe	Normally colonizes colon of humans and animals Spores are found in soil and dust contaminated by feces	Enterotoxin (heat-labile) α toxin (phospholipase C) β toxin ε toxin (permease) ι toxin	Watery diarrhea; acute midgastric cramping; incubation period is 8–24 h; and duration of illness is 24 h
Giardiasis	*G. lamblia* Teardrop-shaped flagellated protozoan Cyst and trophozoite stages	Transmitted by ingestion of cysts found in lake or river water contaminated by feces due to infected beavers, muskrats, or humans Food contaminated with feces Oral–anal sex	Cysts are resistant to chlorine, so water should be treated with filtration, boiling, or iodine Ventral sucking disc	Sudden onset of foul-smelling, watery diarrhea; abdominal cramps; flatulence; steatorrhea; temporary lactose intolerance; incubation period is 1–4 weeks (average of 10 days); duration of illness is 10–14 days; multiple relapses may occur; and some infections may be asymptomatic (i.e., a carrier) Common in hikers

3. *C. perfringens* Type C produces lethal β **toxin** that has necrotizing activity. This results in a hemorrhagic necrosis of the jejunum (enteritis necroticans or pig bel).
4. *C. perfringens* produces lethal ε **protoxin (a permease)** that is activated by trypsin. This results in an increased vascular permeability of the GI wall.
5. *C. perfringens* produces lethal ι **toxin** that has necrotizing and ADP ribosylating activity.

IX Giardiasis Caused by *Giardia lamblia* (Figure 7-2H)

A. **General Features.** *G. lamblia* infection causes giardiasis that is initiated with the ingestion of ≈10 to 25 cysts. Gastric acid stimulates ex-cystation whereby the trophozoites are released into the small intestine. *G. lamblia* attaches to the microvillus border of enterocytes via a ventral sucking disc and blocks absorption. *G. lamblia* is the most frequent cause of waterborne diarrhea in the United States and the most common intestinal parasite. Clinical features include sudden onset of foul-smelling, watery diarrhea; abdominal cramps; flatulence; steatorrhea; temporary lactose intolerance; incubation period is 1 to 4 weeks (average of 10 days); duration of illness is 10 to14 days; multiple relapses may occur; and some infections may be asymptomatic (i.e., a carrier).

B. **Causative Agent (*G. lamblia*).** *G. lamblia* is a pear-shaped flagellated protozoan that replicates by binary fission. *G. lamblia* has both **trophozoite** and **cyst** (the infectious form) stages. Trophozoites are bilaterally symmetrical, pear-shaped, have two nuclei with large central karyosomes, two oblong parabasal bodies located below the nucleus, four pairs of flagella, a rodlike axostyle that runs the length of the organism, a ventral sucking disc, and do not survive outside the GI tract. Cysts are oval-shaped and have four nuclei, four parabasal bodies, and a thick protective wall. One cyst can produce two trophozoites.

C. **Reservoir.** *G. lamblia* is transmitted by ingestion of cysts found in lake or river water contaminated with fecal matter due to infected beavers, muskrats, or humans. *G. lamblia* is also transmitted by food contaminated with fecal matter (e.g., day care diaper changing) or oral–anal sex. Giardiasis is common in hikers who drink untreated water in the wilderness. Cysts are resistant to chlorine, so drinking water should be treated with filtration, boiling, or iodine.

Large Intestine (Table 7-2)

I Infectious Colitis Caused by *Shigella* (Shigellosis) (Figure 7-3A,B)

A. **General Features.** *Shigella dysenteriae, S. boydii, S. flexneri, and S. sonnei* cause infectious colitis. Clinical findings include frequent low-volume stools with blood and pus; fever; tenesmus (painful straining at defecation); abdominal cramping; invasion of mucosa produces local inflammation (neutrophils) and ulceration; does not cause bacteremia; positive methylene blue staining of stool sample indicates the presence of neutrophils; incubation period is 1 to 4 days; no predominant season of infection; duration of untreated disease is 1 to 30 days; most common in children 1 to 4 years of age; mortality occurs in children <15 years of age due to dehydration; and symptoms may vary widely depending on the patient's nutrition or age, the infective strain, or the dose.

B. **Causative Agent *(S. dysenteriae, S. boydii, S. flexneri, and S. sonnei)*.** The genus *Shigella* belonging to the **Enterobacteriaceae family (Gram-negative facultative anaerobic bacilli**; See Small Intestine V B) is a Gram-negative bacillus, facultative anaerobic, nonmotile, catalase positive, oxidase negative, ferments glucose, does not ferment lactose (except *S. sonnei*, which is a slow lactose fermenter), and does not produce H_2S gas. *S. dysenteriae* is rare in the United States and causes the most severe disease. *S. sonnei* is the most common species in the United States and causes mild dysentery (a self-limiting diarrhea).

C. **Reservoir.** Shigella is transmitted by the fecal–oral route primarily by people with contaminated hands. Shigella may also be transmitted in food or by flies (Note: The four Fs: feces, fingers, food, and flies). Humans are the only known reservoir. Shigella epidemics may occur in day care centers, nurseries, and custodial institutions partially due to the extremely low infectious dose of 10 to 100 shigellae.

D. **Virulence Factors**

1. Shigella attaches to and enters the cytoplasm of **M cells** of the Peyer patches, **replicates in the cytoplasm** after escaping the phagolysosome, and **moves laterally** to the adjoining enterocytes through actin polymerization (similar to *Listeria monocytogenes*) which allows Shigella to avoid contact with immune cells in the early stages of infection.
2. Shigella secretes **IpaA, IpaB, IpaC**, and **IpaD bacterial proteins** (a **bacterial Type III secretion system**) which induce membrane ruffling and promote engulfment of Shigella into enterocytes.
3. Shigella **induces apoptosis** of the enterocytes so that it can enter the lamina propria, attract neutrophils and macrophages, and produce the characteristic Shigella ulcers without any vascular invasion (bacteremia is rare).
4. Shigella produces an exotoxin called **Shiga toxin** that consists of **one A subunit** and **five B subunits (an A–B component toxin)**. The B subunits bind to the **Gb_3 glycolipid** on the cell membrane which facilitates the entry of the A subunit into the cell. The A subunit cleaves the 28S rRNA in the 60S ribosomal subunit thereby inhibiting protein synthesis. This results in damage to the intestinal enterocytes and glomerular endothelium. ***S. dysenteriae* Type 1** causes the most severe disease because it produces the most Shiga toxin.
5. **Other virulence factors common to all members of Enterobacteriaceae**. See Small Intestine V B.

II Infectious Colitis Caused by *Salmonella enterica* Serotype *Typhimurium* (Salmonellosis) *(Figure 7-3C,D)*

A. **General Features.** *S. enterica* serotype *Typhimurium* causes infectious colitis. Clinical findings include watery diarrhea; fever; abdominal pain; nausea; vomiting; invasion of mucosa produces local inflammation (neutrophils); does not cause bacteremia; positive methylene blue staining of stool sample indicates the presence of neutrophils; incubation period is 10 to 24 h; duration of disease is 2 to 7 days; and young children and the elderly are particularly susceptible.

B. **Causative Agent (*S. enterica* Serotype *Typhimurium*).** The genus *Salmonella* belonging to the **Enterobacteriaceae family (Gram-negative facultative anaerobic bacilli**; See Small Intestine V B) is a Gram-negative bacillus, facultative anaerobic, motile, catalase positive, oxidase negative, ferments glucose, does not ferment lactose, and produces H_2S gas. Currently, all strains are grouped into a single species called *S. enterica*. This species is further subdivided into >1,500 serotypes based on its cell wall (O), flagellar (H), and capsular (Vi) antigens.

C. **Reservoir.** *S. enterica* serotype *Typhimurium* is transmitted by contaminated raw poultry, raw eggs, raw milk, or reptilian pets (e.g. turtles). There are many animal reservoirs. *S. enterica* serotype *Typhimurium* infection is common in young children, elderly, immunocompromised patients, and individuals with reduced gastric acid production. *S. enterica* serotype *Typhimurium* epidemics may occur in day care centers, nurseries, and custodial institutions. *S. enterica* serotype *Typhimurium* has a very high infectious dose of ≈100,000 salmonellae.

D. **Virulence Factors**

1. Salmonella attaches to (by species-specific fimbriae) and enters the cytoplasm of **M cells** of the Peyer patches and **replicates in the phagolysosome.**
2. Salmonella secretes **Sips or Ssps bacterial proteins** (a bacterial **SPI-1 Type III secretion system**) that induce membrane ruffling and promote engulfment of Salmonella into enterocytes.
3. Salmonella induces apoptosis of the enterocytes so that it can enter the lamina propria and attract neutrophils.
4. Salmonella also secretes other bacterial proteins using a **SPI-2 Type III secretion system**.
5. Salmonella has a **V_i capsular antigen.**
6. Salmonella has an **acid tolerance response (ATR) gene** that protects it from gastric acid and the acid pH of the phagolysosome.
7. Salmonella produces **catalase** and **superoxide dismutase** that protect it from intracellular killing.
8. **Other virulence factors common to all members of Enterobacteriaceae**. See Small Intestine V B.

F. **Other Diseases**

1. **Typhoid Fever. *S. enterica* serotype *Typhi*** causes **typhoid fever** (enteric fever). Typhoid fever is not common in the United States (≈500 cases/year). However, there are ≈17 million cases/year resulting in ≈600 deaths/year worldwide. Clinical findings include gradual onset of a headache, loss of appetite, malaise, lethargy, bacteremia, fever, abdominal pain, constipation in early stages followed by short bouts of diarrhea, hepatosplenomegaly, mesenteric lymphadenopathy, and rose spots on the abdomen.

III Infectious Colitis Caused by *Yersinia enterocolitica* (Figure 7-3E,F)

A. **General Features.** *Y. enterocolitica* causes infectious colitis. Clinical findings include diarrhea with blood and pus; fever; abdominal pain; mesenteric lymphadenitis may mimic appendicitis; reactive arthritis is a late complication that occurs 2 weeks after the GI symptoms; incubation period is 1 to 10 days; winter is the predominant season of infection; duration of disease is 1 to 2 weeks; most common in children; and most commonly seen in Scandinavian countries and colder regions of North America.

B. **Causative Agent (*Y. enterocolitica*).** The genus *Yersinia* belonging to the **Enterobacteriaceae family (Gram-negative facultative anaerobic bacilli**; See Small Intestine V B) is a Gram-negative bacillus, facultative anaerobic, motile, catalase positive, oxidase-negative, ferments glucose, and does not ferment lactose. The genus *Yersinia* consists of 10 species with *Y. pestis*, *Y. enterocolitica*, and *Y. pseudotuberculosis* being the most well-known human pathogens. *Y. enterocolitica* consists of **1A** (does not cause human disease), **1B, 2, 3, 4, and 5 subgroups**. *Y. enterocolitica* is **zoonotic** (transmissible from animals to humans) and **can grow in the cold**.

C. **Reservoir.** *Y. enterocolitica* is transmitted by direct contact with pigs, rodents, livestock, or rabbits. *Y. enterocolitica* may also be transmitted by contaminated meat, raw milk, or water.

D. Virulence Factors

1. The *Yersinia* genus is characterized by its ability to resist phagocytic killing.
2. Yersinia secretes a **YopH gene product** (a **bacterial Type III secretion system**) that dephosphorylates (inactivates) several proteins involved in phagocytosis.
3. Yersinia secretes a **YopE gene product** (a **bacterial Type III secretion system**) that disrupts actin filaments within macrophages.
4. Yersinia secretes a **YopJ/P gene product** (a **bacterial Type III secretion system**) that induces apoptosis in macrophages.
5. **Other virulence factors common to all members of Enterobacteriaceae**. See Small Intestine V B.

E. Other Diseases

1. **Urban Plague (Bubonic Plague; Black Death).** *Y. pestis* causes urban plague which is one of the most devastating diseases in history with at least three major pandemics. Urban plague is spread between rats and humans by infected fleas. It has been effectively eliminated in modern societies by rat control and community hygiene.

IV Infectious Colitis Caused by Enterohemorrhagic *E. coli* Serotype 0157:H7 *(Figure 7-3G,H)*

A. General Features. Enterohemorrhagic *E. coli* serotype 0157:H7 causes infectious colitis that may lead to a hemorrhagic colitis. Pathological findings include enterocytes show microvillus damage and surface effacement; no mucosal invasion; and no predominant neutrophil infiltration. Clinical findings include copious amounts of bloody diarrhea without pus; no prominent fever; severe abdominal cramps; incubation period is 3 to 4 days; summer is the predominant season of infection; duration of disease is 4 to 10 days; most common in children <5 years of age; antibiotic treatment is currently contraindicated; and **hemolytic uremic syndrome** is a serious complication characterized by acute renal failure, thrombocytopenia, platelet aggregation (thrombus formation), and hemolytic anemia (may lead to death).

B. Causative Agent (Enterohemorrhagic *E. coli* serotype 0157:H7). The genus *Escherichia* belonging to the **Enterobacteriaceae family (Gram-negative facultative anaerobic bacilli**; See Small Intestine V B) is a Gram-negative bacillus, facultative anaerobic, motile, catalase positive, oxidase negative, ferments glucose, ferments lactose, phenylalanine positive (produces indole), and reduces nitrites to nitrates. *E. coli* is the most common species. Enterohemorrhagic *E. coli* serotype 0157:H7 is the most common serotype in the United States although >50 serotypes have been identified.

C. Reservoir. Enterohemorrhagic *E. coli* serotype 0157:H7 is transmitted by contaminated **undercooked ground beef (hamburger)**, water, unpasteurized milk or fruit juices (e.g., apple cider made from contaminated apples), or uncooked vegetables. Cattle are the primary reservoir. Enterohemorrhagic *E. coli* serotype 0157:H7 has a low infectious dose of <100 bacteria.

D. Virulence Factors

1. Enterohemorrhagic *E. coli* serotype 0157:H7 produces an exotoxin (or **verotoxin**) called **Shigalike toxin I (SLT-I)** and **Shigalike toxin II (SLT-II)**, both of which consist of **one A subunit** and **five B subunits (an A–B component toxin).** The B subunits bind to the **Gb_3 glycolipid** on the cell membrane which facilitates the entry of the A subunit into the cell. The A subunit cleaves the 28S rRNA in the 60S ribosomal subunit thereby inhibiting protein synthesis. This results in damage to the intestinal enterocytes and glomerular endothelium.
2. **Other virulence factors common to all members of Enterobacteriaceae**. See Small Intestine V B.

V Infectious Colitis Caused by Enteroinvasive *E. coli* (Figure 7-3G,H)

A. **General Features.** Enteroinvasive *E. coli* causes infectious colitis similar to shigellosis. Clinical findings include frequent low-volume stools with blood and pus; fever; tenesmus (painful straining at defecation); abdominal cramping; and invasion of mucosa that produces local inflammation (neutrophils) and ulceration.

B. **Causative Agent (Enteroinvasive *E. coli*).** The genus *Escherichia* belonging to the **Enterobacteriaceae family (Gram-negative facultative anaerobic bacilli**; See Small Intestine V B) is a Gram-negative bacillus, facultative anaerobic, motile, catalase positive, oxidase negative, ferments glucose, ferments lactose, phenylalanine positive (produces indole), and reduces nitrites to nitrates. *E. coli* is the most common species.

C. **Reservoir.** Enteroinvasive *E. coli* is transmitted by contaminated food.

D. **Virulence Factors**
   1. Enteroinvasive *E. coli* has pathogenic properties very closely related to Shigella. Enteroinvasive *E. coli* probably attaches to and enters the cytoplasm of **M cells** of the Peyer patches, **replicates in the cytoplasm** after escaping the phagolysosome, and **moves laterally** to the adjoining enterocytes through actin polymerization (similar to *L. monocytogenes*).
   2. Enteroinvasive *E. coli* expresses the ***pInv* genes** that are carried on a plasmid and mediate invasion of the enterocytes.
   3. **Other virulence factors common to all members of Enterobacteriaceae**. See Small Intestine V B.

VI Pseudomembranous Colitis Caused by *Clostridium difficile* (Figure 7-3I,J)

A. **General Features.** *C. difficile* causes pseudomembranous colitis. Pathological findings include sigmoidoscopy shows white plaques of fibrin, mucus, and inflammatory cells overlying a normal intestinal mucosa. Clinical findings include bloody diarrhea; fever; abdominal pain; dehydration; leukocytosis; associated with patients undergoing antibiotic therapy (most commonly clindamycin, ampicillin, and cephalosporins); discontinuation of the implicated antibiotic is generally sufficient to alleviate mild symptoms; serious disease is treated with metronidazole or vancomycin; and the most common cause of hospital-acquired diarrhea.

B. **Causative Agent (*C. difficile*).** The genus *Clostridium* is a Gram-positive bacillus, obligate anaerobic, and spore forming. *C. difficile* is a Gram-positive bacillus, obligate anaerobic, spore forming, and motile.

C. **Reservoir.** *C. difficile* normally colonizes ≈5% of the healthy adults. Patients undergoing antibiotic therapy may experience an overgrowth of *C. difficile* and subsequent disease (i.e., endogenous infection). After introduction of *C. difficile* to a site, the bedding, toilets, and dust become contaminated with spores and new residents are easily infected (i.e., exogenous infection).

D. **Virulence Factors**
   1. *C. difficile* produces **Toxin A** (an enterotoxin) that is chemotactic for neutrophils. Neutrophils release cytokines that cause hypersecretion of fluids (i.e., diarrhea).
   2. *C. difficile* produces a **Toxin B** (a cytotoxin) that kills enterocytes by actin depolymerization and destruction of the cytoskeleton.

VII Infectious Colitis Caused by *Campylobacter jejuni* (Figure 7-3K,L)

A. **General Features.** *C. jejuni* causes infectious colitis. Pathological findings include enterocytes are damaged; mucosa is ulcerated, edematous, and bloody; and lamina propria is infiltrated with inflammatory cells which is consistent with the invasion of *C. jejuni*. Clinical findings include bloody diarrhea with pus; fever; acute abdominal pain (may resemble appendicitis); malaise; incubation period is 1 to 7 days; summer is the predominant season of infection but occurs throughout the year; duration of disease is <7 days; and most common in preschool children and young adults. *C. jejuni* may cause Guillain–Barre syndrome or reactive arthritis.

B. **Causative Agent (*C. jejuni*).** The genus *Campylobacter* is a **Gram-negative bacillus** that does not ferment carbohydrates and grows only in a reduced level of oxygen (i.e., microaerophilic). *C. jejuni* is a Gram-negative bacillus, does not ferment glucose, microaerophilic, highly motile, small comma shaped, oxidase positive, urease negative, and nalidixic acid sensitive. *C. jejuni* is **zoonotic** (transmissible from animals to humans).

C. **Reservoir.** *C. jejuni* is transmitted by contaminated raw or undercooked poultry, milk, or water. *C. jejuni* can also be transmitted by direct contact with infected animals or pets. Wild and domesticated animals are the primary reservoir.

D. **Virulence Factors**
   1. *C. jejuni* produces an **enterotoxin** that is heat-labile, activates adenylate cyclase, and increases cAMP.
   2. *C. jejuni* has a **LPS** on its outer membrane which serves as a major antigen.

VIII Amebiasis Caused by *Entamoeba histolytica*

A. **General Features.** *E. histolytica* causes amebiasis that is initiated with the ingestion of cysts. Amebiasis is the colonization of the GI tract with or without disease. **Amebiasis with disease (called amebic dysentery)** occurs when the ameba invades the intestinal wall to feed on RBCs and may enter the portal circulation to form **liver abscesses. Amebiasis without disease (i.e., asymptomatic carriers)** occurs when the amebae feed on the intestinal flora (90% of amebiasis cases). Gastric acid stimulates ex-cystation whereby the trophozoites are released into the small intestine. *E. histolytica* attaches to host cell membranes (i.e., enterocytes, neutrophils, monocytes, and lymphocytes) via a **galactose-inhibitable adherence protein** which is required for cytolysis and tissue necrosis. Pathological findings include flask-shaped ulceration, inflammation, and hemorrhage. Clinical findings include signs without systemic involvement are numerous bloody stools per day, abdominal pain, colitis, and cramping; signs with systemic involvement are fever, leukocytosis, rigors, amebic peritonitis with intestinal perforation, pain over the liver, liver abscesses, hepatomegaly (right lobe usually involved), and elevation of the diaphragm.

B. **Causative Agent (*E. histolytica*).** *E. histolytica* is a nonflagellated (but motile) protozoan that replicates by binary fission. Motility is accomplished through the formation of **pseudopodia** causing a snail like movement. *E. histolytica* has both

trophozoite and **cyst** (the infectious form) stages. Trophozoites have a single round nucleus with a central dot (karyosome); a uniform distribution of chromatin at the periphery of the nucleus; pseudopodia; ingested RBCs may be observed in the cytoplasm; and they do not survive outside the GI tract. Cysts are round and have four nuclei and chromatoidal bars (aggregations of ribosomes). One cyst can produce eight trophozoites.

C. **Reservoir.** *E. histolytica* is transmitted by ingestion of cysts found in water and food contaminated with feces due to poor sanitation (i.e., fecal–oral route). Asymptomatic human carriers are the primary reservoir. *E. histolytica* epidemics may occur in day care centers, nurseries, and custodial institutions primarily due to the presence of asymptomatic human carriers. *E. histolytica* is also transmitted through oral–anal sex and is common among homosexual males.

IX Intestinal Schistosomiasis Caused by *Schistosoma mansoni* or *Schistosoma japonicum*

A. **General Features.** *S. mansoni* and *S. japonicum* cause intestinal schistosomiasis which is initiated by skin-penetrating cercaria liberated from snails. Clinical findings include infection causes an intensely itchy rash that disappears in 1 to 3 weeks; diarrhea, fever, and headache occur after the rash disappears; eggs induce an immune response similar to serum sickness 1 to 2 months after initial infection; diarrhea, fever, chills, hepatomegaly, and splenomegaly occur 1 to 2 months after initial infection (called Katayama syndrome); and eggs reach the vasculature of the intestines inducing inflammation, granuloma formation, fibrosis, and scarring.

B. **Causative Agents**

1. ***S. mansoni*** is a trematode (fluke) worm belonging to the Platyhelminthes phylum. *S. mansoni* has separate male and female worms where the female worm lives in a groove on the male worm's body; the female worm is cylindrical-shaped and the male worm is flat-shaped but folds ventrally to hold the female worm; it has both sexual (in the human host) and asexual (in the snail host) reproduction; eggs are large, oval, and have a prominent lateral spine; it is an obligate intravascular parasite; and adult worms reside in the **inferior mesenteric veins** of the descending colon and rectum.
2. ***S. japonicum*** is a trematode (fluke) worm belonging to the Platyhelminthes phylum. *S. japonicum* has separate male and female worms where the female worm lives in a groove on the male worm's body; the female worm is cylindrical-shaped and the male

FIGURE 7-3. **Microbiology of the Large Intestine. (A,B) *Shigella dysenteriae, S. boydii, S. flexneri, and S. sonnei* (Shigellosis). (A)** Light micrograph shows mucosal ulceration and transmural inflammation with many neutrophils. **(B)** Diagram shows the mechanism of action of Shiga toxin. **(C,D) *Salmonella enterica* Serotype *Typhimurium (Salmonellosis) and S. enterica* Serotype. *Typhi* (Typhoid fever). (C)** Light micrograph shows the Gram-negative, flagellated bacillus called *Salmonella enterica* serotype *Typhimurium*. **(D)** Light micrograph of an endoscopic mucosal biopsy from a patient with Salmonellosis. In acute self-limited colitis, the intestinal glands are not distorted (i.e., they remain straight, evenly spaced tubules) and this differentiates it from idiopathic inflammatory bowel disease. The lamina propria contains an inflammatory infiltrate of predominately neutrophils. The neutrophils may accumulate within the intestinal gland lumen to form crypt abscesses. **(E,F) *Yersinia enterocolitica and Y. pestis.* (E)** Light micrograph shows the Gram-negative bacillus called *Yersinia* pestis. Note the bipolar staining. **(F)** Light micrograph shows a prominent necrotizing granuloma (arrow) characteristic of *Y. enterocolitica* infection. The overlying epithelium is atrophic and ulcerated. **(G,H) *Escherichia coli.* (G)** Diagram of *E. coli* shows the O antigens, H antigens, and K antigens. **(H)** Electron micrograph shows enteroinvasive *E. coli* (arrows) within the cytoplasm of an enterocyte. **(I,J) *Clostridium difficile.* (I)** Photograph shows *C. difficile* grown on cycloserine-cefoxitin fructose agar for 48 h. **(J)** Light micrograph shows white plaques (arrow) of fibrin, mucus, and inflammatory cells (predominately neutrophils) along with a normal intestinal mucosa (*). **(K,L) *Campylobacter jejuni.* (K)** Light micrograph shows the Gram-negative bacillus that is small and comma-shaped called *Campylobacter jejuni*. **(L)** Light micrograph shows the lamina propria infiltrated with neutrophils. In addition, neutrophils are found within the lumen of the intestinal gland (arrow) depicting a crypt abscess.

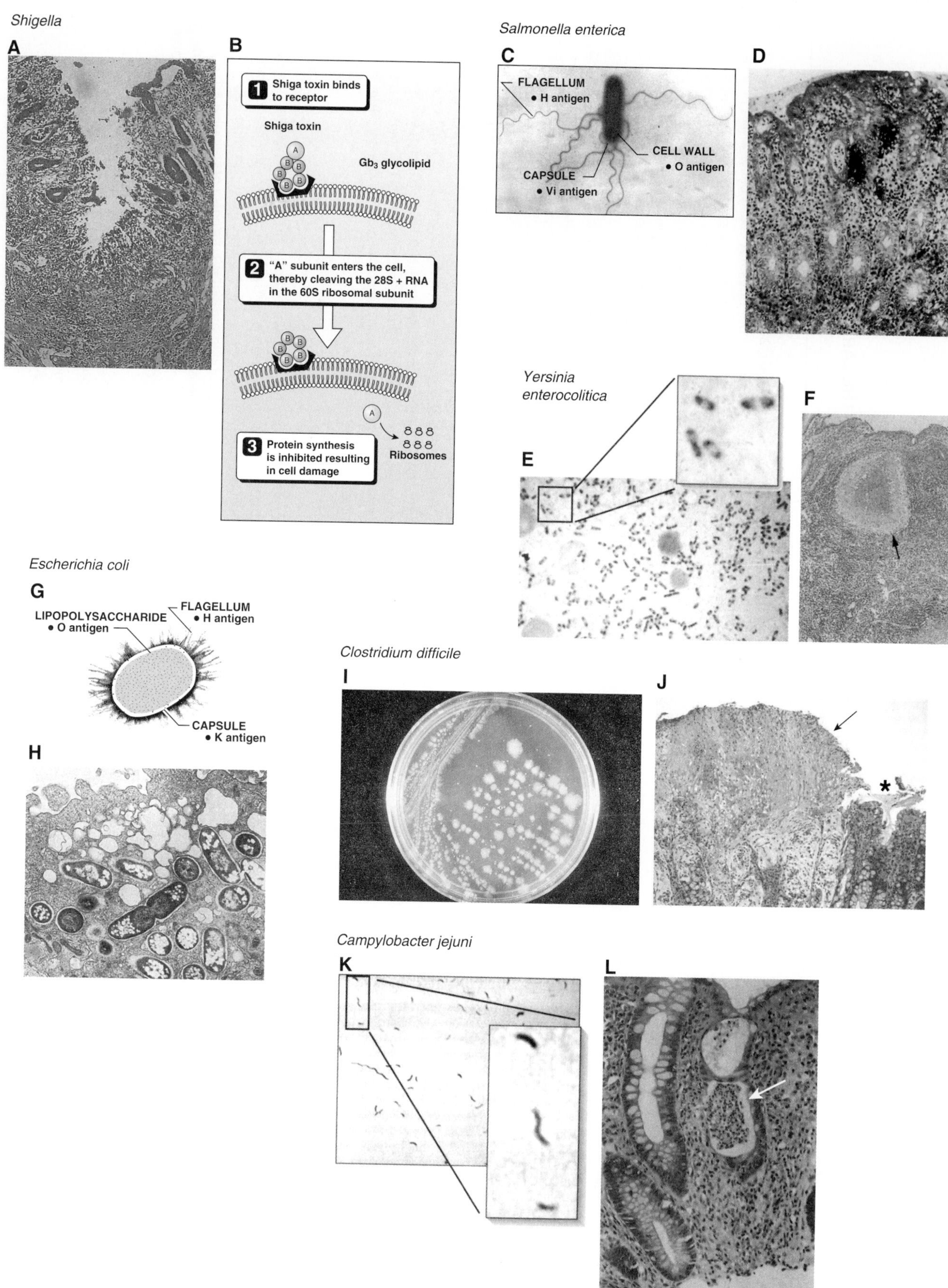
Shigella
A
B
1 Shiga toxin binds to receptor
Shiga toxin
A
B
Gb3 glycolipid
2 "A" subunit enters the cell, thereby cleaving the 28S + RNA in the 60S ribosomal subunit
3 Protein synthesis is inhibited resulting in cell damage
Ribosomes
Salmonella enterica
C
FLAGELLUM
• H antigen
CELL WALL
• O antigen
CAPSULE
• Vi antigen
D
Yersinia enterocolitica
E
F
Escherichia coli
G
LIPOPOLYSACCHARIDE
• O antigen
FLAGELLUM
• H antigen
CAPSULE
• K antigen
H
Clostridium difficile
I
J
Campylobacter jejuni
K
L

TABLE 7-2

SUMMARY TABLE OF MICROBIOLOGIC DISEASES ASSOCIATED WITH THE LARGE INTESTINE

Disease	Causative Agent	Reservoir	Virulence Factors	Clinical Findings
Shigellosis infectious colitis	*S. dysenteriae, S. boydii, S. flexneri, and S. sonnei* Gram-negative bacilli Facultative anaerobe Nonmotile	Transmitted by fecal–oral route by people with contaminated hands Four Fs (feces, fingers, food, and flies)	IpaA, IpaB, IpaC, and IpaD Shiga toxin (A–B component toxin)	Frequent low-volume stools with blood and pus; fever; tenesmus (painful straining at defecation); abdominal cramping; invasion of mucosa produces local inflammation (neutrophils) and ulceration; does not cause bacteremia; positive methylene blue staining of stool sample indicates the presence of neutrophils; incubation period is 1–4 days; no predominant season of infection; duration of untreated disease is 1–30 days; most common in children 1–4 years of age; mortality occurs in children <15 years of age due to dehydration; and symptoms may vary widely depending on the patient's nutrition or age, the infective strain, or the dose
Salmonellosis infectious colitis	*S. enterica* serotype *Typhimurium* Gram-negative bacilli Facultative anaerobe Motile	Transmitted by contaminated raw poultry, raw eggs, raw milk, or reptilian pets (turtles) Many animal reservoirs	Sips and Ssps V_i capsular antigen ATR gene Catalase Superoxide dismutase	Watery diarrhea; fever; abdominal pain; nausea; vomiting; invasion of mucosa produces local inflammation (neutrophils); does not cause bacteremia; positive methylene blue staining of stool sample indicates the presence of neutrophils; incubation period is 10–24 h; duration of disease is 2–7 days; and young children and the elderly are particularly susceptible
Infectious colitis	*Y. enterocolitica* Gram-negative bacilli Facultative anaerobe Motile	Transmitted by direct contact with pigs, rodents, livestock, or rabbits Zoonotic Transmitted by contaminated meat, raw milk, or water	YopH gene product YopE gene product YopJ/P gene product	Diarrhea with blood and pus; fever; abdominal pain; mesenteric lymphadenitis may mimic appendicitis; reactive arthritis is a late complication that occurs two weeks after the GI symptoms; incubation period is 1–10 days; winter is the predominant season of infection; duration of disease is 1–2 weeks; most common in children; and most commonly seen in Scandinavian countries and colder regions of North America
Infectious colitis	Enterohemorrhagic *E. coli* serotype 0157:H7 Gram-negative bacilli Facultative anaerobe Motile	Transmitted by contaminated undercooked ground beef (hamburger), water, unpasteurized milk or fruit juices, or uncooked vegetables Cattle are the primary reservoir	SLT-I (A–B component toxin) SLT-II (A–B component toxin)	Copious amounts of bloody diarrhea without pus; no prominent fever; severe abdominal cramps; incubation period is 3–4 days; summer is the predominant season of infection; duration of disease is 4–10 days; most common in children <5 years of age; antibiotic treatment is currently contraindicated; and **hemolytic uremic syndrome** is a serious complication characterized by acute renal failure, thrombocytopenia, platelet aggregation(thrombus formation), and hemolytic anemia (may lead to death)
Infectious colitis	Enteroinvasive *E. coli* Gram-negative bacilli Facultative anaerobe Motile	Transmitted by contaminated food	*pInv* genes	Frequent low-volume stools with blood and pus; fever; tenesmus (painful straining at defecation); abdominal cramping; and invasion of mucosa produces local inflammation (neutrophils) and ulceration

Pseudo-membranous colitis	*C. difficile* Gram-positive bacilli Obligate anaerobe Spore-forming Motile	Normally colonizes ≈5% of healthy adults Antibiotic therapy may cause overgrowth (endogenous infection) Spores may contaminate bedding, toilet, and dust (exogenous infection)	Toxin A (enterotoxin) Toxin B (cytotoxin)	Bloody diarrhea; fever; abdominal pain; dehydration; leukocytosis; associated with patients undergoing antibiotic therapy (most commonly clindamycin, ampicillin, and cephalosporins); discontinuation of the implicated antibiotic is generally sufficient to alleviate mild symptoms; serious disease is treated with metronidazole or vancomycin; and the most common cause of hospital-acquired diarrhea
Infectious colitis	*C. jejuni* Gram-negative bacilli Microaerophilic Does not ferment glucose Highly motile	Transmitted by contaminated raw or undercooked poultry, milk, or water Transmitted by direct contact with infected animals or pets Wild and domesticated animals are the primary reservoir Zoonotic	Enterotoxin LPS on its outer membrane	Bloody diarrhea with pus; fever; acute abdominal pain (may resemble appendicitis); malaise; incubation period is 1–7 days; summer is the predominant season of infection but occurs throughout the year; duration of disease is <7 days; and most common in preschool children and young adults. *C. jejuni* may cause Guillain–Barre syndrome or reactive arthritis
Amebiasis	*E. histolytica* Protozoa Nonflagellated Motile via pseudopodia Trophozoite and cyst stages	Transmitted by ingestion of cysts found in water and food contaminated with feces due to poor sanitation (fecal–oral route) Asymptomatic human carriers Oral–anal sex		Signs without systemic involvement are numerous bloody stools per day, abdominal pain, colitis, and cramping; signs with systemic involvement are fever, leukocytosis, rigors, amebic peritonitis with intestinal perforation, pain over the liver, liver abscesses, hepatomegaly (right lobe usually involved), and elevation of the diaphragm
Intestinal schistosomiasis	*S. mansoni* *S. japonicum* Trematode (fluke) worm Male and female worms Sexual and asexual reproduction Obligate intravascular parasites	*S. mansoni* is transmitted by cercaria that penetrates the skin; found in Africa, the Middle East, South America, and The Caribbean *S. japonicum* is transmitted by cercaria that penetrates the skin; found in China, Japan, Indonesia, and Philippines		Infection causes an intensely itchy rash that disappears in 1–3 weeks; diarrhea, fever, and headache occur after the rash disappears; eggs induce an immune response similar to serum sickness 1–2 months after initial infection; diarrhea, fever, chills, hepatomegaly, and splenomegaly occur 1–2 months after initial infection (called Katayama syndrome); and eggs reach the vasculature of the intestines inducing inflammation, granuloma formation, fibrosis, and scarring

worm is flat-shaped but folds ventrally to hold the female worm; it has both sexual (in the human host) and asexual (in the snail host) reproduction; eggs are small, spherical, and have a small lateral spine; it is an obligate intravascular parasite; adult worms reside in the **superior mesenteric veins** of the small intestine and ascending colon; and adult worms may also reside in the **choroid plexus** and **venules around the spinal cord** may also be involved.

C. **Reservoir**

1. ***S. mansoni*** is transmitted by the cercaria that penetrates the skin found in contaminated fresh water. *S. mansoni* is found predominately in Africa, the Middle East, South America, and the Caribbean.
2. ***S. japonicum*** is transmitted by the cercaria that penetrates the skin found in contaminated fresh water. *S. japonicum* is found predominately in China, Japan, Indonesia, and the Philippines.

Liver *(Table 7-3)*

I Viral Hepatitis Caused by Hepatitis A Virus *(Figure 7-4)*

A. **General Features.** Hepatitis A virus (HAV) has plagued humankind for centuries and is commonly called "**infectious hepatitis.**" HAV never pursues a chronic course, has **no carrier state**, and infection provides lifelong immunity. Pathological findings include HAV causes a noncytopathic infection within the cytoplasm of hepatocytes; HAV replicates exclusively in the cytoplasm of hepatocytes; and hepatocyte damage is mediated by HAV-specific CD8 + lymphocytes and natural killer cells. Clinical findings include acute, self-limiting disease; fatigue; malaise; nausea; vomiting; anorexia; fever; right upper quadrant pain; dark urine; acholic stools (light-colored stools lacking bilirubin pigment); jaundice; pruritus; marked elevation of serum alanine aminotransferase (ALT) and serum aspartate aminotransferase (AST); HAV IgM is the first detectable antibody in the serum and is the gold standard for acute illness detection; HAV IgG is detectable in the serum during the early convalescent period and remains detectable for decades; incubation period is 2 to 6 weeks; and no predominant season of infection.

B. **Causative Agent (Hepatitis A Virus).** HAV belonging to the **Picornaviridae virus family** is a **nonsegmented, single-stranded, positive sense RNA (ss + RNA) virus**. The virion is a **naked** (nonenveloped) 30-nm **icosahedron**. HAV has tightly fitted capsomers consisting of four virion proteins (**VP1–VP4**) that are involved in binding to the hepatocyte. The HAV genome has a **3′ poly A tail** that enhances infectivity and a **5′ VP_g protein** that plays a role in viral RNA packaging into the capsid and initiating viral RNA synthesis. The HAV genome is comprised of 7,474 nucleotides divided into three regions: a 5′ untranslated region (742 nucleotides), a single open reading frame (6,681 nucleotides), and a 3′ noncoding region (63 nucleotides).

C. **Replication**

1. **Infection and entry.** HAV infects hepatocytes through VP1 capsomer protein binding to hepatocyte **ICAM-1** (intercellular adhesion molecule 1). Upon binding, VP4 is released and the viral genome is injected directly across the cell membrane (called **viropexis**).
2. **Early transcriptional events.** The viral + RNA is used as mRNA and translated within the cytoplasm into one large polypeptide that is cleaved into various viral proteins.

3. **Replication of viral genome.** Viral + RNA replication occurs in the cytoplasm and is mediated by **RNA-dependent RNA polymerase**. The viral + RNA is first transcribed into a –RNA template which then undergoes replication to the viral + RNA genome. VP_g is attached to the 5′ end.
4. **Viral assembly.** The viral proteins (VP1–VP4) associate to form the capsid and the viral + RNA genome is inserted inside the capsid.
5. **Viral release.** The virion is released by cell lysis.

D. **Reservoir.** HAV is transmitted by the fecal–oral route because HAV is released into the stool in high concentrations. HAV is also transmitted by eating contaminated shellfish (Shanghai, China outbreak) and green onions (outbreak traced back to green onions imported from Mexico). HAV is also transmitted by food handlers, day care workers, and children. HAV outbreaks usually arise from a single source and spreads rapidly in a community because most of the infected people become contagious before the symptoms occur.

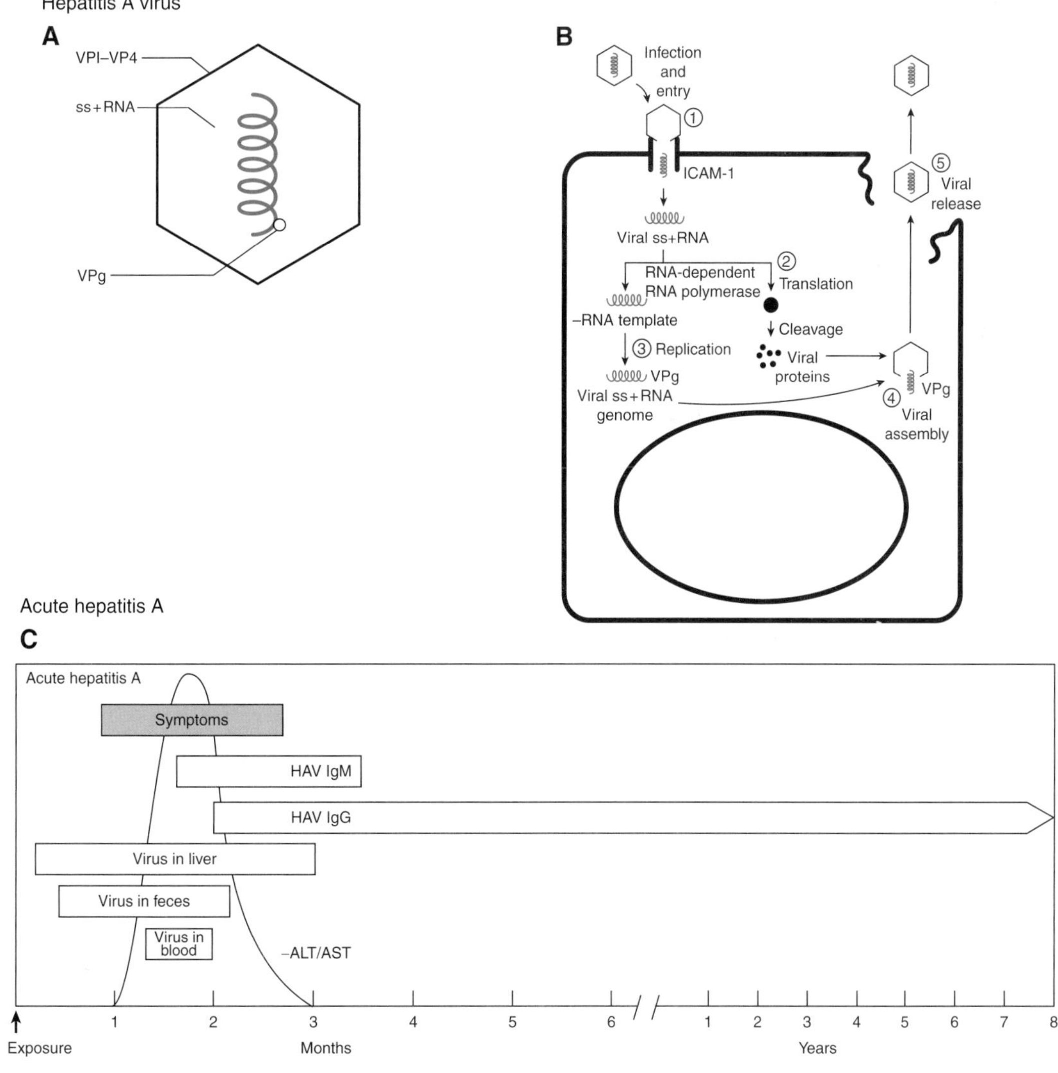

FIGURE 7-4. **Hepatitis A Virus (HAV). (A)** Diagram shows the structure of HAV with its capsid made of VP1–VP4 viral proteins, single-stranded, positive sense RNA (ss + RNA), and VP_g viral protein located on the 5′ end. **(B)** Mechanism of viral replication. See Liver IIC for explanation. **(C) Events Associated with Acute HAV Infection.** Panel shows the temporal sequence of symptoms along with HAV IgM, HAV IgG, ALT/AST, and virus appearance in the liver, feces, and blood.

II Viral Hepatitis Caused by Hepatitis B Virus *(Figure 7-5)*

A. **General Features.** Hepatitis B virus (HBV) hepatitis is a global health problem with >200 million carriers and ≈1 million deaths/year. HBV hepatitis is commonly called "**serum hepatitis.**" HBV is not directly cytopathic to hepatocytes. HBV-related liver disease is related to cytotoxic T-cell-mediated lysis of infected hepatocytes. HBV infection results in two major clinical syndromes called **acute hepatitis B** and **chronic hepatitis B**.

1. **Acute Hepatitis B.** Acute hepatitis B is an acute, self-limiting disease (similar to hepatitis A) in which complete recovery and lifelong immunity generally occurs. Acute hepatitis B may progress to fulminant hepatitis that can be fatal in 7 to 10 days. Clinical findings include acute, self-limiting disease; serum sicknesslike syndrome; fever; rash; arthritis; headache; nausea; jaundice; marked elevation of serum ALT and AST; HBsAg is the first detectable antigen in the serum; HBsAb is detectable in the serum after the disappearance of HBsAg; HBeAg is the second detectable antigen in the serum and correlates with a period of intense viral replication and maximal infectivity of the patient; incubation period is 2 to 6 months; and duration of illness is 8 to 10 weeks.
2. **Chronic Hepatitis B.** Chronic hepatitis B is the presence of necrosis and inflammation in the liver along with the persistence of HBsAg in the serum for >6 months. Pathological findings include a **chronic persistent** type demonstrates minimal necrosis and is associated with a favorable outcome; a **chronic active** type demonstrates piecemeal necrosis and bridging necrosis which can lead to cirrhosis and/or hepatocellular carcinoma. Clinical findings include many patients are asymptomatic (unless they progress to cirrhosis or extrahepatic manifestations); some patients experience nonspecific symptoms like fatigue; extrahepatic manifestations that are caused by circulating immune complexes and include polyarteritis nodosa and a membranous nephropathy; and a **carrier state** may result.

B. **Causative Agent (Hepatitis B Virus).** HBV belonging to the Hepadnavirus family is a **small, circular, partially double-stranded DNA virus**. The +DNA strand is incomplete and the –DNA strand is complete. The virion (called a **Dane particle**) is an **enveloped** (with viral-encoded proteins and host-derived lipids) 42-nm diameter **icosahedron**. The envelope contains the **HBsAg**. The **core** contains **HBcAg** and **HBeAg, a polymerase protein, X protein**, and **circular, partially double-stranded DNA. HBsAg-containing particles** (22-nm diameter) in both filamentous and spherical forms can be released into the serum. The **X protein** is a potent activator of many promoter regions.

C. **Replication**

1. **Infection and entry.** HBV infects hepatocytes through HBsAg on the viral envelope binding to the hepatocyte cell membrane. The virion is uncoated in the cytoplasm and the viral DNA genome enters the nucleus. In the nucleus, synthesis of the +DNA strand is completed to form a closed circular viral DNA.
2. **Early transcription events.** Transcription of the viral genome produces three small mRNAs and one large (3,500 bases) mRNA molecule. The three small mRNAs move into the cytoplasm and are translated into viral proteins. The large 3,500 base mRNA also moves into the cytoplasm.
3. **Replication of the genome.** The large 3,500 base mRNA serves as a template to synthesize the –DNA strand by reverse transcriptase activity. The large 3,500 base mRNA is then degraded by RNase H activity as the +DNA strand is synthesized.
4. **Viral assembly.** The viral proteins surround the large 3,500 base mRNA as the viral DNA genome is being synthesized.
5. **Viral release.** The core is enveloped by Golgi membranes before completion of the +DNA strand yielding a partially double-stranded DNA and then released by exocytosis as HBV (or the 42-nm Dane particle). In addition, HBsAg-containing particles (22-nm diameter) in both filamentous and spherical forms can be released.

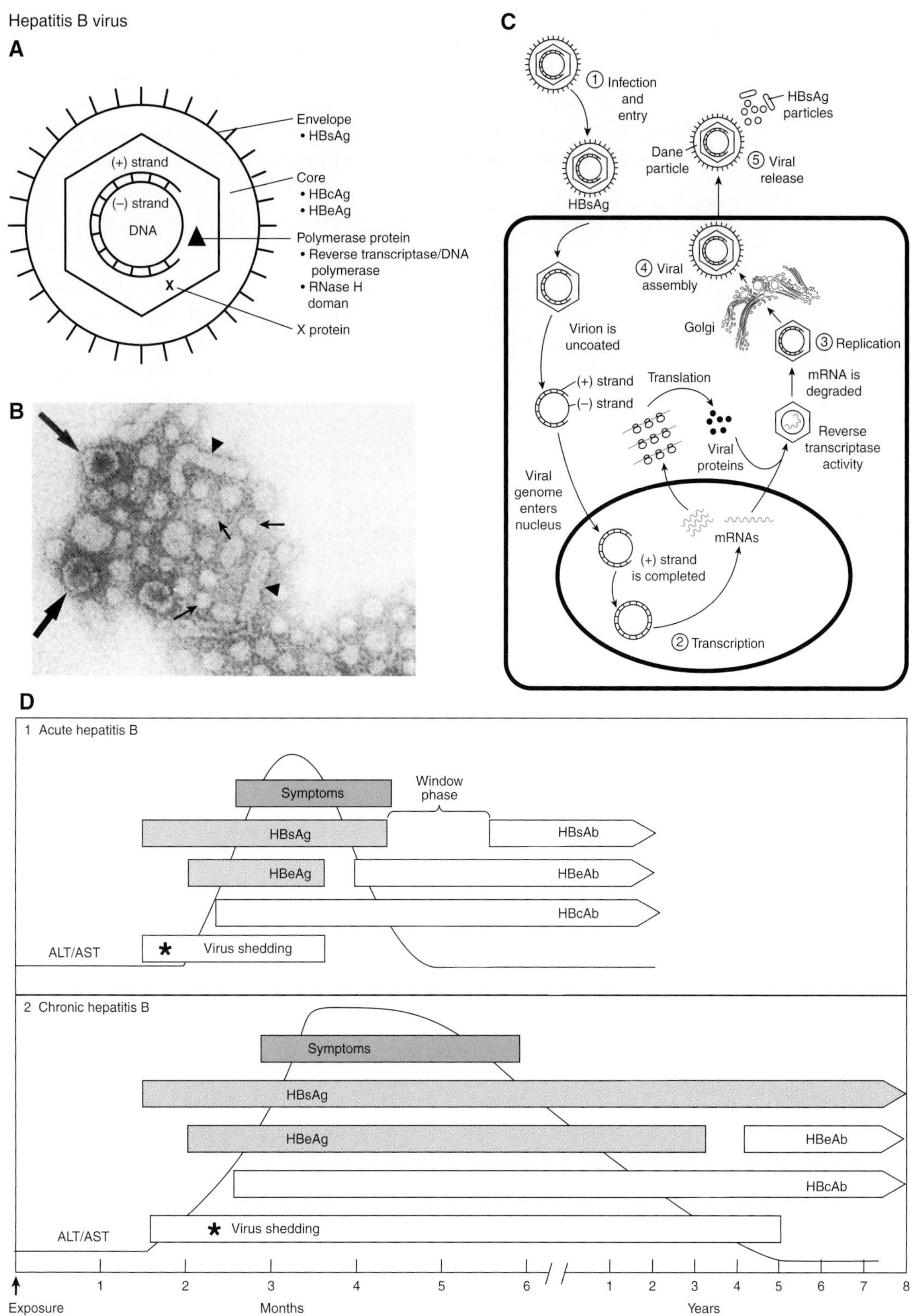

FIGURE 7-5. **Hepatitis B Virus. (A)** Diagram shows the structure of HBV (also called the Dane particle; 42 nm) with its envelope containing HBsAg, core containing HBcAg and HBeAg, a polymerase protein, X protein, and circular, partially double-stranded DNA. **(B)** Electron micrograph of serum from a hepatitis B patient shows the complete HBV (or 42 nm Dane particle; bold arrows) along with HBsAg-containing particles in both filamentous form (arrowheads) and spherical form (arrows). **(C) Mechanism of Viral Replication.** See Liver IIIC for explanation. **(D) Events Associated with Acute and Chronic HBV Infection.** Panel 1 (acute hepatitis) shows the temporal sequence of symptoms along with HBsAg, HBeAg, HBsAb, HbeAb, HBcAb, ALT/AST, and virus shedding. Panel 2 (chronic hepatitis) shows the temporal sequence of symptoms along with HBsAg, HBeAg, HBeAb, HBcAb, ALT/AST, and virus shedding. ALT — serum alanine aminotransferase; AST — serum aspartate aminotransferase;. (*) HBV is being shed; patient is infectious.

D. **Reservoir.** Humans are the only significant reservoir for HBV. HBV is transmitted through **blood** (e.g., accidental needlesticks, IV drug users who share needles, tattooing, etc.). HBV may also be transmitted from **mother-to-baby** (e.g., during passage through the birth canal or during breast feeding). HBV may also be transmitted **sexually** (e.g., homosexual male's sexual practices). HBV begins to replicate within 3 days after infection although symptoms may not appear for >45 days.

III Viral Hepatitis Caused by Hepatitis C Virus *(Figure 7-6)*

A. **General Features.** HCV is a global health problem with >170 million carriers. HCV is the most common indication for liver transplantation and accounts for 50% of patients on the waiting list. After the discovery of HAV and HBV in the early 1970s, it became apparent that a large number of cases of hepatitis were not due to HAV or HBV (i.e., **non-A, non-B hepatitis**). Consequently, another virus was suspected and HCV was isolated in 1989. HCV infection results in two major clinical syndromes called **acute hepatitis C** and **chronic hepatitis C**.

1. **Acute hepatitis C.** Acute hepatitis C is an acute, self-limiting disease. Acute hepatitis C rarely progresses to fulminant hepatitis. Clinical findings include acute, self-limiting disease; asymptomatic or surprisingly mild symptoms; malaise; nausea; right upper quadrant pain; jaundice; marked elevation of serum ALT and AST; HCV-RNA is detectable in the serum by the polymerase chain reaction (PCR) and is the first evidence of HCV infection; HCV-IgG is detectable in the serum; incubation period is 2 to 6 months; and duration of illness is 2 to 12 weeks.
2. **Chronic hepatitis C.** Chronic hepatitis C occurs very frequently after acute hepatitis C infection (≈50% to 70% of the cases). Chronic hepatitis C often progresses to chronic active hepatitis within 10 to 15 years, cirrhosis (20% of the chronic cases), and liver failure (20% of chronic cases). Clinical findings include malaise; nausea; anorexia; myalgia; arthralgia; weakness; weight loss; extrahepatic manifestations include essential mixed cryoglobulinemia, membranoproliferative glomerulonephritis, Type 1 diabetes, non-Hodgkin lymphoma, porphyria cutanea tarda, lichen planus, arthralgia, and sicca syndrome; and a **carrier state** may result.

B. **Causative Agent (Hepatitis C Virus).** Hepatitis C virus (HCV) belonging to the **Flaviviridae virus family** is a **nonsegemented, single-stranded, positive sense RNA (ss + RNA) virus.** The virion is an **enveloped** 30 to 60 nm **icosahedron**. HCV has six major genotypes that vary in their response to interferon therapy: **genotype 1** (most common in the US and Europe), **genotype 2**, **genotype 3** (most common in India, Far East, and Australia), **genotype 4** (most common in Africa and Middle East), **genotype 5** (most common in South Africa), and **genotype 6** (most common in Hong Kong, Vietnam, and Australia). The HCV genome is comprised of 9,500 nucleotides that encode for ≈10 proteins, including the **E1 glycoprotein** and **E2 glycoprotein**. Some HCV proteins inhibit apoptosis and thereby promote persistent infection. The RNA-dependent RNA polymerase **lacks proof-reading ability** which contributes to an observed viral diversity of HCV.

C. **Replication**

1. **Infection and entry**. HCV infects hepatocytes through **E1** or **E2** envelope protein binding to the hepatocyte **CD81** surface receptor or by coating itself with **LDL** (low-density lipoprotein) and binding to the hepatocyte **LDL receptor**. The viral genome enters the hepatocyte cytoplasm by receptor-mediated endocytosis.
2. **Early transcriptional events.** The viral + RNA is used as mRNA and translated within the cytoplasm into one large polypeptide that is cleaved into various viral proteins.
3. **Replication of viral genome.** Viral + RNA replication occurs in the cytoplasm and is mediated by **RNA-dependent RNA polymerase**. The viral + RNA is first transcribed into a –RNA template which then undergoes replication to the viral + RNA genome.

4. **Viral assembly.** The viral proteins associate to form the capsid and the viral + RNA genome is inserted inside the capsid. The virion is enveloped by Golgi membranes.
5. **Viral release.** The virion is released by exocytosis or remains within the hepatocyte cytoplasm.

D. **Reservoir.** HCV is transmitted through **blood** (e.g., accidental needlesticks, IV drug users who share needles, tattooing, etc.). HCV may also be transmitted from **mother-to-baby** (e.g., during passage through the birth canal or during breast feeding). HBV may also be transmitted **sexually** (e.g., homosexual male's sexual practices).

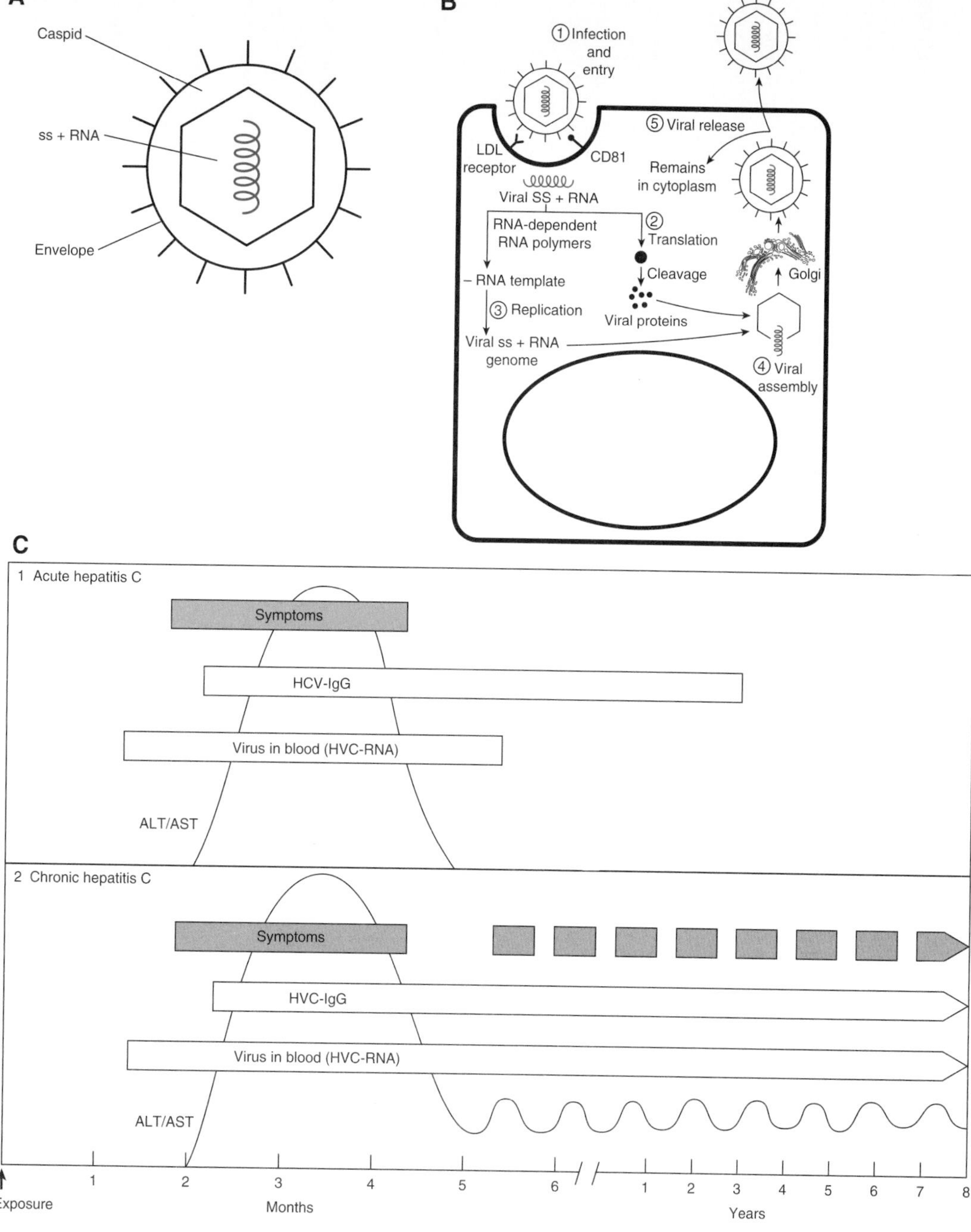

FIGURE 7-6. Hepatitis C Virus. (A) Diagram shows the structure of HCV with its envelope, single-stranded + sense RNA, and capsid. **(B) Mechanism of Viral Replication.** See Liver IVC for explanation. **(C) Events Associated with Acute and Chronic HCV Infection.** Panel 1 (acute hepatitis C) shows the temporal sequence of symptoms along with HCV-IgG, ALT/AST, and virus appearance in the blood (HCV-RNA). Panel 2 (chronic hepatitis C) shows the temporal sequence of symptoms along with HCV-IgG, ALT/AST, and virus appearance in the blood (HCV-RNA).

TABLE 7-3 SUMMARY TABLE OF MICROBIOLOGIC DISEASES ASSOCIATED WITH THE LIVER

Disease	Causative Agent	Reservoir	Clinical Findings
Viral hepatitis A "Infectious Hepatitis"	HAV Single-stranded (+) RNA virus Naked, nonenveloped 30 nm icosahedron ALT/AST HAV IgM HAV IgG	Transmitted by the fecal–oral route Contaminated shellfish and green onions Transmitted by food handlers, day care workers, and children Spreads rapidly in a community	Acute, self-limiting disease; fatigue; malaise; nausea; vomiting; anorexia; fever; right upper quadrant pain; dark urine; acholic stools (light-colored stools lacking bilirubin pigment); jaundice; pruritus; marked elevation of ALT and AST; HAV IgM is the first detectable antibody in the serum and is the gold standard for acute illness detection; HAV IgG is detectable in the serum during the early convalescent period and remains detectable for decades; incubation period is 2–6 weeks; and no predominant season of infection
Viral hepatitis B "Serum Hepatitis" Acute hepatitis B Chronic hepatitis B	HBV Small, circular, partially double-stranded DNA virus Dane particle Enveloped 42 nm icosahedron ALT/AST HBsAg HBcAg HBeAg HBsAb HBeAb HBcAb	Transmitted through blood, mother-to-baby, or sexually	**Acute:** Acute, self-limiting disease; serum sicknesslike syndrome; fever; rash; arthritis; headache; nausea; jaundice; marked elevation of ALT and AST; HBsAg is the first detectable antigen in the serum; HBsAb is detectable in the serum after the disappearance of HBsAg; HBeAg is the second detectable antigen in the serum and correlates with a period of intense viral replication and maximal infectivity of the patient; incubation period is 2–6 months; and duration of illness is 8–10 weeks **Chronic:** Many patients are asymptomatic (unless they progress to cirrhosis or extrahepatic manifestations); some patients experience nonspecific symptoms like fatigue; extrahepatic manifestations that are caused by circulating immune complexes include polyarteritis nodosa and a membranous nephropathy; and a **carrier state** may result
Viral hepatitis C "non-A, non-B hepatitis" Acute hepatitis C Chronic hepatitis C	HCV Single-stranded (+) RNA virus Enveloped 30–60-nm icosahedron Genotypes 1–6 ALT/AST HCV-RNA HCV-IgG	Transmitted through blood, mother-to-baby, or sexually	**Acute:** Acute, self-limiting disease; asymptomatic or surprisingly mild symptoms; malaise; nausea; right upper quadrant pain; jaundice; marked elevation of ALT and AST; HCV-RNA is detectable in the serum by the PCR and is the first evidence of HCV infection; HCV-IgG is detectable in the serum; incubation period is 2–6 months; and duration of illness is 2–12 weeks **Chronic:** Malaise; nausea; anorexia; myalgia; arthralgia; weakness; weight loss; extrahepatic manifestations include essential mixed cryoglobulinemia, membranoproliferative glomerulonephritis, Type 1 diabetes, non-Hodgkin lymphoma, porphyria cutanea tarda, lichen planus, arthralgia, and sicca syndrome; and a **carrier state** may result

IV Viral Hepatitis Caused by Hepatitis D Virus

Hepatitis D virus (HDV) is an incomplete RNA virus transmitted by contaminated blood and body fluids (percutaneous and sexual contact). HDV is a defective RNA virus whose assembly in the hepatocyte requires HBsAg produced by HBV. Consequently, HDV infection is limited to persons with HBV infection. Infection with HDV may occur simultaneously with HBV (coinfection) or following HBV infection (superinfection). Superinfection with HDV of a HBV carrier will typically increase the severity of the existing chronic hepatitis.

V Viral Hepatitis Caused by Hepatitis E Virus

Hepatitis E virus (HEV) is an RNA virus (calicivirus) transmitted primarily person-to-person by the fecal–oral route. HEV has an incubation period of 2 to 9 weeks after which the patient develops clinical signs similar to hepatitis A. Hepatitis E is a self-limiting disease that does not lead to fulminant hepatitis or chronic hepatitis. A characteristic feature of hepatitis E is a high mortality rate among pregnant women.

Chapter **8**

Pharmacology

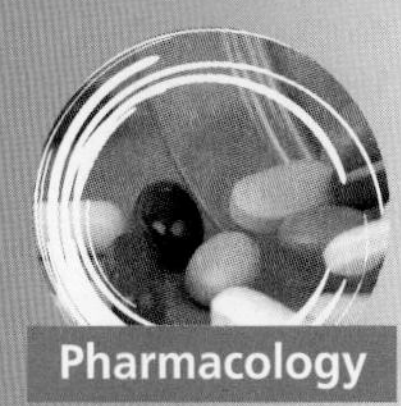

I Prokinetic Drugs

Prokinetic drugs promote upper gastrointestinal (GI) tract motility. Diseases that damage nerves to the viscera (e.g., diabetes) frequently result in a loss of motility in the esophagus and stomach. This results in delayed GI emptying, nausea, and severe bloating. Prokinetic drugs include:

A. **Metoclopramide (Apo-Metoclop, Clopra).** Metoclopramide is a **D_2 (dopamine) and 5-HT_3 (hydroxytryptamine) receptor antagonist. The mechanism of action:** metoclopramide blocks D_2 and 5-HT_3 receptors located on GI smooth muscle, which results in an acceleration of GI emptying and intestinal transit time (i.e., prokinetic activity). Metoclopramide also facilitates acetylcholine (ACh) release from cholinergic nerve terminals in the myenteric plexus. Metoclopramide also affects dopaminergic neurons in the basal ganglia and substantia nigra producing Parkinson disease as a side effect. **Clinical uses:** GI radiography, intestinal intubation, gastroparesis resulting from diabetes, gastroesophageal reflux, and reduced postoperative and chemotherapy induced vomiting. **Side effects:** Parkinsonism, extrapyramidal effects, and diarrhea.

II Laxative Drugs

A. **Bulk-Forming Laxatives (Dietary Fiber, Methylcellulose, Psyllium [Metamucil, Serutan]).** Bulk-forming laxatives are **undigestible plant, fruit, or vegetable products (i.e., high fiber products). The mechanism of action:** Bulk-forming laxatives form gels within the GI lumen, which results in H_2O retention, distention, and increased peristaltic activity. **Clinical uses:** constipation (one of the most preventive and therapeutic treatment for common constipation). **Side effects:** flatulence and reduced drug absorption (e.g., cardiac glycosides).

B. **Saline Laxatives (Magnesium Hydroxide [Milk of Magnesium], Magnesium Citrate).** Saline laxatives are **hypertonic solutions** of poorly absorbable salts (e.g., magnesium, citrate, sulfate, and phosphate). **The mechanism of action:** saline laxatives cause H_2O accumulation within the GI lumen which results in distention and increased peristaltic activity. **Clinical uses:** constipation; colonic lavage prior to surgery, radiology, or colonoscopy; elimination of parasites, and poisoning. **Side effects:** dehydration and electrolyte imbalance, contraindicated in patients with congestive heart failure or impaired renal function.

C. **Osmotic Laxatives (Sorbitol, Lactulose [Chronulac, Cephulac], Polyethylene Glycol [GoLYTELY, CoLyte], and Glycerin).** Osmotic laxatives are hyperosmotic agents.
   1. **Sorbitol and lactulose** are **nonabsorbable sugars** that increase osmolarity within the GI lumen. **The mechanism of action:** sorbitol and lactulose cause H_2O accumulation within the GI lumen which results in distention and increased peristaltic activity. **Clinical uses:** constipation and chronic hepatic encephalopathy (reduces ammonia absorption). **Side effects:** flatulence, abdominal cramps, and nausea.
   2. **Polyethylene glycol** is a **nonabsorbable polymer** in an isotonic solution which increases osmolarity within the GI lumen. **The mechanism of action:** polyethylene glycol causes H_2O accumulation within the GI lumen which results in distention

and increased peristaltic activity. **Clinical uses:** colonic lavage prior to colonoscopy (patient must drink 3 to 4 L of the solution). **Side effects:** diarrhea.

3. **Glycerol** is a clear, colorless, **syrupy liquid** ($C_3H_8O_3$) that increases osmolarity within the GI lumen when given as a suppository (glycerol is metabolized when given orally). **The mechanism of action:** glycerol causes H_2O accumulation within the GI lumen which results in distention and increased peristaltic activity, softens the stool, and lubricates the bowel. **Clinical uses:** constipation.

D. **Stimulant Laxatives (Phenolphthalein [Modane, ExLax], Bisacodyl [Ducolax], Senna [Senokot], and Casara sagrada).** Stimulus laxatives are various agents that stimulate GI H_2O secretion, electrolyte transport, and peristaltic activity. **The mechanism of action:** stimulant laxatives cause H_2O accumulation within the GI lumen (by inhibiting Na^+–K^+ ATPase which increases H_2O secretion and electrolyte transport into the GI lumen) and increased peristaltic activity (by stimulating Auerbach plexus). **Clinical uses:** constipation and colonic lavage prior to surgery, radiology, or colonoscopy. **Side effects:** fluid and electrolyte deficiencies, abdominal cramps, and pink-colored urine.

E. **Emollient Laxatives (Docusate Sodium [Colace] and Poloxamers).** Emollient laxatives are **docusate salts** that act as anionic surfactants. **The mechanism of action:** emollient laxatives soften the stool which facilitates passage and increases H_2O secretion and electrolyte transport into the GI lumen. Emollient laxatives do not stimulate GI motility. **Clinical uses:** constipation. **Side effects:** diarrhea, nausea, abdominal cramps, and rash.

F. **Castor Oil.** Castor oil is a **distasteful oil** that is metabolized to glycerol and **ricinoleate** (an anionic surfactant and active agent). **The mechanism of action:** ricinoleate decreases H_2O and electrolyte absorption and increases peristalsis in the small intestine causing rapid evacuation. **Clinical uses:** severe constipation and colonic lavage prior to radiology. Castor oil is too powerful of a laxative to treat common constipation. **Side effects:** dehydration, electrolyte imbalance, colic, and contraindicated in pregnant women.

III Antidiarrheal Drugs

A. **Loperamide (Imodium, Imodium-AD).** Loperamide is an **opioid receptor agonist**; a meperidine analog. **The mechanism of action:** loperamide stimulates opioid receptors in the enteric nervous system which results in a decreased peristaltic activity. **Clinical uses:** diarrhea. **Side effects:** abdominal cramps.

B. **Diphenoxylate HCl (Lomotil, Motofen).** Diphenoxylate HCl is an **opioid receptor agonist**; a meperidine analog. Diphenoxylate is metabolized to difenoxin (the active agent). **The mechanism of action:** difenoxin stimulates opioid receptors in the enteric nervous system which results in a decreased peristaltic activity. **Clinical uses:** diarrhea; Lomotil and Motofen contain atropine to discourage abuse. **Side effects:** dry mouth and blurred vision due to the presence of atropine (anticholinergic effects).

IV Antiemetic Drugs

A. **Dronabinol (Marinol).** Dronabinol (δ-9HTC) is the psychoactive agent found in **marijuana** (i.e., the legal form of marijuana). **The mechanism of action:** dronabinol acts on the chemoreceptor trigger zone of the medulla. **Clinical uses:** chemotherapy-induced nausea and vomiting and AIDS-associated anorexia. **Side effects:** dizziness, drowsiness, and nausea.

B. **Ondansetron (Zofran) and Granisetron (Kytril).** Ondansetron and Granisetron are **5-HT$_3$ receptor antagonists. The mechanism of action**: Ondansetron and Granisetron block 5-HT$_3$ receptors located on the nerve terminals of the vagus nerve (CN X) and in the chemoreceptor trigger zone of the medulla. **Clinical uses:** chemotherapy-induced, postoperative, and radiation-induced nausea and vomiting. **Side effects:** headache, constipation, dizziness, and somnolence.

C. **Hydroxyzine (Vistaril).** Hydroxyzine is a **H$_1$ (histamine) receptor antagonist. The mechanism of action**: hydroxyzine blocks H$_1$ receptors located in the chemoreceptor trigger zone of the medulla. **Clinical uses:** nausea and vomiting, antihistamine, antianxiety, and a sedative. **Side effects:** drowsiness, blood dyscrasias, dry mouth, and blurred vision (anticholinergic effects).

D. **Prochlorperazine (Compazine).** Prochlorperazine is a **D$_2$ (dopamine) receptor antagonist. The mechanism of action**: prochlorperazine blocks D$_2$ receptors located on the nerve terminals of the vagus nerve (CN X) and in the chemoreceptor trigger zone of the medulla. **Clinical uses:** nausea and vomiting. **Side effects:** drowsiness, hypotension, and extrapyramidal effects.

V Emetic Drugs

A. **Apomorphine.** Apomorphine is a dopamine receptor agonist. **The mechanism of action**: apomorphine induces vomiting by stimulating the chemoreceptor trigger zone of the medulla. **Clinical uses:** treatment of drug overdose in patients found within 30 min of drug ingestion.

VI Pharmacology of Gastroesophageal Reflux Disease (GERD) and Gastric/Duodenal Ulcers

A. **Cimetidine (Tagamet), Ranitidine (Zantac), Famotidine (Pepcid), and Nizatidine (Axid).** These drugs are **H$_2$ receptor antagonists. The mechanism of action**: these drugs block the stimulatory effect of histamine released from EC cells or mast cells on HCl secretion from the parietal cell (i.e., ↓gastric acid). **Clinical uses:** promote healing of gastric and duodenal ulcers and prophylaxis for patients at risk for recurrent ulcers. **Side effects of cimetidine:** sedation, headache, dizziness, GI distress, and muscle pain; slurred speech, delirium, and confusion in elderly patients; galactorrhea in women; and gynecomastia and low sperm count in men.

B. **Propantheline (Pro-Banthine), Isopropamide (Darbid), and Scopolamine.** These drugs are **muscarinic ACh receptor antagonists. The mechanism of action:** these drugs block the stimulatory effect of ACh on HCl secretion from the parietal cell (i.e., ↓gastric acid). **Clinical uses:** promote healing of gastric and duodenal ulcers, rarely used alone to treat ulcers, and required dose produces systemic anticholinergic effects.

C. **Omeprazole (Losec, Prilosec).** Omeprazole is a **covalent, irreversible inhibitor of the H^+-K^+ATPase** proton pump located in the parietal cell. **The mechanism of action:** omeprazole blocks both basal and stimulated HCl secretion from the parietal cell (i.e., ↓gastric acid). **Clinical uses:** promotes healing of gastric and duodenal ulcers, reduces gastric damage caused by nonsteroidal anti-inflammatory drug (NSAID) therapy, and used in treatment of Zollinger–Ellison syndrome. **Side effects:** nausea, diarrhea, and abdominal colic.

D. **Misoprostol (Cytotec).** Misoprostol is a **PGE$_1$ analog. The mechanism of action:** misoprostol inhibits HCl secretion from the parietal cell and stimulates mucus and HCO_3^- secretion. **Clinical uses:** reduction of gastric damage caused by NSAID therapy. **Side effects:** diarrhea, contraindicated in pregnant women (potential abortifacient).

E. **Calcium Carbonate (Tums), Aluminum Hydroxide, Magnesium Hydroxide (Milk of Magnesia), Maalox, Mylanta II, Gelusil, and Sodium Bicarbonate.** These drugs are **weak bases** (a combination of hydroxide and metallic cations) that act as **antacids. The mechanism of action:** these drugs neutralize HCl and reduce pepsin activity. **Clinical uses:** promote healing of gastric and duodenal ulcers, GERD, and hyperacidity.

F. **Sucralfate (Carafate, Sulcrate).** Sucralfate is a **complex polysaccharide** complexed with aluminum hydroxide. **The mechanism of action:** sucralfate forms a polymer in an acid environment that binds to normal gastric mucosa and ulcers to prevent further acid damage. **Clinical uses:** promotes healing of gastric and duodenal ulcers.

G. **Bismuth Subsalicylate (Pepto-Bismol), Tetracycline, and Metronidazole or Amoxicillin and Clarithromycin Regimens.** These drugs are **antibiotic regimens. The mechanism of action:** these antibiotic regimens eradicate *Helicobacter pylori* (bacteria implicated in the etiology of ulcers). **Clinical uses:** promote healing of gastric and duodenal ulcers.

VII Pharmacology of Crohn Disease

A. **Corticosteroids**

1. **Prednisone** is a synthetic glucocorticoid derived from cortisone. Prednisone is the mainstay of treatment for patients with mild Crohn symptoms who are unresponsive to other treatments or for patients who present with severe initial symptoms.
2. **Controlled ileal release budesonide.** Controlled ileal release (CIR) budesonide is a synthetic glucocorticoid with low systemic activity due to a high first-pass hepatic metabolism. CIR budesonide is used in many steroid-responsive illnesses since it has similar efficacy to conventional steroid therapy but less steroid toxicity. CIR budesonide seems to be effective in inducing remission of Crohn disease.

B. **Antibiotics.** Antibiotics are commonly used to treat Crohn disease although their efficacy in the treatment of the primary disease process involved in Crohn disease is not well established. The relationship between bacterial targets of antibiotics and their therapeutic efficacy remains obscure.

1. **Metronidazole.** Metronidazole is a mainstay drug for the treatment of anaerobic bacterial diarrhea caused by *Clostridium difficile* and protozoan infections. **The mechanism of action:** metronidazole is reduced by **pyruvate ferredoxin oxidoreductase (PFOR)** in the mitochondria of obligate anaerobic bacteria which produces toxic intermediate compounds and toxic free radicals that cause DNA breakage. PFOR is absent in eukaryotic cells. **Side effects:** nausea, vomiting, abdominal discomfort, dizziness, headache, metallic taste, dry mouth, discoloration of urine, contraindicated in pregnant women (may be teratogenic)
2. **Ciprofloxacin (Cipro).** Ciprofloxacin is a fluoroquinolone that belongs to the DNA replication and transcription inhibitor class of antibiotics. Fluoroquinolones are fluorinated analogs of nalidixic acid. **The mechanism of action:** fluoroquinolones are transported across the bacterial cell membrane by transport proteins, enter the bacterial cytoplasm, and inhibit DNA replication by inhibiting **DNA gyrase** (an enzyme similar to DNA topoisomerase II present in human cells). **Side effects:** nausea, dizziness, headaches, arthralgia in children, rash, photosensitivity, contraindicated in pregnant women and neonates.
3. **Combination of metronidazole and ciprofloxacin.**

C. **Azathioprine and 6-Mercaptopurine.** Azathioprine (AZA) is the 1-methyl-4-nitro-5-imidazolyl derivative thioguanine which is a purine mimic antimetabolite. AZA is a prodrug that is converted to **6-mercaptopurine** by glutathione in red blood cells and serves as an **immunomodulator. The mechanism of action:** 6-mercaptopurine is metabolized to **thioinosinic (TS)** and **thioguanylic acid (6TG)** by hypoxanthine guanine phosphoribosyltransferase. TS and 6TG inhibit intracellular inosinic acid synthesis which reduces adenine ribonucleotide and guanine ribonucleotide production. This reduction results in reduced numbers of **circulating B and T lymphocytes** and **reduced immunoglobulin synthesis. Side effects:** bone marrow suppression, leukopenia, megaloblastic anemia, nausea, vomiting, increased incidence of skin cancer, and lymphomas with prolonged use.

D. **Sulfasalazine and 5-Aminosalicylic Acid.** Sulfasalazine is a prodrug that is reduced by the bacterial enzyme azoreductase to **sulfapyridine** and **5-aminosalicylic acid (5-ASA)**. Sulfapyridine has antibacterial properties and accounts for its side effects. 5-ASA has anti-inflammatory properties. **The mechanism of action of 5-ASA:** the precise mechanism of action is not known although in vitro studies have shown an inhibition of prostaglandin and leukotriene synthesis, free radical scavenging, and inhibition of cytokine synthesis. **Side effects:** rash, Steven–Johnson syndrome, skin eruptions, photosensitivity, kernicterus in newborns, contraindicated in pregnant women and newborns. 5-ASA that is orally ingested undergoes rapid absorption in the jejunum so that 5-ASA has limited efficacy in the distal small intestine and colon. Therefore, delayed release formulations of 5-ASA have been developed as indicated below:

1. **Mesalamine (Asacol, Pentasa, and Salofalk).** Mesalamine is a 5-ASA that is coated with acrylic resins or encapsulated in ethylcellulose to enhance drug delivery to the distal small intestine and colon.
2. **Olsalazine (Dipentum).** Olsalazine is a 5-ASA that is dimerized to prepare delayed compounds.
3. **Balsalazide (Colazal).** Balsalazide is 5-ASA that is linked to an inert unabsorbed carrier molecule.

E. **Antitumor Necrosis Factor Therapy.** Tumor necrosis factor (TNF)-α seems to play a central role in Crohn disease. For example, patients with Crohn disease have elevated stool levels of TNF-α and TNF-α correlates with disease activity. Therefore, a number of drugs have been developed that ameliorate the effects of TNF-α as indicated below:

1. **Infliximab (Remicade).** Infliximab is a **chimeric IgG1 monoclonal antibody** (human and murine sequences) directed against TNF-α. **The mechanism of action:** infliximab neutralizes the biological activity of TNF-α probably by destroying activated effector cells through apoptosis.
2. **Adalimumab (Humira).** Adalimumab is a **recombinant human IgG1 monoclonal antibody** directed against TNF-α.
3. **Certolizumab pegol (Cimzia).** Certolizumab pegol is **humanized monoclonal antibody Fab fragment** linked to polyethylene glycol directed against TNF-α. Certolizumab does not have an F_c region so that the complement pathway is not activated.

F. **Anti-Integrin Therapy**

1. **Natalizumab (Tysabri).** Natalizumab is a **humanized monoclonal antibody** directed against α-4 integrin. **The mechanism of action:** natalizumab impedes leukocyte migration to inflammation sites by binding to α-4 integrin on the leukocyte cell membrane.

VIII Pharmacology of Ulcerative Colitis

A. **Mild Cases.** In mild cases, patients are treated with 5-ASA suppositories and/or steroid foams or suppositories. Systemic steroids (e.g., prednisone) are rarely required in mild cases.

1. **Sulfasalazine and 5-aminosalicylic acid.** Sulfasalazine is a prodrug that is reduced by the bacterial enzyme azoreductase to **sulfapyridine** and **5-ASA.** Sulfapyridine has antibacterial properties and accounts for its side effects. 5-ASA has

anti-inflammatory properties. **The mechanism of action of 5-ASA:** the precise mechanism of action is not known although in vitro studies have shown an inhibition of prostaglandin and leukotriene synthesis, free radical scavenging, and inhibition of cytokine synthesis. 5-ASA that is orally ingested undergoes rapid absorption in the jejunum so that 5-ASA has limited efficacy in the distal small intestine and colon. Therefore, delayed release formulations of 5-ASA have been developed as indicated below:

a. **Mesalamine (Asacol, Pentasa, and Salofalk).** Mesalamine is a 5-ASA that is coated with acrylic resins or encapsulated in ethylcellulose to enhance drug delivery to the distal small intestine and colon.
b. **Olsalazine (Dipentum).** Olsalazine is a 5-ASA that is dimerized to prepare delayed compounds.
c. **Balsalazide (Colazal).** Balsalazide is a 5-ASA that is linked to an inert unabsorbed carrier molecule.

2. **Steroid foam (Cortifoam).** Cortiform is **hydrocortisone acetate.**

B. **Moderate to Severe Cases.** In moderate to severe cases, patients are treated by adding systemic steroids to the treatment regime.

1. **Prednisone** is a synthetic glucocorticoid derived from cortisone. Prednisone is the mainstay of treatment for patients with mild Crohn symptoms who are unresponsive to other treatments or for patients who present with severe initial symptoms.
2. **Controlled ileal release budesonide.** CIR budesonide is a synthetic glucocorticoid with low systemic activity due to a high first-pass hepatic metabolism. CIR budesonide is used in many steroid-responsive illnesses since it has similar efficacy to conventional steroid therapy but less steroid toxicity. CIR budesonide seems to be effective in inducing remission of Crohn disease.

C. **Refractory Cases.** In refractory cases, patients may be treated with anti-TNF therapy. TNF-α may play a role in ulcerative colitis.

1. **Infliximab (Remicade).** Infliximab is a **chimeric IgG1 monoclonal antibody** (human and murine sequences) directed against TNF-α. **The mechanism of action:** infliximab neutralizes the biological activity of TNF-α probably by destroying activated effector cells through apoptosis.

IX Pharmacology of Hypercholesterolemia

A. **Lovastatin (Mevacor), Simvastatin (Zocor), Pravastatin (Pravachol), and Fluvastatin (Lescol).** These drugs are reversible and competitive inhibitors of **3-hydroxy-3-methylglutaryl-coenzyme A reductase (HMG-CoA).** HMG-CoA is an enzyme that catalyzes the rate-limiting step in cholesterol synthesis (HMG-CoA → mevalonate). This results in an **increased low density lipoprotein (LDL) receptors in the liver** and **increased catabolism of LDL. Clinical uses:** Type IIa and Type IIb hyperlipidemia. **Side effects:** constipation, diarrhea, stomach pain, nausea, myalgia, and an increase in liver enzymes, contraindicated in pregnant and nursing women, children, and patients with hepatic disease.

B. **Cholestyramine (Questran) and Colestipol (Colestid).** These drugs are resins that promote the excretion of bile salts by forming an insoluble complex in the small intestine. This results in an **increased conversion of cholesterol → bile, increased LDL receptors in the liver,** and **increased catabolism of LDL. Clinical uses:** Type IIa and Type IIb hyperlipidemia. **Side effects:** constipation, steatorrhea, stomach pain, and decreased absorption of fat soluble vitamins and certain drugs.

C. **Niacin (Nicotinic Acid, Vitamin B_3).** Niacin is a vitamin that decreases production of very low density lipoprotein leading to a decreased LDL level and an increase in high-density lipoprotein (HDL) levels by an unknown mechanism. **Clinical uses:** Type IIb, III, IV, and V hyperlipidemia, niacin deficiency, and pellagra. **Side effects:** intense cutaneous flush, pruritus, nausea, vomiting, and contraindicated in patients with hepatic disease, diabetes, peptic ulcers, and gout.

D. **Ezetimibe.** Ezetimibe is an inhibitor of intestinal absorption of cholesterol. A single dose lowers LDL by 14% which is additive to the effects of statin drugs. Patients with familial hypercholesterolemia may experience greater LDL reduction.

X Pharmacology of Gallstones

A. **Chenodiol (Chenix).** Chenodiol is a **chenodeoxycholic acid**, which is a primary bile acid. **The mechanism of action**: chenodiol increases secretion of bile acids and decreases secretion of cholesterol into the bile, both of which result in the reduction of cholesterol in the bile. **Clinical uses:** effective only against cholesterol gallstones, requires 3 months to 2 years for complete gallstone dissolution, high incidence of diarrhea, and ineffective against radiopaque gallstones.

B. **Ursodiol (Actigall).** Ursodiol is an **ursodeoxycholic acid**, which is a minor secondary bile acid. **The mechanism of action**: ursodiol has no effect on the secretion of bile acids but does decrease the secretion of cholesterol into the bile. **Clinical uses:** effective only against cholesterol gallstones, requires 3 months to 2 years for complete gallstone dissolution, low incidence of diarrhea and other side effects, is combined with sonic lithotripsy to dissolve gall stones, and ineffective against radiopaque gallstones.

C. **Methyl ter-Butyl Ether.** Methyl ter-butyl ether (MTBE) is a potent cholesterol **organic solvent. The mechanism of action**: MTBE directly dissolves cholesterol gallstones. **Clinical uses**: effective only against cholesterol gallstones, infused directly into the gall bladder or bile duct, and ineffective against radiopaque gallstones.

XI Pharmacology of Hepatitis

A. **Hepatitis A Virus**

1. HAV infection in children is usually a minor and self-limiting disease that requires no specific therapy.
2. **HAVRIX** is a vaccine derived from the HM175 virus strain that has been formaldehyde inactivated. Primary immunization in children and adolescents consists of a single dose and a booster dose 6 to 12 months later.
3. **VAQTA** is a vaccine derived from the CR326 virus strain that has been formalin inactivated. Primary immunization in children and adolescents consists of a single dose and a booster dose 6 to 18 months later.

B. **Hepatitis B Virus**

1. **Lamivudine** (3TC). Lamivudine (3TC) is the (–) enantiomer of 2′,3′-dideoxy 3′-thiacytidine which becomes phosphorylated to 3TC-triphosphate (3TC-TP). 3TC-TP competes with dCTP for incorporation into the viral DNA during viral DNA replication and thereby terminates viral DNA replication.
2. **Lamivudine and interferon-α.** Interferon-α (IFN-α) is a cytokine, which is secreted by viral-infected cells, and it acts not only on the viral-infected cell but also on the neighboring uninfected cells. IFN-α binds to cell membrane receptors and acts through the JAK-STAT pathway. This leads to the transcription of 300 gene products that play a role in the amelioration or elimination of the viral infection. IFN-α also activates a latent ribonuclease that degrades ssRNA and inactivates a protein

synthesis initiation factor that inhibits protein synthesis. Apparently, destroying most of its RNA and shutting down protein synthesis allows the viral-infected cell to inhibit viral replication without killing itself.

3. **Entecavir.** Entecavir is a cyclopentyl guanosine analogue which competes with natural substrates and thereby reduces viral DNA replication.
4. **First generation HBV vaccine.** The first generation HBV vaccine is a vaccine derived by concentrating and purifying plasma from HBsAg carriers to isolate HBsAg 22-nm diameter viral particles. Due to concerns about transmitting bloodborne infections from the HBsAg carriers to the vaccine recipients, this vaccine is no longer used in developed countries but is still widely used on a global scale because of the low cost of production.
5. **Recombivax and Engerix-B (thimerosal-free).** Recombivax and Engerix-B are vaccines derived by cloning the HBV S gene into yeasts forming yeast recombinants. These vaccines contain the nonglycosylated HBV small S envelope protein. These vaccines do not contain the large L envelope protein or the middle M envelope protein.
6. **Other HBV vaccines.** The other HBV vaccines are vaccines derived by cloning various combinations of the HBV pre-S1 (large L envelope protein), pre-S2 (middle M envelope protein), and S (small S envelope protein) regions into mammalian cells forming mammalian cell recombinants. Three vaccines have been developed by this technique.
   a. **Vaccine 1.** This vaccine contains the HBV small S envelope protein and the middle M envelope protein.
   b. **Vaccine 2 and 3.**These vaccines contain the HBV small S envelope protein, the large L envelope protein, and the middle M protein.
7. **Twinrix.** Twinrix is a combination vaccine of both Engerix-B and HAVRIX.

C. Hepatitis C Virus

1. **Ribavirin.** Ribavirin is a nucleoside analog which inhibits RNA virus replication in vitro and decreases HCV infectivity in a dose-dependent manner. **The mechanism of action**: the mechanism of action is not completely understood but probably includes depletion of intracellular triphosphate pools, inhibition of 5′ cap structure of viral RNA, inhibition of viral-dependent RNA polymerases, and induction of mutations into the viral RNA. Ribavirin does not achieve a sustained virologic response and therefore has a limited role as a primary treatment of HCV.
2. **Interferon α-2b (Intron A).** Interferon α-2b is produced by recombinant DNA techniques.
3. **Interferon α-2a (Roferon).** Interferon α-2a is produced by recombinant DNA techniques but differs from interferon α-2b by a single amino acid. A high proportion of patients develop neutralizing antibodies to interferon α-2a.
4. **Interferon αcon-1 (consensus interferon; Infergen).** Interferon αcon-1 is a non-natural recombinant interferon developed by scanning subtypes of interferon α and assigning the most frequently observed amino acid at each position to form a consensus molecule.
5. **Interferon α-n1 (Wellferon).** Interferon α-n1 is a mixture of nine interferon subtypes produced from a human B lymphoblastoid cell line.
6. **Pegylated interferon.** Pegylated interferon is an interferon covalently bound to polyethylene glycol which has the advantage of sustaining more uniform interferon concentrations.
7. **Ribavirin plus interferon.** Ribavirin improves the rate of sustained virus clearance when given in combination with a standard of pegylated interferon α.
8. **HCV vaccine.** No prophylactic or therapeutic vaccine for HCV is available.

XII Summary Table of Drugs *(Table 8-1)*

TABLE 8-1 SUMMARY TABLE OF DRUGS

Drug Class	Drug
Prokinetic drugs	Metoclopramide (Apo-Metoclop, Clopra) Cisapride (Propulsid)
Laxatives	Bulk-forming laxatives (dietary fiber, methylcellulose, and psyllium [Metamucil, Serutan]) Saline laxatives (magnesium hydroxide [milk of magnesium] and magnesium citrate) Osmotic laxatives (sorbitol, lactulose [Chronulac, Cephulac], polyethylene glycol [GoLYTELY, CoLyte], and glycerin) Stimulant laxatives (phenolphthalein [Modane, ExLax], bisacodyl [Ducolax], senna [Senokot], and casara sagrada) Emollient laxatives (docusate sodium [Colace], poloxamers) Castor oil
Antidiarrheal drugs	Loperamide (Imodium, Imodium-AD) Diphenoxylate HCl (Lomotil, Motofen)
Antiemetic drugs	Dronabinol (Marinol) Ondansetron (Zofran) and Granisetron (Kytril) Hydroxyzine (Vistaril) Prochlorperazine (Compazine)
Emetic drugs	Ipecac Apomorphine
GERD and ulcer drugs	Cimetidine (Tagamet), Ranitidine (Zantac), Famotidine (Pepcid), and Nizatidine (Axid) Propantheline (Pro-Banthine), Isopropamide (Darbid), and Scopolamine Omeprazole (Losec, Prilosec) Misoprostol (Cytotec) Calcium carbonate (Tums), aluminum hydroxide, magnesium hydroxide (milk of magnesia), Maalox, Mylanta II, Gelusil, and Sodium Bicarbonate Sucralfate (Carafate, Sulcrate) Bismuth Subsalicylate (Pepto-Bismol), Tetracycline, and Metronidazole or Amoxicillin and Clarithromycin Regimens
Pharmacology of Crohn disease	Corticosteroids (Prednisone, CIR budesonide) Antibiotic Therapy: Metronidazole, Ciprofloxacin (Cipro), and a combination of Metronidazole and Ciprofloxacin AZA and 6-mercaptopurine Sulfasalazine and 5-ASA (Mesalamine[Asacol, Pentasa, and Salofalk], Olsalazine [Dipentum], and Balsalazide [Colazal]) Anti-TNF Therapy: (Infliximab [Remicade], Adalimumab [Humira], and Certolizumab pegol [Cimzia) Anti-integrin therapy: Natalizumab (Tysabri)
Pharmacology of ulcerative colitis	Mild cases: Sulfasalazine and 5-ASA (Mesalamine [Asacol, Pentasa, and Salofalk], Olsalazine [Dipentum], and Balsalazide [Colazal]) Steroid foam (Cortifoam) Moderate to severe cases: Corticosteroids (Prednisone, CIR budesonide) Refractory cases: Infliximab (Remicade)
Pharmacology of hypercho-lesterolemia	Lovastatin (Mevacor), Simvastatin (Zocor), Pravastatin (Pravachol), and Fluvastatin (Lescol) Cholestyramine (Questran), Colestipol (Colestid) Niacin (nicotinic acid, vitamin B_3)

(Continued)

TABLE 8-1 CONTINUED

Drug Class	Drug
Pharmacology of gallstones	Chenodiol (Chenix) Ursodiol (Actigall) MTBE
Pharmacology of viral gastroenteritis	Pentavalent human–bovine reassortment rotavirus vaccine (ROTATEQ) Attenuated human rotavirus vaccine (Rotarix)
Pharmacology of cholera	Oral rehydration therapy: Oral rehydration solutions (ORS) Intravenous volume repletion (IVR): Isotonic solution, Ringer's lactate Antibiotic therapy: Tetracycline (Achromycin) Doxycycline (Vibramycin) Cholera vaccine (rBS-WC, Dukoral)
Pharmacology of diarrhea caused by enterotoxigenic *Escherichia coli* or enteropathogenic *E. coli*	IVR: Isotonic solution or Ringer's lactate No antibiotic therapy
Pharmacology of food poisoning caused by *Staphylococcus aureus* or *Clostridium perfringens*	Only the symptoms are treated
Pharmacology of infectious colitis caused by *Shigella*	Oral rehydration therapy: ORS Antibiotic therapy: Trimethoprim–sulfamethoxazole (TMP–SMX) and Ampicillin
Pharmacology of infectious colitis caused by *Salmonella enterical* serotype *Typhimurium*	Oral rehydration therapy: ORS Antibiotic therapy: TMP–SMX and Fluoroquinolones (Ciprofloxacin, Ofloxacin, and Norfloxacin)
Pharmacology of infectious colitis caused by *Yersinia enterocolitica*	Oral rehydration therapy: ORS Antibiotic therapy: TMP–SMX and Fluoroquinolones (Ciprofloxacin, Ofloxacin, and Norfloxacin)
Pharmacology of infectious colitis caused by Entero-hemorrhagic *E. coli* and Enteroinvasive *E. coli.*	The only current treatment is supportive Monitor for hemolytic uremic syndrome
Pharmacology of pseudomem-branous colitis caused by *C. difficile*	Stoppage of the inciting antibiotic as soon as possible Antibiotic therapy: Metronidazole and Vancomycin

Pharmacology of infectious colitis caused by *Campylobacter jejuni*	Oral rehydration therapy: ORS Antibiotic therapy: Erythromycin
Pharmacology of *Giardiasis*	Metronidazole Tinidazole Nitazoxanide
Pharmacology of *Entamoeba histolytica*	Metronidazole Iodoquinol
Pharmacology of *Schistosomiasis*	Praziquantel (Biltricide)
Pharmacology of HAV	No specific therapy HAVRIX vaccine VAQTA vaccine
Pharmacology of HBV	Lamivudine (3TC) Lamivudine and interferon-α (IFN-α) Entecavir First generation HBV vaccine Recombivax and Engerix-B (thimerosal-free) vaccines Other HBV vaccines: Vaccine 1 (contains the HBV small S and middle M envelope protein) Vaccine 2 and 3 (contain the HBV small S, middle M, and large L envelope protein) Twinrix
Pharmacology of HCV	Ribavirin Interferon α-2b (Intron A) Interferon α-2a (Roferon) Interferon αcon-1 (consensus interferon; Infergen) Interferon α-n1 (Wellferon) Pegylated Interferon Ribavirin plus Interferon No prophylactic or therapeutic vaccine for HCV is available

Credits

Figure 1-1: From Dudek RW, Fix J. BRS Embryology. 3rd Ed. Philadelphia: Lippincott Williams & Wilkins, 2005, p. 102.

Figure 1-2: **A–C** From Dudek RW. High-Yield Lung. Philadelphia: Lippincott Williams & Wilkins, 2006, p. 2. **D-F** From Dudek RW. High-Yield Embryology. 3rd Ed. Philadelphia: Lippincott Williams & Wilkins, 2007, p. 41. **Original Sources: D** Fenoglio-Preiser CM. Gastrointestinal Pathology: An Atlas and Text. 2nd Ed. Philadelphia: Lippincott Williams & Wilkins, 1999, p. 33. **E** Fenoglio-Preiser CM. Gastrointestinal Pathology: An Atlas and Text. 2nd Ed. Philadelphia: Lippincott Williams & Wilkins, 1999, p. 31. (Courtesy of Dr Cooley Butler, Scripps Memorial Hospital, La Jolla, CA.) **F** Fenoglio-Preiser CM. Gastrointestinal Pathology: An Atlas and Text. 2nd Ed. Philadelphia: Lippincott Williams & Wilkins, 1999, p. 36.

Figure 1-3: **A–C** From Dudek RW. High-Yield Embryology. 3rd Ed. Philadelphia: Lippincott Williams & Wilkins, 2007, p. 42. **Original Sources: A** Johnson K. NMS Human Developmental Anatomy. Baltimore: Williams & Wilkins, 1989, p. 211. **B** Yamada T, Alpers DH, Laine L, et al. Textbook of Gastroenterology, vol 1, 3rd Ed. Philadelphia: Lippincott Williams & Wilkins, 1999, p. 1331.

Figure 1-4: From Dudek RW. High-Yield Embryology. 3rd Ed. Philadelphia: Lippincott Williams & Wilkins, 2007, p. 44. **Original Sources: A** Johnson K. NMS Human Developmental Anatomy. Baltimore: Williams & Wilkins, 1989, p. 215. **B** Yamada T, Alpers DH, Laine L, et al. Textbook of Gastroenterology, vol 1, 3rd Ed. Philadelphia: Lippincott Williams & Wilkins, 1999, p. 2250.

Figure 1-5: From Dudek RW. High-Yield Embryology. 3rd Ed. Philadelphia: Lippincott Williams & Wilkins, 2007, p. 45. **Original Sources: A** Johnson K. NMS Human Developmental Anatomy. Baltimore: Williams & Wilkins, 1989, p. 215. **A1** Henrikson RC. NMS Histology. Baltimore: Williams & Wilkins, 1991, p. 368. **B–D** Redrawn and modified from Cubilla AL, Fitzgerald PJ. Tumors of the exocrine pancreas. In: Hartmann WH, Sobin LH, eds. Atlas of Tumor Pathology. 2nd series; fascicle 19. Washington DC: Armed Forces Institute of Pathology, 1984. **E** Yamada T, Alpers DH, Laine L, et al. Textbook of Gastroenterology, vol 2, 3rd Ed. Philadelphia: Lippincott Williams & Wilkins, 1999, p. 2118. (Courtesy of Dr. Peter B. Cotton; Durham, NC.) **F** Yamada T, Alpers DH, Laine L, et al. Textbook of Gastroenterology. 3rd Ed. Philadelphia: Lippincott Williams & Wilkins, 1999, p. 1338. **Original Source:** Misiewicz JJ, Bartram CI, Cotton PB, et al. Atlas of Clinical Gastroenterology. London: Gower Medical Publishing, 1981. **G** Swischuk LE. Imaging of the Newborn, Infant, and Young Child. 5th Ed. Philadelphia: Lippincott Williams & Wilkins, 2004, p. 392.

Figure 1-6: From Dudek RW. High-Yield Embryology. 3rd Ed. Philadelphia: Lippincott Williams & Wilkins, 2007, p. 47. **Original Sources: A** Johnson K. NMS Human Developmental Anatomy. Baltimore: Williams & Wilkins, 1988, p. 218. **B** Feniglio-Preiser CM. Gastrointestinal Pathology: An Atlas and Text. 2nd Ed. Philadelphia: Lippincott Williams & Wilkins, 1999, p. 311. **C** Feniglio-Preiser CM. Gastrointestinal Pathology: An Atlas and Text. 2nd Ed. Philadelphia: Lippincott Williams & Wilkins, 1998, p. 312. **D** Swischuk LE. Imaging of the Newborn, Infant, and Young Child. 5th Ed. Philadelphia: Lippincott Williams & Wilkins, 2004, p. 410. **G** Feniglio-Preiser CM. Gastrointestinal Pathology: An Atlas and Text. 2nd Ed. Philadelphia: Lippincott Williams & Wilkins, 1999, p. 315. **H, inset** Feniglio-Preiser CM. Gastrointestinal Pathology: An Atlas and Text. 2nd Ed. Philadelphia: Lippincott Williams & Wilkins, 1999, p. 318. **I** Swischuk LE. Imaging of the Newborn, Infant, and Young Child. 5th Ed. Philadelphia: Lippincott Williams & Wilkins, 2004, p. 425.

Figure 1-7: From Dudek RW. High-Yield Embryology. 3rd Ed. Philadelphia: Lippincott Williams & Wilkins, 2007, p. 50. **Original Sources: A (drawings)** Adapted from Sadler TW. Langman's Medical Embryology. 8th Ed. Philadelphia: Lippincott Williams & Wilkins, 2000, p. 299. **A (photo)** Sternberg SS. Histology for Pathologists. 2nd Ed. Philadelphia: Lippincott-Raven, 1997, p. 554. **B** Swischuk

LE. Imaging of the Newborn, Infant, and Young child. 5th Ed. Philadelphia: Lippincott Williams & Wilkins, 2004, p. 448.

Figure 1-8: A From Swischuk LE. Imaging of the Newborn, Infant, and Young Child. 5th Ed. Philadelphia: Lippincott Williams & Wilkins, 2004, p. 460. **Original Source:** Santulli TV, Schullinger JN, Amoury RA, et al. Malformations of the anus and rectum. Surg Clin North Am 1965;45:1253–1271. **B** From Swischuk LE. Imaging of the Newborn, Infant, and Young Child. 5th Ed. Philadelphia: Lippincott Williams & Wilkins, 2004, p. 461. **Original Source:** Santulli TV, Schullinger JN, Amoury RA, et al. Malformations of the anus and rectum. Surg Clin North Am 1965;45:1253–1271. C From Avery GB, Fletcher MA, MacDonald MG. Neonatology: Pathophysiology and Management of the Newborn. 5th Ed. Philadelphia: Lippincott Williams & Wilkins, 1999, p. 1033.

Figure 2-1: A From Dudek RW. High-Yield Gross Anatomy. 2nd Ed. Philadelphia: Lippincott Williams & Wilkins, 2002, p. 64. **B** From Erkonen WE, Smith WL. Radiology 101: The Basics and Fundamentals of Imaging. 2nd Ed. Philadelphia: Lippincott Williams & Wilkins, 2005, p. 111. C From Moore KL, Dalley AF. Clinically Oriented Anatomy. 5th Ed. Philadelphia: Lippincott Williams & Wilkins, 2006, p. 338.

Figure 2-4: A From Sternberg SS. Histology for Pathologists. 2nd Ed. Philadelphia: Lippincott-Raven, 1997, p. 463.

Figure 2-5: A From Dudek RW. High-Yield Gross Anatomy. 3rd Ed. Philadelphia: Lippincott Williams & Wilkins, 2008, p. 116. **Original Source:** Cromack DH. Clincally Integrated Histology. Philadelphia: Lippincott Williams & Wilkins, 1998, p. 193. **B** From Sauerland EK. Grant's Dissector. 12th Ed. Philadelphia: Lippincott Williams & Wilkins, 1999, p. 66.

Figure 2-6: A From Agur AMR, Dalley AF. Grant's Atlas of Anatomy. 11th Ed. Philadelphia: Lippincott Williams & Wilkins, 2005, p. 132. **B** From Agur AMR, Dalley AF. Grant's Atlas of Anatomy. 11th Ed. Philadelphia: Lippincott Williams & Wilkins, 2005, p. 136.

Figure 2-7: A From Moore KL, Dalley AF. Clinically Oriented Anatomy. 5th Ed. Philadelphia: Lippincott Williams & Wilkins, 2006, p. 272. **B** From Moore KL, Dalley AF. Clinically Oriented Anatomy. 5th Ed. Philadelphia: Lippincott Williams & Wilkins, 2006, p. 274.

Figure 2-8: A From Moore KL, Dalley AF. Clinically Oriented Anatomy. 5th Ed. Philadelphia: Lippincott Williams & Wilkins, 2006, p. 445. **B** From Dudek RW. High-Yield Gross Anatomy. 3rd Ed. Philadelphia: Lippincott Williams & Wilkins, 2008, p. 140.

Figure 2-9: A From Agur AMR, Dalley AF. Grant's Atlas of Anatomy. 11th Ed. Philadelphia: Lippincott Williams & Wilkins, 2005, p. 142. **B** From Agur AMR, Dalley AF. Grant's Atlas of Anatomy. 11th Ed. Philadelphia: Lippincott Williams & Wilkins, 2005, p. 142. C From Agur AMR, Dalley AF. Grant's Atlas of Anatomy. 11th Ed. Philadelphia: Lippincott Williams & Wilkins, 2005, p. 143. D From Dudek RW. High-Yield Gross Anatomy. 3rd Ed. Philadelphia: Lippincott Williams & Wilkins, 2008, p. 127.

Figure 2-10: A From Snell RS. Clinical Anatomy by Systems. Philadelphia: Lippincott Williams & Wilkins, 2007, p. 781. **B** From Moore KL, Dalley AF. Clinically Oriented Anatomy. 5th Ed. Philadelphia: Lippincott Williams & Wilkins, 2006, p. 303.

Figure 2-11: A Modified from Moore KL, Dalley AF. Clinically Oriented Anatomy. 5th Ed. Philadelphia: Lippincott Williams & Wilkins, 2006, p. 283. **B** From Moore KL, Dalley AF. Clinically Oriented Anatomy. 5th Ed. Philadelphia: Lippincott Williams & Wilkins, 2006, p. 284.

Figure 3-1: A Redrawn from Erkonen WE, Smith WL. Radiology 101: The Basics and Fundamentals of Imaging. 2nd Ed. Philadelphia: Lippincott Williams & Wilkins, 2005, p. 78. **B** From Daffner RH. Clinical Radiology: The Essentials. 3rd Ed. Philadelphia: Lippincott Williams & Wilkins, 2007, p. 236. C Redrawn from Erkonen WE, Smith WL. Radiology 101: The Basics and Fundamentals of Imaging. 2nd Ed. Philadelphia: Lippincott Williams & Wilkins, 2005, p. 78. **D** Redrawn from Erkonen WE, Smith WL. Radiology 101: The Basics and Fundamentals of Imaging. 2nd Ed. Philadelphia: Lippincott Williams & Wilkins, 2005, p. 78.

Figure 3-2: **A1** and **A2**: From Moore KL, Dalley AF. Clinically Oriented Anatomy. 5th Ed. Philadelphia: Lippincott Williams & Wilkins, 2006, p. 247. **B** From Sternberg SS. Histology for Pathologists. 2nd Ed. Philadelphia: Lippincott-Raven, 1997, p. 463. **C** From Erkonen WE, Smith WL. Radiology 101: The Basics and Fundamentals of Imaging. 2nd Ed. Philadelphia: Lippincott Williams & Wilkins, 2005, p. 91. **D** From Erkonen WE, Smith WL. Radiology 101: The Basics and Fundamentals of Imaging. 2nd Ed. Philadelphia: Lippincott Williams & Wilkins, 2005, p. 92. (Courtesy of Bruce Brown, MD.)

Figure 3-3: **A and B** From Daffner RH. Clinical Radiology: The Essentials. 3rd Ed. Philadelphia: Lippincott Williams & Wilkins, 2007, p. 278. **C** From Erkonen WE, Smith WL. Radiology 101: The Basics and Fundamentals of Imaging. 2nd Ed. Philadelphia: Lippincott Williams & Wilkins, 2005, p. 93. (Courtesy of Bruce Brown, MD.) **D** From Yamada T, Alpers DH, Laine L, et al. Textbook of Gastroenterology, vol 2, 3rd Ed. Philadelphia: Lippincott Williams & Wilkins, 1999, p. 2956. **E** From Yamada T, Alpers DH, Laine L, et al. Textbook of Gastroenterology, vol 2, 3rd Ed. Philadelphia: Lippincott Williams & Wilkins, 1999, p. 2959. **F** From Moore KL, Dalley AF. Clinically Oriented Anatomy. 5th Ed. Philadelphia: Lippincott Williams & Wilkins, 2006, p. 280.

Figure 3-4: **A and B** From Daffner RH. Clinical Radiology: The Essentials. 3rd Ed. Philadelphia: Lippincott Williams & Wilkins, 2007, p. 273. **C** From Yamada T, Alpers DH, Laine L, et al. Textbook of Gastroenterology, vol 2, 3rd Ed. Philadelphia: Lippincott Williams & Wilkins, 1999, p. 3102. **D** From Yamada T, Alpers DH, Laine L, et al. Textbook of Gastroenterology, vol 2, 3rd Ed. Philadelphia: Lippincott Williams & Wilkins, 1999, p. 3103.

Figure 3-5: **A–C** From Erkonen WE, Smith WL. Radiology 101: The Basics and Fundamentals of Imaging. 2nd Ed. Philadelphia: Lippincott Williams & Wilkins, 2005, p. 102.

Figure 3-6: **A–C** From Erkonen WE, Smith WL. Radiology 101: The Basics and Fundamentals of Imaging. 2nd Ed. Philadelphia: Lippincott Williams & Wilkins, 2005, p. 103.

Figure 3-7: **A–C** From Erkonen WE, Smith WL. Radiology 101: The Basics and Fundamentals of Imaging. 2nd Ed. Philadelphia: Lippincott Williams & Wilkins, 2005, p. 104.

Figure 4-1: **A–D** Courtesy of Dr Ron Dudek, PhD.

Figure 4-2: **A–D** Courtesy of Dr Ron Dudek, PhD.

Figure 4-3: **A–D** Courtesy of Dr Ron Dudek, PhD.

Figure 4-4: **A** From Fenoglio-Preiser CM. Gastrointestinal Pathology: An Atlas and Text. Philadelphia: Lippincott Williams & Wilkins, 1999, p. 749. **B** Courtesy of Dr. Ron Dudek, PhD.

Figure 4-5: **A** From Sternberg SS. Histology for Pathologists. 2nd Ed. Philadelphia: Lippincott-Raven, 1997, p. 542. **B** From Sternberg SS. Histology for Pathologists. 2nd Ed. Philadelphia: Lippincott-Raven, 1997, p. 541.

Figure 4-6: **(Photograph of the anal canal)** From Sternberg SS. Histology for Pathologists. 2nd Ed. Philadelphia: Lippincott-Raven, 1997, p. 554. **A** From Sternberg SS. Histology for Pathologists. 2nd Ed. Philadelphia: Lippincott-Raven, 1997, p. 559. **B** From Fenoglio-Preiser CM. Gastrointestinal Pathology: An Atlas and Text. Philadelphia: Lippincott Williams & Wilkins, 1999, p. 1072. **C** From Sternberg SS. Histology for Pathologists. 2nd Ed. Philadelphia: Lippincott-Raven, 1997, p. 563. **D** From Sternberg SS. Histology for Pathologists. 2nd Ed. Philadelphia: Lippincott-Raven, 1997, p. 564. **E** From Sternberg SS. Histology for Pathologists. 2nd Ed. Philadelphia: Lippincott-Raven, 1997, p. 556.

Figure 4-7: From Dudek RW. High-Yield Histopathology. Philadelphia: Lippincott Williams & Wilkins, 2008, p. 183.

Figure 4-8: **A–D** Courtesy of Dr Ron Dudek, PhD.

Figure 4-9: Courtesy of Dr Ron Dudek, PhD.

Figure 4-10: **A, B** Courtesy of Dr Ron Dudek, PhD. **C** From Sternberg SS. Histology for Pathologists. 2nd Ed. Philadelphia: Lippincott-Raven, 1997, p. 623.

Figure 5-1: **A** From Dudek RW. High-Yield Physiology. Philadelphia: Lippincott Williams & Wilkins, 2008, p. 138. **Original Source:** Redrawn from Johnson L. Gastrointestinal Physiology. 6th Ed. St. Louis: Mosby, 2000. **B** From Dudek RW. High-Yield Physiology. Philadelphia: Lippincott Williams & Wilkins, 2008, p. 138. **Original Source:** Bullock J, Boyle J III, Wang MB. NMS Physiology. 4th Ed. Philadelphia: Lippincott Williams & Wilkins, 2001, p. 525. **C** From Dudek RW. High-Yield Physiology. Philadelphia: Lippincott Williams & Wilkins, 2008, p. 138. **Original Source:** Redrawn from Pasley JN. USMLE Road Map Physiology. New York: Lange, 2003, p. 119.

Figure 5-2: **A** From Dudek RW. High-Yield Physiology. Philadelphia: Lippincott Williams & Wilkins, 2008, p. 139. **B** From Dudek RW. High-Yield Physiology. Philadelphia: Lippincott Williams & Wilkins, 2008, p. 139. **Original Source:** Modified from Dudek RW. High-Yield Histology. 3rd Ed. Philadelphia: Lippincott Williams & Wilkins, 2004, p. 137. (Also see page 136, Figure 15-1 for a digitized figure of the parietal cell.) **C** From Dudek RW. High-Yield Physiology. Philadelphia: Lippincott Williams & Wilkins, 2008, p. 139.

Figure 5-3: From Dudek RW. High-Yield Physiology. Philadelphia: Lippincott Williams & Wilkins, 2008, p. 152.

Figure 5-4: From Dudek RW. High-Yield Physiology. Philadelphia: Lippincott Williams & Wilkins, 2008, p. 153.

Figure 5-5: From Dudek RW. High-Yield Physiology. Philadelphia: Lippincott Williams & Wilkins, 2008, p. 153.

Figure 5-6: From Dudek RW. High-Yield Physiology. Philadelphia: Lippincott Williams & Wilkins, 2008, p. 153.

Figure 5-7: **A** From Dudek RW. High-Yield Physiology. Philadelphia: Lippincott Williams & Wilkins, 2008, p. 160. **B** From Dudek RW. High-Yield Physiology. Philadelphia: Lippincott Williams & Wilkins, 2008, p. 160. **Original Source:** From Kamath PS, Phillips SF, OConnor MK, et al. Colonic capacitance and transit in man: Modulation by luminal contents and drugs. Gut 1990;31:443. **C** From Dudek RW. High-Yield Physiology. Philadelphia: Lippincott Williams & Wilkins, 2008, p. 160. **Original Source:** Redrawn from Despopoulos A, Silbernagl S. Color Atlas of Physiology. 5th Ed. New York: Thieme, 2003, p. 265.

Figure 5-8: From Dudek RW. High-Yield Physiology. Philadelphia: Lippincott Williams & Wilkins, 2008, p. 162.

Figure 5-9: From Dudek RW. High-Yield Physiology. Philadelphia: Lippincott Williams & Wilkins, 2008, p. 173.

Figure 5-10: From Dudek RW. High-Yield Physiology. Philadelphia: Lippincott Williams & Wilkins, 2008, p. 174.

Figure 5-11: From Dudek RW. High-Yield Physiology. Philadelphia: Lippincott Williams & Wilkins, 2008, p. 183.

Figure 5-12: From Dudek RW. High-Yield Physiology. Philadelphia: Lippincott Williams & Wilkins, 2008, p. 184.

Figure 6-1: **A** From Sternberg SS. Histology for Pathologists. 2nd Ed. Philadelphia: Lippincott-Raven, 1997, p. 467. **B** From Gartner LP, JL Hiatt. Color Atlas of Histology. 4th Ed. Philadelphia: Lippincott Williams & Wilkins, 2006, p. 291. **C** From Sternberg SS. Histology for Pathologists. 2nd Ed. Philadelphia: Lippincott-Raven, 1997, p. 475. **D** From Sternberg SS. Histology for Pathologists. 2nd Ed. Philadelphia: Lippincott-Raven, 1997, p. 476.

Figure 6-2: **A** From Rubin R, Strayer DS. Rubin's Pathology: Clinicopathologic Foundations of Medicine. 5th Ed. Philadelphia: Lippincott Williams & Wilkins, 2008, p. 567. **B** From Erkonen

WE, Smith WL. Radiology 101: The Basics and Fundamentals of Imaging. 2nd Ed. Philadelphia: Lippincott Williams & Wilkins, 2005, p. 113. **C** From Rubin R, Strayer DS. Rubin's Pathology: Clinicopathologic Foundations of Medicine. 5th Ed. Philadelphia: Lippincott Williams & Wilkins, 2008, p. 567. **D** From Erkonen WE, Smith WL. Radiology 101: The Basics and Fundamentals of Imaging. 2nd Ed. Philadelphia: Lippincott Williams & Wilkins, 2005, p. 113.

Figure 6-3: **A** From Yamada T, Alpers DH, Laine L, et al. Atlas of Gastroenterology. 2nd Ed. Philadelphia: Lippincott Williams & Wilkins, 1999, p. 282. **B** From Dudek RW. High-Yield Histopathology. Philadelphia: Lippincott Williams & Wilkins, 2008, p. 172. **Original Source:** Damjanov I. Histopathology: A Color Atlas and Textbook. Baltimore: Williams & Wilkins, 1996, p. 197. **C** From Rubin R, Strayer DS. Rubin's Pathology: Clinicopathologic Foundations of Medicine. 5th Ed. Philadelphia: Lippincott Williams & Wilkins, 2008, p. 588.

Figure 6-4: **A** From Dudek RW. High-Yield Histology. 3rd Ed. Philadelphia: Lippincott Williams & Wilkins, 2004, p. 143. **Original Source:** Yamada T, Alpers DH, Laine L, et al. Atlas of Gastroenterology. 2nd Ed. Philadelphia: Lippincott Williams & Wilkins, 1999, p. 334. **B** From Erkonen WE, Smith WL. Radiology 101: The Basics and Fundamentals of Imaging. 2nd Ed. Philadelphia: Lippincott Williams & Wilkins, 2005, p. 114. **Original Source:** Yamada T, Alpers DH, Laine L, et al. Textbook of Gastroenterology, vol 1, 3rd Ed. Philadelphia: Lippincott Williams & Wilkins, 1999, p. 1484. **C** From Rubin E, Farber JL. Pathology. 3rd Ed. Philadelphia: Lippincott Williams & Wilkins, 1999, p. 731. **D** From Erkonen WE, Smith WL. Radiology 101: The Basics and Fundamental of Imaging. 2nd Ed. Philadelphia: Lippincott Williams & Wilkins, 2005, p. 115.

Figure 6-5: **A** From Rubin R, Strayer DS. Rubin's Pathology: Clinicopathologic Foundations of Medicine. 5th Ed. Philadelphia: Lippincott Williams & Wilkins, 2008, p. 593. **B** From Yamada T, Alpers DH, Laine L, et al. Atlas of Gastroenterology. 2nd Ed. Philadelphia: Lippincott Williams & Wilkins, 1999, p. 27. **C** From Yamada T, Alpers DH, Laine L, et al. Atlas of Gastroenterology. 2nd Ed. Philadelphia: Lippincott Williams & Wilkins, 1999, p. 417.

Figure 6-6: **A** From Yamada T, Alpers DH, Laine L, et al. Atlas of Gastroenterology. 2nd Ed. Philadelphia: Lippincott Williams & Wilkins, 1999, p. 382. **B** From Dudek RW. High-Yield Histology. 3rd Ed. Philadelphia: Lippincott Williams & Wilkins, 2004, p. 148. (Courtesy of Dr Ron Dudek.) **C** From Yamada T, Alpers DH, Laine L, et al. Atlas of Gastroenterology. 2nd Ed. Philadelphia: Lippincott Williams & Wilkins, 1999, p. 404. **D** From Dudek RW. High-Yield Histology. 3rd Ed. Philadelphia: Lippincott Williams & Wilkins, 2004, p. 148. (Courtesy of Dr Ron Dudek.)

Figure 6-7: **A** From Rubin R, Strayer DS. Rubin's Pathology: Clinicopathologic Foundations of Medicine. 5th Ed. Philadelphia: Lippincott Williams & Wilkins, 2008, p. 652. **B** From Damjanov I. Histopathology: A Color Atlas and Textbook. Baltimore: Williams & Wilkins, 1996, p. 224. **C** From Damjanov I. Histopathology: A Color Atlas and Textbook. Baltimore: Williams & Wilkins, 1996, p. 225. **D** From Rubin R, Strayer DS. Rubin's Pathology: Clinicopathologic Foundations of Medicine. 5th Ed. Philadelphia: Lippincott Williams & Wilkins, 2008, p. 656.

Figure 6-8: **A** From Yamada T, Alpers DH, Laine L, et al. Atlas of Gastroenterology. 2nd Ed. Philadelphia: Lippincott Williams & Wilkins, 1999, p. 474. **B** From Rubin R, Strayer DS. Rubin's Pathology: Clinicopathologic Foundations of Medicine. 5th Ed. Philadelphia: Lippincott Williams & Wilkins, 2008, p. 669. **C** From Yamada T, Alpers DH, Laine L, et al. Atlas of Gastroenterology. 2nd Ed. Philadelphia: Lippincott Williams & Wilkins, 1999, p. 475. **D** From Damjanov I. Histopathology: A Color Atlas and Textbook. Baltimore: Williams & Wilkins, 1996, p. 241. **E** From Damjanov I. Histopathology: A Color Atlas and Textbook. Baltimore: Williams & Wilkins, 1996, p. 241.

Figure 6-9: **A** From Rubin R, Strayer DS. Rubin's Pathology: Clinicopathologic Foundations of Medicine. 5th Ed. Philadelphia: Lippincott Williams & Wilkins, 2008, p. 679. **B** From Rubin R, Strayer DS. Rubin's Pathology: Clinicopathologic Foundations of Medicine. 5th Ed. Philadelphia: Lippincott Williams & Wilkins, 2008, p. 680. **C** From Yamada T. Alpers DH, Laine L, et al. Atlas of Gastroenterology. 2nd Ed. Philadelphia: Lippincott Williams & Wilkins, 1999, p. 442.

Figure 7-1: **A** From Yamada T, Alpers DH, Laine L, et al. Atlas of Gastroenterology. 2nd Ed. Philadelphia: Lippincott Williams & Wilkins, 1999, p. 216. **B** Yamada T, Alpers DH, Laine L, et al. Atlas of Gastroenterology. 2nd Ed. Philadelphia: Lippincott Williams & Wilkins, 1999, p. 216. (Courtesy of H. Appelman, MD.)

Figure 7-2: **A** From Strohl WA, Rouse H, Fisher BD. Lippincott's Illustrated Reviews: Microbiology. Philadelphia: Lippincott Williams & Wilkins, 2001, p. 185. **Original Source:** Volk WA, Gebhardt BM, Hammarskjold M, et al. Essentials of Microbiology. 5th Ed. Philadelphia: Lippincott-Raven, 1996, p. 373. **B** From Strohl WA, Rouse H, Fisher BD. Lippincott's Illustrated Reviews: Microbiology. Philadelphia: Lippincott Williams & Wilkins, 2001, p. 186. **C** From Yamada T, Alpers DH, Laine L, et al. Atlas of Gastroenterology. 2nd Ed. Philadelphia: Lippincott Williams & Wilkins, 1999, p. 270. **D** From Rubin R, Strayer DS. Rubin's Pathology: Clinicopathologic Foundations of Medicine. 5th Ed. Philadelphia: Lippincott Williams & Wilkins, 2008, p. 313. **Original Source:** Farrar WE, Wood MJ, Innes JA, et al. Infectious Diseases Text and Color Atlas. 2nd Ed. New York: Copyright Gower Medical Publishing, 1992. **E** From Burton GRW, Engelkird PG. Microbiology for the Health Sciences. 7th Ed. Philadelphia: Lippincott Williams & Wilkins, 2004, p. 2. **F** Koneman EW, Allen SD, Janda WM, et al. Color Atlas and Textbook of Diagnostic Microbiology. 5th Ed. Philadelphia: Lippincott-Raven, 1997, Color Plate 14-3B. **G** From Fenoglio-Preiser CM. Gastrointestinal Pathology: An Atlas and Text. 2nd Ed. Philadelphia: Lippincott Williams & Wilkins, 1999, p. 352. (Courtesy of Robin Cooke, MD, Department of Pathology, Royal Brisbane Hospital, Brisbane, Australia.) **H1** From Koneman EW, Allen SD, Janda WM, et al. Color Atlas and Textbook of Diagnostic Microbiology. 5th Ed. Philadelphia: Lippincott-Raven, 1997, Color Plate 20-2B.

Figure 7-3: **A** From Fenoglio-Preiser CM. Gastrointestinal Pathology: An Atlas and Text. 2nd Ed. Philadelphia: Lippincott Williams & Wilkins, 1999, p. 828. **C** From Strohl WA, Rouse H, Fisher BD. Lippincott's Illustrated Reviews: Microbiology. Philadelphia: Lippincott Williams & Wilkins, 2001, p. 179. **Original Source:** Volk WA, Benjamin DC, Kadner RJ, et al. Essentials of Microbiology. 4th Ed. Philadelphia: JB Lippincott Company, 1991, p. 250. **D** From Yamada T, Alpers DH, Laine L, et al. Atlas of Gastroenterology. 2nd Ed. Philadelphia: Lippincott Williams & Wilkins, 1999, p. 668. **E** From Strohl WA, Rouse H, Fisher BD. Lippincott's Illustrated Reviews: Microbiology. Philadelphia: Lippincott Williams & Wilkins, 2001, p. 205. **Original Source:** Hart T, Shears P. Color Atlas of Medical Microbiology. London: Mosby-Wolfe; 1996, p. 133. **F** From Fenoglio-Preiser CM. Gastrointestinal Pathology: An Atlas and Text. 2nd Ed. Philadelphia: Lippincott Williams & Wilkins, 1999, p. 378. **G** From Strohl WA, Rouse H, Fisher BD. Lippincott's Illustrated Reviews: Microbiology. Philadelphia: Lippincott Williams & Wilkins, 2001, p. 176. **H** From Rubin R, Strayer DS. Rubin's Pathology: Clinicopathologic Foundations of Medicine. 5th Ed. Philadelphia: Lippincott Williams & Wilkins, 2008, p. 313. **Original Source:** Farrar WE, Wood MJ, Innes JA, et al. Infectious Diseases Text and Color Atlas. 2nd Ed. New York: Copyright Gower Medical Publishing, 1992. **I** From Koneman EW, Allen SD, Janda WM, et al. Color Atlas and Textbook of Diagnostic Microbiology. 5th Ed. Philadelphia: Lippincott-Raven, 1997, Color Plate 14-4F. **J** From Rubin R, Strayer DS. Rubin's Pathology: Clinicopathologic Foundations of Medicine. 5th Ed. Philadelphia: Lippincott Williams & Wilkins, 2008, p. 592. **K** From Strohl WA, Rouse H, Fisher BD. Lippincott's Illustrated Reviews: Microbiology. Philadelphia: Lippincott Williams & Wilkins, 2001, p. 181. **Original Source:** Koneman EW, Allen SD, Janda WM, et al. Color Atlas and Textbook of Diagnostic Microbiology. 5th Ed. Philadelphia: Lippincott-Raven, 1997, Plate 6-1A. **L** From Yamada T, Alpers DH, Laine L, et al. Atlas of Gastroenterology. 2nd Ed. Philadelphia: Lippincott Williams & Wilkins, 1999, p. 372.

Figure 7-4: **B** From Dudek RW. High-Yield Lung. Philadelphia: Lippincott Williams & Wilkins, 2006, p. 117.

Figure 7-5: **B** From Rubin R, Strayer DS. Rubin's Pathology: Clinicopathologic Foundations of Medicine. 5th Ed. Philadelphia: Lippincott Williams & Wilkins, 2008, p. 637.

Index

Page numbers followed by an "f" indicate figures; those followed by a "t" denote tables.

A

B

C

D

E